Straw into Gold

"A beautifully written, searingly honest, and profoundly moving account of one woman's journey through chronic illness and suffering, and the life lessons she learned."
—**Jim Dreaver**, author of *End Your Story, Begin Your Life*

"I had the unique privilege of working closely with Diane during the last year of her life as part of her integrative health care team. Diane was a gifted writer and poet, an out-of-the-box spirit who would come in for her vitamin infusion dressed in a long blue wig with wild sunglasses. She never lost her sense of humor throughout the ravages of dealing with chronic illness and then cancer. In her last month of life, she presided over her 'living' wake, a wild and wonderful dress-up party outdoors, with Diane in her bed on the throne under the spreading oak tree. Her unique talents make her story not only touching, but exquisitely and subtly expressed. During her last days, we took turns reading to her aloud to put the final touches on her editing, with many tears of sadness and joy being shed. This book is a treasure."
—**Elaine Weil**, Nurse Practitioner, Amitabha Medical Clinic and Healing Center, Sebastopol, CA

"Many years of illness and pain prepared Diane for her last adventure with friends to the Sonoma Coast. Propped up on many pillows and blankets she ate dark chocolate and ripe raspberries while singing 'Give yourself to Love' and experienced the total joy we shared with her so often throughout her dying process."
—**Tom Meyskens**, lover of spoken poetry, fellow Love Choir member and friend

"Diane fully engaged in her life and her death. She didn't want to miss anything. Though debilitated, weak, and living with chronic pain, she traveled with us to Mexico and went on by herself to another retreat, sending us home with a suitcase of homeopathic drugs and other heavy items. She camped, canoed, and attended musical festivals during her last throws with cancer with a 'little' help from her friends. At her request, we have spread her ashes in beautiful places where the people she loves go and can be with her. She was a great teacher. She shared her joy and her tears, her life and her death with grace, honesty, and openness. Straw into Gold shares Diane's amazing journey and imparts the wisdom of a woman who inspired many with the way she moved beyond illness, hardship, and dying to embrace love and life."
—**Linda Mollenhauer-Meyskens**, Life coach and close friend

Straw into Gold

*Illness, Loss and Hardship
as a
Path to Inner Peace*

Diane LaRae Bodach

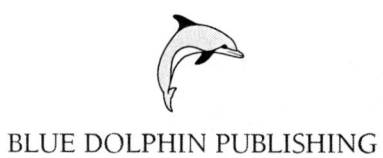

BLUE DOLPHIN PUBLISHING

Copyright © 2011 Diane LaRae Bodach
All rights reserved.

Published by Blue Dolphin Publishing, Inc.
P.O. Box 8, Nevada City, CA 95959
Orders: 1-800-643-0765
Web: www.bluedolphinpublishing.com

ISBN: 978-1-57733-223-7 paperback
ISBN: 978-1-57733-332-6 e-book

Library of Congress Cataloging-in-Publication Data

Bodach, Diane LaRae, 1946-2007.
  Straw into gold : illness, loss, and hardship as a path to inner peace / Diane LaRae Bodach.
      p. cm.
  Includes bibliographical references.
  ISBN 978-1-57733-223-7 (pbk. : alk. paper) — ISBN 978-1-57733-332-6 (e-book)
  1. Bodach, Diane LaRae, 1946-2007—Health. 2. Breast—Cancer—Psychological aspects. 3. Chronic diseases--Psychological aspects. 4. Adjustment (Psychology) 5. Death. 6. Life. I. Title.
  RC280.B8B595 2011
  616.99'449—dc22
                                                            2010054338

Printed in the United States of America

10   9   8   7   6   5   4   3   2   1

Contents

Foreword	xi
Introduction	1
1. Attention Means Attention	9
2. Opening to Grief	15
The Princess and the Pea	15
The Soul Knows What to Do	16
"All Dreams Come in the Service of Healing"	18
Our Bodies Carry the Crisis State with Us	20
Despair Can Be a Gateway	23
All Losses Must Be Grieved	26
We Must Give up Our Demand to Be Happy	29
It's Only Too Late If You Don't Start Now	30
The Dark Night of the Soul	33
3. Alien	36
Fifteen Words for Snow	37
Planet Scleroderma	39
The Wish to Be Understood	39
The Language of Disability	41
The Push–Pull of Shame	43
The Difficulty of Partnering	45
Though Our Bodies Have Changed, Our Souls Have Not	47
Hidden Prejudice	49
A Small Gesture Goes a Long Way	50
The Loneliness of Living with a Chronic Illness	52
The Paradox of Living with Illness	53
We Are All Aliens	54
The Reed Flute's Song	55
Forgiveness Begins at Home	55
What Helps and What Doesn't	57

The Hard and Icy Couch	59
The Eye with Which I See God	61
4. Opportunity	62
Our Obsession with Freedom	62
The Hindrance Will Become the Lens	64
The Usefulness of Restriction	65
Illness and Restriction as Agents of Change	66
Being Lucky	68
The Gift of Choicelessness	69
Our Main Job: To Be	70
5. Sickness As Path—Getting to Yes	74
Loss of Identity	76
The Picture Does Not Match	79
The Shadow	80
Phantom Feelings	81
"The Bus Hit"	83
Breaking Through Attachment	84
The List Dragon	85
Spiritual Poverty	87
Death as Teacher	88
Getting to Yes	91
Mindfulness	92
Being Present in the Now	94
Surrender	96
6. Practicing with Loss, Illness and Dying	98
Practicing with Loss	103
Practicing with Illness and Death	104
7. The Function of Emotions	110
A Bum Rap	111
A New Paradigm of Healing	113
The Ecology of the Soul	114
We Are Programmed for Joy	115
Brother Donkey	117
8. Working with Negative Emotions	119
9. Loving Kindness	122
The Alpha and the Omega	123
The Shadow	124
This Is No Accident and No Dirty Trick	126
The "Catch–22" of Spiritual Practice	128

A Saving Nightmare	129
Having an Intention Is the First Step	130
Somewhere in Us We Know Love	131
The Truth Is, We Are Love	133
I Met Myself Face to Face and Didn't Like What I Saw	133
10. Practicing with Negative Emotions	135
How We Avoid Experiencing	135
The Shadow "I" and the Impartial Observer	136
No More Important Task	137
The Past Is Where We Live	138
Experiencing	140
We Need to Unwrap Our Pain Slowly	143
Deep Inquiry	145
The Longing Itself IS the Connection We Seek	148
Pre-verbal Experience	149
Allow	151
Release	152
11. Dialoguing with the Inner Child	158
Re-parenting the Inner Child	159
Meeting Your Inner Sorrow with Mercy and Kindness	160
Telling the Child the Truth	162
Lack of Feelings Can Signal Trouble	163
Having Our Buttons Pushed	165
12. Getting to Yes and No—Taking a Stand Against False Beliefs	167
Sometimes Getting to Yes Means Accepting That You're Saying No	167
God Save Me from God	169
My "Yes" Religion	170
Beliefs Are Not Feelings	171
We Usually Have It Backwards	173
Illness Can Begin to Eat Away at Our Self-Esteem	174
You Have Not Sinned	176
False Beliefs and Fears	178
Labeling Thoughts	179
Special Circumstances in Relationship	181
Turning It Around	181
Working with the "No" in Small Ways	185
The Myth of Consistency	186

13. The Peace That Surpasseth Understanding	189
14. The Warrior Path	201
15. On Not Being Able to Do	208
Life in the Slow Lane	209
New Look at Priorities	212
Writing the Book	216
Lightening the Load	218
Hard Truths	219
What Is the Essence of Being Human?	221
The Longing for Purpose	222
Learning to Receive—Being Love	225
Doing Versus Being—The Practice of Being a Tree	228
16. The Practice of Being Without	229
17. The Way to Be Happy	236
18. The Inner Healer	243
The Divine Child	244
Practices for Connecting with the Inner Child or Creative Self	250
Challenges of Tuning into the Inner Healer	262
The Dangers of a "Teaching"	263
Trust Yourself—Developing Your Intuitive Self	267
Actualizing a Teaching	269
The Wise One	270
The Devil and God Are in the Details	271
Small Efforts	275
The Relationship Between Play and Practice	276
Healing Exercises	277
19. New Order	282
A New Way of Looking	282
Create Your Own Myth	283
A Different Set of Laws	285
Putting Your Life on Hold	288
Hitting the Wall	289
Changing from a Goal-Oriented to a Feeling-Oriented Life	289
Yearning for a "Normal Life"	291
The Paradox of Illness: Nourishment of the Soul vs. Taking Care of the Body	292
Inventing Your Life	294
Tectonic Plates Are Moving	295

Finding New Resources	*299*
The Smile	*301*
20. Moving On	303
Impermanence	*303*
The Usefulness of a New Identity (and Giving It Up)	*307*
Letting Go of the Messenger	*308*
Life as Teacher	*313*
Appendix	315
A Simple Loving Kindness Meditation	*315*
The Forgiveness Meditation	*318*
Notes	323
Bibliography	324
About the Author	327

Foreword

I WOULD LIKE TO DEDICATE THIS BOOK TO ITS AUTHOR—my mother—Diane LaRae Bodach, who died of cancer on September 18, 2007. I feel it is important to recognize that she died knowing her book would be published.

In ways, my mom was like a saint—never in my life have I known a person more kind and compassionate than she, nor more pure in good intention. However, I chuckle (tenderly) to call her a saint because she was indeed as human as any other, challenging at times to those who knew her well, and with as many demons and self-judgments as the rest of us. But through the years, Diane LaRae Bodach learned to see clearly, to examine her relationship to herself, to others, and to all things in life with complete honesty. In so doing, she lived (and died) with her heart wide open and free.

Although her body suffered physically, weakened by chronic illness and often overcome by indescribable pain due to cancer, I would not say that my mom suffered. In fact, she died in peace, in her own home, with acceptance and true love and joy in her heart. She was, even on her deathbed, more alive than many of us will ever be.

Through years of spiritual practice, my mom cultivated the willingness to open to herself and others, to life, and ultimately to her own death. It took her dying for me to finally see clearly something I had previously only understood on an intellectual leve—what it means to JUST BE—and then to actually practice it in my own daily life. Her death was my wake-up call, my opportunity to discover joy and love in the most unlikely place—or in any place—right here, right now, inside of me.

Particularly, in the months together before my mom died, I learned from her not only how to accept death as a part of life, with dignity and grace, but also how to live, how to live fully with life as it is in each moment, even in the most painful moments I have ever experienced. She taught me what it means to spin straw into gold.

And so I offer this book to you on her behalf. I believe these pages unlock a glimmer of the wisdom she gathered throughout her lifetime. I believe they hold riches beyond measure from which we may all benefit, learn, and grow.

—Jenessa Bayda

Introduction

Come, come whoever you are,
Wanderer, worshiper, lover of leaving, (it doesn't matter.)
Ours is not a caravan of despair.
Come, come even if you have
broken your vows a thousand times.
Come, come yet again, come.

—Rumi

THE ALCHEMISTS USED LEAD; Rumplestiltskin's heroine used straw; Parsival found the sacred cup hidden amidst a wasteland. These stories of turning what is base or ordinary into gold and finding the prized cup of salvation in a place of desolation are metaphors for the journey of the soul, our path to the heart, to the final prize—Love. We are all given, at some time in our lives, the raw materials necessary for our journey. They come in the forms of illness, loss, deprivation, hardship, insufferable people or situations. These base materials or experiences, the dregs of our lives, the things we despise and strive desperately to avoid or be rid of, are the very things that have the potential, if we let them, to lead us finally to the Promised Land.

On August 15, 1980, the day before my oldest daughter's seventh birthday, I was an active mother of two, overseeing a small homestead with my husband. I co-tended a half-acre garden, canned and froze produce for the winter, milked goats, cared for chickens we had raised from baby chicks, cooked everything from scratch, baked bread, made cheese, yogurt, sprouts, pickles, and crafted soft leather shoes to gently enclose my daughters' feet, in addition to all the normal chores required to maintain a household with two small children. I played guitar, painted, sewed and organized crafts for the children; I took long bike rides, and for vacation, loved nothing more than camping at a beautiful wild spot and taking long adventurous hikes.

On August 16, I awoke feeling ill, and from that day forward I was a person debilitated by chronic illness, incapable for many years of anything but the most rudimentary tasks required for a subsistence level of life. Of course at the time, I, like the teen who thinks herself invincible, assumed my body would heal itself as it always had. But as the months wore on, doubt crept in, then fear. The unthinkable seeped into my consciousness like a heavy fog gradually soaks the clothes of the unprepared hiker. "Suppose I never get well? Suppose I'm like this for the rest of my life?"

My doctor told me I was depressed. I came home in a rage and screamed at him in my head, "You'd be depressed, too, if you were sick for three months and saw no signs of getting better!" I thought I might as well be dead. I thought August 16, 1980, marked the end of my life. But in truth, that was the day I really began to learn how to live.

When I was well, what thought I gave to those who were sick or disabled was often superficial and fleeting. I felt sorry for them, but they just weren't part of my life or consciousness—so I thought. But underneath, there was something more going on, something that I wasn't willing to or didn't want to acknowledge. In retrospect, I see that these people represented to me pain and suffering. By marginalizing them, I was marginalizing my own pain and suffering, and the pain and suffering of the whole world. Hovering in the background, just out of consciousness or perhaps just barely in, was the thought, "I'm so glad that is not me."

It was as though by not giving too much attention, too much juice, to those suffering in the world, I could keep suffering out of my life. It was like going through life with blinders on, the kind they use with horses to keep them from being distracted or frightened by things happening on the sides. The problem with this approach is that it gave me a very narrow view of life. And contrary to the belief that suffering could be kept at bay in this way, I discovered the opposite to be true: by blocking out the pain, the suffering in myself and others, I was actually cutting myself off from connection with my own deepest self, fragmenting myself and thus making true joy impossible. Before we begin to truly open to life as it is, and to our innermost self, we are living in a make-believe world. We think that somehow we are going to avoid the calamity we see all around us.

I think we all do this in one way or another. Some, depending on personality type, might take the opposite tack—putting lots of attention on others who are suffering, spending inordinate amounts of time and energy helping them—in order to avoid facing what they don't want to face in themselves. When I was very sick, a woman from my daughter's school befriended me and brought me meals—beautifully prepared works of art, always with a flower on top and often mixed into the food as well, along with a lovely handwritten artistic note. I marveled at her way of being: how selflessly she seemed to offer herself to others. When I told her this, she replied, "Actually, I do this out of selfishness. It's for me. It helps me to avoid my own deep emotional suffering."

When we are well, we think, somehow magically, that that kind of devastating illness and loss will not happen to us. We think it only happens to other people. I *used* to be one of those people that disability and loss didn't happen to. Then it happened to me. I became ill and never got well again. After working with my chronic illness for many years, I finally saw I was no different from anyone else. And that chronic illness can happen to anyone. But I was still one of those people that cancer didn't happen to. I was going to live a long life, albeit a limited one. Then cancer happened to me.

Now I see that anything can happen to anyone. How can we go through life in such denial? It seems unfathomable, really. People are sick and dying and suffering all around us, and we never think it can happen to us.

Illness, pain or suffering gives us another chance to reconnect with the deepest part of ourselves and with others, to rejoin the human race. It is a great burden to be privileged. To lose our privileged place, to come down to the lowest common denominator—the level of a common person, to be poor, to suffer, to be sick—can be a great relief. At some point the question becomes not so much "Why me?" but "Why not me?".

When we can finally, willingly, take our share of the great pie of human suffering, we discover, to our amazement, that this pie is filled with the most luscious fruit. And we can finally relinquish our fear that some devastation will come our way—because it already has. If we have opened to the experience and allowed it to teach us, we see, if we are honest, that not only have we survived, but also that our lives may, in many ways, be better or richer than they were before. Of course, in the case of terminal illness the path ends in death, as does each human life. And thus we are given the opportunity, as each human ultimately will be, to experience the ultimate teaching and opening.

Although the thrust of this book is positive, and the underlying message is the joy that can come out of hardship and suffering, it is not a Pollyanna story, and there is much here that may be difficult to read. The utter terror and despair that confronts each person when much of what he has held dear is taken away, or when he is indeed facing death itself, is very real. But as Robert Frost said, "The only way out is always through," and if we have tools, if we don't feel so alone, if we understand what is happening in a larger context, if we can see some light at the end of the tunnel, the way may begin to seem more tenable.

The stories, exercises, meditations and insights gathered together in this book represent the wisdom of many who have learned from their illnesses, disabilities, and hardships. Though not everyone can be thankful for illness, pain or suffering, you may at least not feel so alone. As you open to your journey and connect more deeply with your own heart and with others also exploring the depths to which suffering can lead, you begin to find some peace in life. Those not directly dealing with loss or illness may gain some insight into the hearts and minds of partners, friends or children who are suffering.

And even the so called "ordinary" people, those whose lives have been seemingly untouched by such hardship or personal tragedy, whether happy or unhappy with their lives, may find benefit here. I have found that beneath the veneer of a happy person often lies some deep sadness or fear, or simply a vague unease of something amiss. There may be thoughts or feelings, almost unformed, that life is passing by without ever having been truly experienced, that the thing or person that could make one truly happy is forever out of reach.

Jane, a young friend of mine whose real name (along with the names of others who requested anonymity) I have changed, suffered from agoraphobia that didn't really surface until her second year of college. She told me about her life before illness:

> I was a college student and I was doing all the things that I loved to do, but I couldn't allow myself to really be in them and ... this scene that actually came back to me was ... getting on my bike and going up into the redwoods and just bringing a book and sitting in the meadow. I just remember in particular, I knew it would be a wonderful thing to do.
> And as I was doing it, I couldn't allow myself to be with my experience, and that sitting in that meadow even felt alienated. Part of me feels like before my illness ... there was such a distance from experience....
> I was so far removed. And actually this is what came to me—this "badness" just overwhelmed me the other night. Here was this person who was so afraid of herself to not be able to sit in the meadow and enjoy that experience. And there was this longing to be able to go back to that time and that person and be able to re-experience those things that I couldn't then and I wanted so badly.

And buried more deeply, in a place that never sees the light of day or any spoken word, or perhaps even any conscious thought at all, may be the belief that at the base of it all there is something dreadfully wrong, or that at one's core, one is really a bad, incompetent or unlovable person—the feeling that says, "If they knew who I really am inside, they wouldn't love me."

I grew up having many of these thoughts and feelings and believed them. I used to think that I was the only one in the world who felt that way. But in my journey, I have met many who have admitted to having these kinds of feelings at least fleetingly, and I have come to believe that these are very common human experiences. During one very difficult time when Jane was struggling with some deep and troubling inner demons, she shared some of her thoughts and fears with me. "I trusted," she said,

> that on some level ... I was dealing with it. But there was also another level that knew it was absolutely nuts. And that if anyone really, really, knew I had [these] fears, I'd get locked up.

I shared with my friend my own wondering if everybody doesn't have these same kinds of thoughts and feelings, these same fears that are so deeply hidden because we're afraid to tell people about them.

"I had so many of those same thoughts," I said. "If people really knew what was going on inside me, they'd think I was crazy or they'd see that 'I'm so fucked up,' you know, maybe not that they'd lock me away, but just...." I paused for a moment to collect my thoughts.

"They'd reject me." Jane finished my sentence for me. So there you have it. And there was silence between us as we allowed ourselves to experience the realization that it mostly boils down to the underlying fear of rejection that has condensed in most human hearts.

Our inner desperation or despair may be covered over by the happy face we put on to meet the world. How often we read in the newspaper a story of someone who has committed suicide. Those who knew the person may say he or she seemed happy. They just didn't see it coming. No judgment. Mercy. Mercy on the souls who, for whatever reason, were not able to continue the journey in this lifetime. May they be blessed. May they have peace. Most of us aren't going to go so far, though many may have considered it. We limp along often pretending everything is fine.

Sharon, a woman in my wellness support group for people with chronic illnesses, talked about how she puts out a certain self to the world, a well self. So people always think she's doing well. When she's really bad, she stays home. Another woman said she also does that. She thinks that if she's happy, people will like her—and if she's not, if she's hurting or sick, they won't like her.

But even happiness, at least as we usually know it, is almost always accompanied by its companion, the fear of the end of happiness. So we carry with us, even in happiness, the seeds of sorrow. To me, these afflictions are more disabling than any illness.

There has been no single phrase that has affected me so profoundly in my illness and my spiritual path as Steven Levine's response to a woman in great pain from a body wracked with cancer, when she asked him if she should stop trying to heal and just let herself die:

> Her question penetrated my body and froze my mind in place. I looked into her eyes, unable to respond from anything I knew or had ever experienced.
>
> Clearly it was a question only the heart could answer. And my heart, knowing deeper, whispered, "The real question is, 'Where is healing to be found?'" It is the question life asks itself: "What is completion?" It

brings into focus the no-man's-land between the heart and mind. Where is wholeness to be found in the seemingly separate? Where is the heart of healing in which all duality is resolved? (1987, 1)

What I realized when I read his words was that there were parts of me that needed healing much more than my body, and if those were healed, it wouldn't matter if my body was cured or not. What a huge relief that was—to give myself permission to stop chasing after bodily health, to open to the possibility that I could be healed and whole regardless of my physical condition, and that I wasn't a failure if I didn't heal in the body.

This was news—good news. And though the path before me looked long and difficult, it somehow didn't seem hopeless. It seemed almost do-able. My illness had cracked me open, made me humble enough to be receptive to whatever kind of healing was in store for me. I was ready—ready for healing into love. I thought of the Christian story of the paralytic whose friends were so devoted that they took apart the roof of the building in which Jesus was teaching, and lowered their friend into the room on his pallet so Jesus could heal him. And what did Jesus do? He said, "Son, your sins are forgiven." He did actually later heal the man physically as well, but that was sort of an aside—an afterthought. The primary healing was one of the heart.

I write and offer this book with deep humility from my limited understanding in the hope that someone may benefit from these words. Yet even if I were a completely enlightened being, anything I or anyone can speak or put on paper is only a partial truth. Though the truth may be beyond our knowing in any kind of intellectual way, it is not beyond knowing experientially—of this I am certain.

Many have shared this journey with me, who have been my teachers, pupils, lovers and friends. I hope to share some of what we have learned in our travels through chronic illness and cancer, disability, and unimaginable losses, about truly living life fully and openly in each moment, embracing the totality of our experience, and about healing in the largest possible sense.

I want to affirm with them now that living in Love and Joy *is* possible, even in the midst of tremendous physical or emotional pain or loss; that we can at last have mercy on ourselves, even after a lifetime of castigation; we can welcome our banished selves back into our hearts; we can regain the wholeness we lost in that first moment when someone in our world reflected back to us that we weren't okay; and we can heal the split from our true hearts that was brought on by our pain and our fear that through that rejection, we would be left alone forever. We are all on a journey—the journey of a lifetime, the journey home.

CHAPTER 1

Attention Means Attention

I asked myself if I could wake up tomorrow, have [my illness] be gone, be completely well, would I do it? And the answer was no.
—Member of Attitudinal Center Wellness Group

I DIVIDE MY LIFE UP INTO TWO PARTS: before suffering and after suffering. In reality, that's backwards because the first section labeled before suffering was actually the period in which I consider myself to have *really* been suffering. I affectionately refer to these parts as BS and AS.

It's amazing how much suffering we can endure before we begin to pay attention and realize we need to, or are motivated enough, to do something about it. The old Zen master Ichu said, "Attention means attention" (Kapleau, 1967, 10-11). Something needs to get our attention—unfortunately that something for many people comes in the form of a devastating life event or health crisis.

Now that I have a chronic illness, one *could* say that I am *really* suffering. I ache and am in pain much of the time. I can't work or do ninety percent of the activities I used to enjoy. Even talking to people is often impossible. Yet, I have more joy and am more at peace than at any other time of my life. Before the joy and peace, however, sandwiched between the BS and AS came a time of severe suffering. The little sufferings from the first part of my life paled in comparison.

This division of life into BS and AS (before suffering and after suffering) is, of course, a gross oversimplification, for, to be human is to suffer. The Buddha said, "Life is suffering." But to be fully alive we must open to our suffering, and it is the rare individual who can truly open to the pain of life.

Jesus said, "Behold, I stand at the door and knock; if any man hear my voice, and open the door, I will come in to him, and will sup with him, and he with me." (Rev. 3:20) Why do so few people open the door? Perhaps it is because we sense that to do so is to open the door to our deepest suffering and the suffering of the whole world, to give up our own little private world as we have arranged it and the control that we think we have over it. The Desert Fathers have warned us to be sure we really want what we are asking for when we ask the Holy Spirit to enter, for, they say, He will not leave us until He has broken our hearts and bones.

So we see that to open the door to Jesus, the Holy Spirit, God, Buddha, Nirvana, our True Hearts, Life As It Is—whatever name you put on it—is not a thing to be taken lightly. To open the door is to suffer; to not open the door is to suffer. So what are we to do? For people who are sincerely seeking the truth in their lives, it becomes obvious at some point that the second option is a dead end. The question then becomes, not so much *if* they will open the door, but *when*. This is a question each person must answer for him- or herself.

We may know deep in our hearts that our lives are untenable but have become so enmeshed in the web of lies and half truths that we have told ourselves and others for so many years, and the resultant life that has solidified around these descriptions, that opening to the truth may bring up anguish and the possibility of the kind of loss we are not ready for or even capable of handling. This is okay—as the first and most important thing to learn on this journey is to have loving kindness for ourselves.

When I was reading Steven Levine's book, *Healing Into Life and Death* for the first time, I came to the chapter on grief and closed the book. Our family was planning a trip to the East Coast to visit in-laws, and somehow I knew that if I read the chapter on grief, my life would unravel and I would never make it through the trip. That's because I was already so close to opening the door, I felt the vibrations behind it. My marriage was in trouble. I had known this for years. Also, I had been chronically ill for years with no signs of ever getting better. If I did decide to leave my husband, I had no idea how I would make it on my own.

My illness had exacerbated the problems in the marriage and vice versa, or may even, in part, have been triggered by the stress of living in a dysfunctional relationship. Our oldest daughter, a bright, creative and willful child, seemed to be taking the brunt of the dysfunction between my husband and I. We fought frequently over how to deal with her behavior and she was alienating herself from us all. I worried about her constantly. Add to this the stress of trying to keep a lid on all the pain from my own childhood, and one can see that the ice was pretty thin for me. When I came home, I read the chapter and my life fell apart. *I* fell apart—broken into a thousand pieces in a puddle of tears on the bedroom floor.

Opening to the grief of a lifetime is heady business. But what a relief: the truth at last allowed. And putting Humpty Dumpty together again in a new order could at last begin. Of course, Humpty Dumpty can never *really* be put back together, because he is the false self that has been held together through the years only with smoke and mirrors. And so one wouldn't *want* to put him back together. But the falling apart is the first step in opening to a new life—a more authentic and joyous life. There can be no real change until we are willing to fall apart. There can be no new order until we are willing to let go of the old order—the false self we have constructed over all the years of our lives.

In this process, suffering can be our ally. We cling to the belief that suffering is bad, but suffering is "good medicine." We are stuck like glue to our false view of reality—to become unstuck requires strong medicine. When the suffering has become so intense that it is no longer possible to ignore it, when it is breaking the door down, then we will open it.

Usually the kind of suffering that brings us to this point is not the kind of self-imposed suffering we all put ourselves through in our day-to-day lives—feeling inferior, put upon, rejected or abandoned—though it can. All these petty fears and hurts we encounter and carry with us through our lives are more easily tucked beneath the covers of our persona or projected outward onto others as anger or resentment. The real and severe physical or mental suffering brought on by a life-threatening or chronic illness rendering a person temporarily or permanently disabled, or a tragedy such as the death or disappearance of a child, or any other prolonged or severe hardship or loss, is harder to ignore or to rationalize away.

Those who have crossed over the threshold of the normal pains and disappointments of an ordinary life into extraordinary pain and suffering are often changed dramatically and irrevocably. They are forced to give up their view of life as they had previously seen it and have the opportunity to embark upon a path of profound healing and peace.

People who, in health or in what we might call a "normal" life, would probably never have been drawn to spiritual practice, are given an opportunity through their illness or loss. Because they are brought to the edge of despair, which is exactly where one needs to be to begin real work, they are delivered by grace, so to speak, to the very place at which serious spiritual seekers arrive only after years of effort or may never reach at all. When pain or suffering have battered us enough, we will finally surrender our stranglehold on life, and become soft and pliant as abalone beneath the cook's mallet.

These are the lucky ones. Some see their good fortune in a relatively short period of time, but usually it takes years or even a lifetime. Some may die never realizing what an extraordinary opportunity they have allowed to pass by.

This is not to say that an ill person or someone who has suffered a tragedy does not have to try or that it is easy for him. And it is certainly not to be implied that there is any kind of guarantee of spiritual opening simply because one has suffered a great loss. It is just that the choices for an ill or dying person, or someone who has lost a child for example, are so starkly drawn that he may begin to realize that, in a sense, he really has no choice. That is, he can choose to be utterly miserable or he can choose the path of acceptance, the path of peace. As the Zen master Suzuki Roshi put it, "Strictly speaking, for a human being, there is no other practice than this practice; there is no other way of life than this way of life." (1983, 23)

The same is true for a well or "normal" person; his life is full of pain and dead-end paths, and he is as surely on that one-way track toward death as the very sick or terminally ill person, but the diversions are so prolific and so tempting that making the choice to work on oneself is more likely to be put off for a long time, or even for a lifetime.

The grace of the situation, for me at least, is that I'm not at all sure I'd have had the courage or the fortitude to stay on the road and not turn back, had I not been given a one-way ticket via my illness. The title of Pema Chodron's wonderful book, The *Wisdom of No Escape*, expresses this truth beautifully.

It is a great leap for the ordinary person facing the possibility of a lifetime of debilitating illness to imagine that he may one day be thankful for this experience. Yet, as unbelievable and illogical as it may seem, this is often exactly what happens. I have seen it time and time again in the chronically ill people I have known, as well as in myself. And the same holds true for people who have endured other extreme hardships or loss, or are indeed facing the ultimate loss—life itself.

I remember sitting in my wellness group one sunny afternoon, having a discussion and a sharing about this topic. Every group member shared that in one way or another he or she had become a better, more compassionate, more joyful person because of his illness and had experienced a profound gratitude for this and a new, deeper appreciation for his life. Out of nine people sharing the circle that day, all but one agreed that, if they could choose to be well again, but had to give up what they had learned, they would not do it. One man had just finished telling us all the things that were wrong with his body. Then he added,

> I asked myself if I could wake up tomorrow, have it all be gone, be completely well, would I do it? And the answer was "no." Somehow all these aches and pains are an opening into my soul. When I was growing up, there were so many things, so many feelings that were taboo. I put them all in a box. Now I'm starting to open that box. The biggest problem is loneliness. But I had that problem before I got sick. Actually I was even more lonely before I got sick.

Another woman, Denise, had been through a long series of acute and chronic conditions over a period of years: first a car accident that permanently debilitated her knee, then a series of operations and a long drawn-out criminal trial in which she tried in vain to get back medical expenses and some recompense for the suffering she had endured and the life she had forgone.

Meanwhile the painkillers and steroids her doctors were prescribing were slowly eating away at her stomach and immune system. She contracted endometriosis, which further debilitated her. She tried to keep up, but had incredible stress with her job and her family. Finally at the end of her rope, she gave in to repeated urges from doctors to have a hysterectomy—dashing her long-held dreams of bearing children.

But somehow all these dark years were fertile for Denise. Through her pain and loss she was learning valuable lessons. I had watched her blossom from a woman with low self-esteem and a victim mentality, to a vibrant and loving being very much in touch with her inner spirituality. She had gone through huge swings in her state of health. At one point, though still dealing with significant health problems, things improved to the point where she was back to work full-time and able to do things that hadn't been possible for many years. At that time (in an earlier circle) she had told us that doors were opening faster than she could even keep up with them. Her life was zooming ahead full speed. "I was working ten-hour days," she had said.

> I had my nieces and nephews with me. I was trying to make up for all the fun I missed in the last eleven years. I was very close to life as it was before I got sick and suddenly realized I didn't want it. I was driving down the freeway with two kids in my car at eighty-five miles an hour and I said to myself, "This is crazy."

So on the day of the sharing about gratitude for the teachings our illnesses had brought us, Denise said,

> Illness is a gift because, if I didn't have those wake up calls, I would be back to my old life of compulsion and addiction to doing. What I am learning is so completely contrary to old beliefs, that it is something I'm going to have to keep learning over and over again.

The stories went on around the circle as we shared the bittersweet blessings of our individual losses. This teaching of course is not a magic bullet. Illness or personal tragedy is an event, and like all of life's events, it is, in its essence, neutral. It is not out to get us or to save us. It is just life living itself. How we react to it and whether we benefit or lose depends mainly on our openness and our willingness to let life, our experiences, our feelings in—to let them work on us, mold us. In that sense, all of life's experiences are out to save us.

CHAPTER 2

Opening to Grief

The soul would have no rainbow if the eyes had no tears.
—Native American Proverb

USUALLY, IN OUR LIVES, we're too busy to pay much attention to the inner life. We pay it lip service: some may go to church on Sundays or take up a meditation practice; others may seek occasional help from a therapist. But mostly, the pressing concerns of life seem to demand our attention—and we give in a little too quickly, without really questioning the necessity of the things and activities that seem to spring up like weeds to fill our lives. Subconsciously, I think, we're not only glad for them, but actually create more and more distractions and busyness to keep ourselves from experiencing the gnawing pain inside, the one we hoped to quiet or mollify with that little dose of religion, meditation, or therapy. We're trying desperately to stem the tide of the inevitable that is constantly threatening to wash over us and sweep us away into the dark depths of we know not what.

The Princess and the Pea

There is a fairy tale about a princess who couldn't sleep because she had a pea under her mattress. She kept piling up mattresses to try to keep from feeling the pea. But no matter how many she piled up, the morning found her bleary-eyed from lack of sleep because of the discomfort of that pea. Our busyness is the padding we put between ourselves and our pain to keep from feeling it. We glide along in our lives, ignoring all the little signs sent to us from our subconscious telling us that all is not well. But no matter how busy we make ourselves, something deep inside keeps poking at us. And when these pokes can no longer be ignored, we use religion, meditation, or therapy to try to fix things up: get *more* mattresses, *thicker* mattresses, *softer* mattresses, *harder* mattresses, sleep on your side, sleep on your stomach, visualize the pea as a snowball melting, and on and on and on we go seeking more and more solutions.

Man is a tinkerer and a fusser. He always thinks he can make things better by changing them. Our species has introduced a witch's brew of pesticides, atomic bombs, plastics, fiberglass, and all manner of pills and synthetic hormones to fix or improve things. We have built dams to restrict the natural flow of water, fences to restrict the natural flow of wildlife, and drugs to restrict the natural healing powers of the human body. But the human body and Mother Earth, both of which have evolved swimmingly over centuries, changing from the inside out and outside in to adapt to each other and the cosmos, don't have a clue about what to do with these new substances and structures suddenly thrust upon them. And this tinkering, this seemingly endless proclivity of man to fix things up or make them better does not end with the physical world or the body. We think we can fix up our souls as well—make them better or more spiritual—more "pure."

There are several systems of healing, such as homeopathy and chi gung, that are based on the premise that the body *does* know what to do with itself. These gentle healing methods teach that sometimes, because of all the unnatural substances in the world, the body gets a little confused and needs a nudge to get back on the right track—that is, tuned back into its own wisdom. One of these, the anthroposophical approach to homeopathy, goes so far as to say that certain illnesses are *necessary* in order for us to enter a new phase of growth, either physically or on a spiritual level. It has been noted that children often make a big shift after intense childhood illnesses such as measles or chickenpox, that they are more well or more robust or have had a positive psychological movement.

The Soul Knows What to Do

And on an even deeper level, the soul knows what to do with itself. While we have been busy tinkering—piling up bigger and better mattresses—our souls have been working in conjunction with the

Great Wisdom underlying all creation, to bring us to a point where we will finally pay attention. As the famous words from a Rolling Stone's song remind us, "You can't always get what you want, but if you try sometimes, you just might find you get what you need." And what we may need to get back on track, if we have wandered far from our spiritual path, is a big jolt—something which may, on the level of everyday life, seem very bad.

It may seem like an unfortunate (to our limited thinking mind) coding in our genetic make-up that makes humans pay a higher level of attention to negative or powerful experiences (burn = pain = "stay away from fire") than we do to more pleasurable ones. We are biological beings, and we are subject to biological laws under which the highest level of good is survival. When we encounter something that may be dangerous, fear kicks in, which can be a very useful emotion under certain conditions. The body is flooded with hormones that get the heart beating, the blood flowing, and energy to every part of the body. When there is physical danger, we need these hormones flowing to give us the super-strength we may need to run from danger, to lift a boulder, to swim for our lives.

In the modern world, however, the dangers we perceive are more often psychological in nature. In our more sedentary lives, the "fight or flight" hormones that flood our bodies, when we need to work everyday with a boss we hate or our children develop a mysterious illness that won't go away, can be a double-edged sword. They make us pay attention—yes, but unless we know how to use this surging energy, it can wreak havoc on the body, perhaps even contributing to a serious long-term illness. This would normally be looked on in the world of everyday thinking as a bad thing—a "negative outcome."

The year before I contracted my long-term chronic illness was the most stressful year of my life. I recognized that my body was in a "fight or flight" condition a majority of the time. I knew it was bad for my body, but didn't know what to do, how to deal with it. I thought I could deal with it by doing lots of meditation. As I sat in meditation, I felt like a kettle of boiling oil with the lid on. I thought, if I could only get to the peaceful core, I would be all right. But I couldn't do it. Day after day I boiled in the pot, trying desperately to avoid being boiled.

I didn't know about "experiencing" the process that was later to become the mainstay of my spiritual practice.[1] I think I had an inkling about it at this point, but I was still trying to some extent to jump over the painful part—the transformational cooking—into what I thought I "should" be. I didn't know that to simply allow myself to "be the boiling" could cook me into some delectable delight. Finally I think, the raging hormones in the boiler, along with exposure to several toxic pesticides and a far from stellar genetic inheritance, led to a major collapse of my body from which it has never quite recovered. And from this outcome, originally perceived as negative, has flowed an incredible outpouring of learning, light and love. I have learned to be the boiling. I have learned to trust life in a way I never thought possible.

"All Dreams Come in the Service of Healing"

It seems the penchant for the psyche to pay more attention to dangerous stimuli than to more pleasurable ones, as a survival mechanism, carries over into the dreaming world as well. Jeremy Taylor, a Jungian psychologist who specializes in dreams, says that "all dreams come in the service of healing"—even nightmares. He claims, in fact, that if the psyche really wants us to pay attention to some valuable information, it will be presented as a nightmare. The great spiritual teachers often speak of life as a dream from which we are called to awake. I asked myself if perhaps all of our waking dreams also come in the service of healing? I believe they do, even our worst nightmares. Sometimes, I think, we even energetically create or bring to ourselves that which we need to work on, or the conditions that will bring us to the stuck or wounded places in ourselves that need healing.

Ezra Bayda, a teacher at the San Diego Zen Center, keeps a picture on his wall of a skater gliding along on the ice with one leg out behind her, and her arms and head thrown up in a grand gesture, blissfully ignorant of the sign she is speeding past, which warns of thin ice. He says, "It's like we're skating on the ice—the momentum of life almost carries us along on automatic pilot. But even when we're gliding along, something inside of us knows that we're ignoring things that we'll ultimately have to face. Yet we glide along, even knowing that the ice is thin."

This ice is another analogy for the separation we put between ourselves and the unpleasant parts of ourselves or life that we don't want to experience. The skater gliding along obliviously on top of the ice represents us sailing along in our lives in what we consider to be our "good" selves, when life is going fairly smoothly. We're feeling okay about ourselves in general—having fun, being successful, or successful "enough"; we have friends, we may have a mate or are at least dating. In the case of spiritual practitioners, we may feel that our practice is going well, or at least that we're dealing with our difficulties in a positive way. Our lives are good, or at least okay, according to whatever definition we have of that.

Lurking beneath the ice, however, is all the unconscious baggage that we carry from a lifetime of inexperienced, and consequently unhealed, pain, and all the wounded "I"s that think of themselves as bad, wrong, flawed, or unlovable, and see life as too hard, too painful, or too frightening. Falling through the ice is what happens when our world falls apart in big or little ways, causing us to come face-to-face with that pain and often with one or more of our wounded selves. One might conclude, when contemplating the picture of the skater near the thin ice, that the idea or "moral to the story" would be to avoid the thin ice, to steer clear of that place where we would fall through into the freezing water.

But this is not necessarily the case. That world on the other side of the ice is part of our own Self—the part we have rejected—the part without which we cannot be whole. In the Gurdjieffian system, there are things called "buffers," insulating shields between the various selves and belief systems that keep us from seeing any but the one we're inhabiting at the moment, thus giving us the illusion of a unified self. However, when something happens that threatens that self or worldview, the shield is sometimes penetrated and we see what's on the other side. These buffers may be looked at as the ice between the skater and her darker unacknowledged side—the shadow side. Though our life has brought us plenty of opportunities to wake up, to see what's on the other side, we have missed most of them.

Actually, we fall through the ice in little ways every day. Perhaps just a foot breaks through, and we feel the icy water for a few moments. We find ourselves in a crisis, which we think has been caused by someone or something. We tell ourselves this is an unusual state, that usually we are calm and that this is something different. We wonder what hit us when suddenly, without warning, a song or a few casual words spoken by a friend, a co-worker, or even a total stranger bring tears or throw us suddenly into catastrophe.

Our Bodies Carry the Crisis State with Us

The truth is that our bodies carry the crisis state with us all the time. We are so used to it, that most of the time we don't even notice it is there. Someone criticizes us (or says something we perceive as critical), we're called upon to give a presentation or simply to talk in an unfamiliar situation, we're not invited to an affair to which we expected an invitation, a friend doesn't treat us in the way we think we should be treated, a contractor messes up a job at our house and refuses to take responsibility, or, in a moment of anger, we say something hurtful to a loved one, and in a heartbeat, the composure and the upbeat attitude we thought we had toward life is suddenly gone, replaced with anger, resentment, insecurity, shame, guilt, fear, or a combination of any number of negative feelings.

And under these negative feelings, if we care to look, are all of our false beliefs about life, and all the selves we refuse to acknowledge in our "normal" state. A person in my meditation group once shared how someone she had never met, or even heard of, triggered in her all kinds of negative feelings, including the feeling that she didn't belong on this earth, simply by leaving a very nasty note on her car. In this case, it may seem obvious to spiritual practitioners that these feelings were already there and the note was merely a tool (ice pick) to enable her to access these feelings. These occurrences are actually excellent opportunities to practice. They're more manageable than the big-time "fall throughs," and can help prepare us for the major crises in our lives.

For many people, the idea of falling through the ice may be easier to relate to when they think of it as a result of some big crisis such as the death of a loved one, the loss of a job, divorce, or serious illness. But even this is still just an idea. We don't really, in our actual experience, "get it." In our magical thinking, we don't *really* see ourselves as subject to that devastation, unless it is actually happening to us or sometimes to someone very close to us. However many chances we get in our everyday life, or how clear in theory the idea may be, some of us may just not get it. We may actually need to fall through the ice into the freezing water, before we will pay attention. Maybe it will be an incurable illness, paralysis, or the death of a child that finally wakes us up.

Ken, a man in my meditation group, had experienced several run ins with what would later prove to be a serious and debilitating illness. These preliminary experiences didn't impact him much on an emotional or spiritual level. Ken said,

> I was a little concerned, but I wasn't really afraid, and I just had the attitude that I would beat my illness. So even though there was probably some fear there, there was more the attitude that I'm not really sick. And so I did this special diet, I took special vitamins, I did healing meditations, and I just decided I would make myself better and that was all there was to it. And the truth is I did get better—I don't know if any of those three things worked, but mostly I didn't have a lot of emotion around it and I didn't learn very much from it.

It wasn't until a few years later, when the illness returned with a vengeance, that Ken could no longer maintain his illusion of control and of not really being sick.

> After around three weeks I started to have all the classic emotional reactions following the denial that I was going to stay sick, when I realized that I was just getting weaker and weaker. There was very definitely anger, why is this happening to me? It was very definitely self-pity, big doses of self-pity—about poor me. There was a lot of fear, because the fear was, "What's going to happen to me? Will I ever be able to make a living?" I was losing my ability to relate to my wife as a husband. I was losing my ability to relate to my children as a father. I couldn't work anymore. I couldn't be a Zen person anymore. I couldn't play music.
>
> And basically I had the fear and the sense of groundlessness of losing all my identities, and along with that there was a sense of isolation. It was difficult to talk, even to my close friend who already understood about this, because I felt inwardly isolated. There was also the sense of grief, of life no longer being the way I expected it to be.
>
> This tremendous sense of loss, especially around my physical body—the realization that I couldn't be physical, and that maybe I wouldn't be able to be physical again, although there was a part of me

that didn't even really believe it, but I couldn't really pretend, like [I had earlier], that I could just make myself better, because it was obvious that I couldn't. In general my initial experiences of being ill really had no depth. When it returned in full force and didn't go away, it had a great deal of depth, but in the beginning I only saw it in negative terms, because I only saw it through the filter of fear and self-pity.

When a person feels him/herself spiraling downward into a seemingly hopeless situation such as a fatal disease, incurable long-term illness or progressive disorder, or suffers an "insufferable" loss, the resultant feeling of loss of control, hopelessness and despair can bring about a crisis. You may feel as if you're falling off the face of the earth. There were times in my illness when I thought I might as well be dead, because for all intents and purposes it seemed I already was. Not that I ever contemplated suicide, but the feeling of total uselessness that I felt, and that many in similar circumstances experience, can lead to depression. And that depression can turn to despair. At that point we may totally lose our grounding.

My friend Jane, who fell into a severe episode of agoraphobia in college, experienced this groundlessness in a very literal way. She described her descent into fear and hopelessness culminating in a sense of alienation from the earth itself:

> I'd had a lot of fear most of my life, or probably all of my life, but I never had a way to understand it. Or, I never put it in terms of an illness, I guess, because it was just me; it was what I dealt with. I had all my little strategies for coping with it. And then in 1993, I was a sophomore in college, and all of my coping mechanisms just weren't doing the trick, and so things that I could do sort of uncomfortably before were now just becoming impossible ... I wasn't able to ride the bus anymore ... there were so many seats in a classroom that I couldn't sit in, and so everything, just everything, had become harder and harder.
>
> And then I saw [a friend of mine] after several months and she said that, during the time I hadn't seen her, she had actually tried to commit suicide and was in the hospital ... and told me the story. Well, something about that traumatized me. It was horrifying to imagine. I had never considered suicide literally, but I think something about life is unbearable, like getting to that place was really resonating, and to realize that it could go all the way.... Something just broke in me.
>
> All these things just started collecting really fast. I was in such an enormous state of panic. Of course I didn't recognize it as panic. I

thought of it as "I'm leaving the planet," but I literally couldn't function at all, couldn't leave my room, couldn't do anything, and called my mom in the middle of the night from school. And she came down immediately and got me. And I never went back.

I just didn't feel like there was anything in me ... NOTHING in me that I could count on, not from one breath to the next, not that I could decide that my left leg was going to move and take a step.

I really felt that somehow I didn't have a legitimate place on the earth, that the fear was so deep about just existing, but that at one moment in particular I remember standing on the ground and feeling like the earth could just decide to kick me off. So there was this mixed up feeling ... [that] tied in with the fear of existing and also the feeling that I did't fit in any social order any more, like I did't have a social universe to hold myself in; and I was also just terrified of existing, so I felt like I did't have a physical universe to exist in.

If we do have a spiritual practice, nothing that we've learned may seem to apply. The reason for this is that the "I" we are experiencing is not the "I" who practices. If we have fallen through big-time, we may actually be under the ice, and have no access to our world or our belief system as we knew them when we were the skater on top of the ice.

"I was lost," Ken remembers.

I couldn't do my regular meditation practice, because I couldn't sit in zazen. I didn't realize at the time that you could meditate even if you didn't have any energy. I was really floundering in that I had lost all sense of practice and all sense of direction.

Despair Can Be a Gateway

This is the groundlessness that can cause panic or despair. This is a crucial point. Despair can be the gateway to a new way of seeing and being, a downward spiral into self-pity and bitterness, or an escape into mind-numbing activities and addictions. Worse, this can be the point where some contemplate or actually commit suicide. Jane, like me, never consciously considered suicide, but it nevertheless played a huge part in her subconscious world.

I hadn't had enough life experience yet to have a sense of who I was. And this was the time where I was trying to figure out what that was,

[to] find out for myself, but at the time, I couldn't even think about tomorrow. I couldn't even imagine anything but eating breakfast, so there was just a huge void [in terms of] relating to myself as a person. "What kind of person am I? Am I really a person?"

I never allowed [the process] to be fully conscious [but] somewhere, below consciousness I struggled a lot with [questions like,] "Should I stay alive?" And I think that partly because I had a friend who tried to commit suicide, which scared me so, so, so, much, any thought that even remotely had anything to do with my thinking that way, I just couldn't let it surface. But I know that sense of meaninglessness and void that wonders, "Do I have a future of any kind?"—I know those [stem from] extreme fear and exhaustion from the fear of life. I am afraid to be alive. I know all of those things played in some subconscious way [with the question of] whether I should keep living.

I was definitely afraid of knives at that time. I could hardly look at them. The thought would just uncontrollably pop into my mind, almost like a filmstrip of myself taking a knife and slitting my wrist, but I could never consciously think those thoughts through.

At least three people that I know of from our chronic illness support group contemplated suicide. One of my best friends from the group struggled with the urge to end her life for years as she dealt with unbelievable daily pain, which continued virtually unabated during that difficult time. She could not tolerate any of the powerful pain medications that might have provided relief. When, in desperation, she tried, on a doctor's recommendation, having a morphine pump implanted, it caused her Responsive Sympathetic Dystrophy (RSD)[2] to get worse, consequently increasing the pain she experienced. Another woman, unable to find any light or hold on to any hope of better times, committed suicide when she reached the end of her ability to cope with the seemingly endless pain and difficulty in her life.

The tragedy in suicide is that this point of hopelessness, when we have hit rock bottom, is precisely the point at which something real can happen. At this point, a person is presented with a choice. What all this loss is really bringing up for us is grief. But we don't want the grief, so we often fall into despair instead. Despair is what happens when we hold our grief at arm's length—when we block it from entering the heart. Grief has movement to it—it is authentic healing. Despair is a dead end. Despair is a signal telling us that we are closed.

We are resisting our life. The choice is to stay closed or to open to that grief—the grief of a lifetime—and begin healing.

Ken's attitude toward his illness shifted when he began to see it as his path.

> I started to understand what Stephen Levine meant about the difference between being healed and being cured, because even when I didn't know what direction the physical symptoms were going to take in terms of actually getting cured, I started to understand what it meant to become healed, in the sense of becoming a more whole person by going much more deeply into myself, allowing the force of quieting down to become a positive force.

My friend with RSD, after going through several extremely dark and difficult years, began to open to many aspects of her true self that she hadn't been acknowledging. She turned many things in her life to go in a new direction and her pain eventually became more manageable. She now feels satisfied with her life, happy to be alive and very grateful she didn't succumb to her desire to commit suicide during those extremely difficult times.

Though each person's path to healing is different, what is amazing is the similarity of the states and experiences people report on their journeys, whatever the source of their grief. Elisabeth Kubler-Ross has done a great service by developing and teaching the five stages of grief, which are described in her ground-breaking book, *On Death and Dying*, and have helped untold numbers of people deal with the final stages of dying, and grief-stricken parents, lovers, and friends all over the world to understand and process the feelings that arise with the profound loss of a loved one. They have also become valuable tools used by bereavement workers to help others deal with such loss. The stages of grief identified by Elisabeth Kubler-Ross are:

Denial (this isn't happening to me!)
Anger (why is this happening to me?)
Bargaining (I promise I'll be a better person *if...*)
Depression (I don't care anymore.)
Acceptance (I'm ready for whatever comes.)

I think these descriptions are very useful as far as they go and to the extent that it is extremely helpful to know that most of the feelings we are experiencing when we go through such losses are common to many in similar circumstances—that we are not freaks and not necessarily lost or doomed because we are experiencing such dark or negative emotions. It is also useful to have information that at least points to the idea that these are stages or states that are likely to change (even though we may not believe it at the time we are feeling lost in denial, anger or despair.)

All Losses Must Be Grieved

Though I have found these descriptions extremely useful when dealing with my own extensive grief, they are, in my opinion, somewhat limited and incomplete. One limitation is the implication that grief and the grieving process belong to the realm of death and dying. While this is, I think, true in a very fundamental way—that is, in the sense that all experience of loss and all fears stem from the fear of death—our daily griefs, which seem to pop up like weeds in the gardens of our souls, need to be addressed as they present themselves.

We experience losses daily—some huge, some tiny, and everything in between. These losses can take many forms: the loss of a job, a pet or a friend, the loss of an ideal such as "til death do us part" when our marriage is shattered by divorce, or the loss of our home or a treasured keepsake. And there are the losses having to do with our bodies: the loss of bodily function and the resulting loss of many beloved activities through accident, illness or age, the loss or disfigurement of an actual part of our body, a limb or our face, and thus perhaps our image of ourselves as desirable. These losses can be as devastating as facing death or perhaps more so because they do not have an end. They go on and on.

On some level we must grieve all of our losses in order to integrate them and move on with our lives. I love Lucille Clifton's ode to her breast before having it removed:

> lumpectomy eve
>
> > all night I dream of lips
> > that nursed and nursed
> > and the lonely nipple

> lost in loss and the need
> to feed that turns at last
> on itself that will kill
>
> its body for its hunger's sake
> all night I hear the whispering
> the soft
>
> love calls you to this knife
> for love for love
>
> all night it is the one breast
> comforting the other

(*Contemporary American Poetry*, p. 82, used without permission)

What a beautiful and loving way to grieve the loss of her breast. We may not all be as graceful in our grieving process. Sometimes it is messy and ugly. But it is important for us to reassure ourselves and others that grieving for the things we have lost is a necessary and positive step. Though most mental health professionals are coming to see that grief is much wider, deeper, and more pervasive in the human psyche than previously thought, and that it is a normal response to many kinds of loss or change not limited to death and dying, some still cling to more antiquated ideas.

This is not surprising, considering that as recently as 1974 the *Handbook of Psychiatry* defined grief as "... the normal response to the loss of a loved one by death," while responses to other kinds of losses were categorized as "Pathological Depressive Reactions." Since many therapists trained during that era would still be practicing today, and understanding that we were all raised in the traditions of bygone eras, it would be surprising if this mindset did not still pervade, or at least color, the attitudes of current practice. However, until we come to accept loss and grief as inextricable and perhaps necessary aspects of everyday life, we will go through our lives feeling that there's something wrong with us for having these completely normal human experiences. We make the movement through grief harder than it needs to be by adding guilt or shame to an already difficult process.

The second major limitation or, as I see it, "missing part," in the commonly accepted stages of grief is the implication that we can go from depression/despair directly into acceptance. Simply because someone has depression/despair does not mean that they will automatically move to acceptance. I understand that Dr. Kubler-Ross cautioned followers not to expect a linear or orderly progression through the five stages, and most grief counselors now say it is very common to skip around and backtrack in the grieving process.

Still, I think, there is an additional stage in the process of grieving that is essential to experience before it is actually possible to move on to true acceptance. I would call this stage simply "grief" or "opening to grief" and place it between depression/despair and acceptance. Before we can really move to acceptance, we must, in my opinion, first move from depression/despair *into* grief. The key here, I think, is willingness. We must be willing to have our depression or despair, our sickness or our loss, despite the intense pain it may bring. We must be willing to truly experience the bodily pain and the emotional pain. When we become willing to participate in our lives in whatever form they take, things begin to shift.

Jane's condition seemed to get worse when she got her diagnosis of agoraphobia, but in allowing herself to be who she was and stop resisting her life, a new healing force came into her life.

> And interesting, as soon as I got the agoraphobia book, I couldn't even leave the house. But I think in realizing that this is what I have, there was almost a letting go or giving up or resting. I know I've been white knuckling it my whole life and in order to learn another way, I've gotta let that go. I feel like through all of this, there [has been] a lot of wisdom that kind of just surrounded me [when] I would be experiencing all the fear. Then there would be a perspective that saw it as a process. I guess that's why I was saying there were several levels I could get so hysterical, despondent, terrified, ashamed, depressed, and all these things that, "oh my God, I have no life and what if I never have one again and I'm only twenty years old and my God, I'm a shut-in" and, you know, all of that stuff. And, at the same time there was also the perspective that this is a process that was the underlying voice, but it didn't keep me from feeling all those other feelings.

We Must Give up Our Demand to Be Happy

Krishnamurti says that in order to be free we must give up our demand to be happy. And if we hold onto a demand that we need to be well in order to be happy, we'll never be free either, *or* happy. His words are tricky because even the word "freedom," in the way that we normally think of it, has implications that may not be what Krishnamurti meant. Perhaps "love" might be a word I would choose, but both love and freedom are words which have connotations in everyday life that are too small and limiting for the meaning implied here, which is a state beyond freedom, hope or happiness as we normally think of them.

We can wish for our illness to be gone, we can prefer that it be gone, but if we hold onto it as a demand for our happiness, we're trapped forever in being unhappy until our demand is met. We must move into our grief completely. We must give ourselves to our grief. We must be willing to have our grief. We must *be* our grief. Only then can we truly move to the stage of acceptance, or acceptance will emerge of its own as a natural outcome.

Ken slowly learned to be with his illness in a new way, no longer needing to fight or conquer it, but opening to whatever it would bring and whatever his life would bring. "Probably the most valuable part of being sick," he said,

> was, along with slowing down and gradually feeling the texture of life and gradually learning to appreciate life more in its details, was the gradual understanding of what it means to just let life be—to not have to try to change or do anything about anything. Instead, whatever comes up, including the experience of illness or other difficulties, to learn how to just acknowledge that they are there, acknowledge my reactions to them, even if they're negative, and then just let it all be there.

The Chinese character for crisis is made up of two other characters—the character for danger and the character for opportunity. There seems to be a message embedded in the Chinese language that opportunity walks hand-in-hand with danger. But opportunity for what? The word "opportunity" implies action. We tend to think that when opportunity arises, we don't need to act on it right away. That's the old trick of the mind again—telling us we have time. "What's the hurry?" it tells us. "It will be there tomorrow, next week, next year." We think we can put it off. We have something else we want to do first. But opportunity is a strange thing—it doesn't work like that.

It's Only Too Late If You Don't Start Now

I remember a book I saw recently titled, *It's Only Too Late If You Don't Start Now*. That seems true. There are windows of opportunity that open—and then close again—while we're getting sidetracked with that something we wanted to do first. These openings go by like ducks in a shooting gallery. If we see one we like or that is useful, we'd better shoot it or grab it or enter it or be it now, because soon enough it will fall off the edge of the track. Truly each moment is one of these windows, and in a moment it is gone.

Kabir said,

> If you don't break your ropes while you're alive,
> do you think ghosts will do it after?
> The idea that the soul will join with the ecstatic
> just because the body is rotten—
> That is all fantasy.
>
> *The Kabir Book,* versions by Robert Bly, p. 24

My sense is that this being human—simply being born into a real physical flesh and blood body—is a rare opportunity, an opportunity to do something that the unembodied celestial beings cannot do. Sometimes when one is really present, the experience of this world is so exquisite, so beautiful or tender or poignant that we want to tell others about our experience, record it, share it somehow in words, in pictures, in song. But there is no way really to do this because nothing can really capture that experience in its totality.

I was having one of those moments one night alone in my bed before sleep. Touching my own arm was like making love; and the walls, the very air between me and those walls, seemed alive, vibrant with beauty. I thought, "If God wanted to create an instrument capable of having such an experience, He would create a being exactly like me." This may sound incredibly redundant, but it was actually a huge epiphany—that these seemingly imperfect physical bodies are the perfect instrument through which being-ness can be experienced. And that when illness or grief or some great calamity comes along to crack us open, this too is a rare opportunity and we should take it—for all things pass.

Don Juan, the Yaqui Indian teacher from the books of Carlos Castaneda, talked about twilight as being the crack between the worlds—the crack between the noetic spiritual world and the physical world, an opening, a way to bridge these two, or perhaps a doorway through which one can enter the noetic world from the physical.

When I have been very ill, and this illness goes on for a very long time, I feel sometimes that I am living in a twilight zone—half dead, or perhaps half alive; sometimes I don't know which. At these times I don't know which world I belong in—the world of the dead or the world of the living. I now see this as an opportunity, a crack between the worlds—an opening. I know that this window too will close. This opportunity will exist only for a time. This very body, this form, is exactly right for me in this moment. It is a metaphor for the spiritual landscape. In some mysterious way, there seems to be an interface, that how we relate to our physical world is reflected in the spiritual realm.

Metaphor

I live in two bodies like the river
with her silent sister
beneath the earth. Each invisible
truth has its manifest shadow,
the dream mistaken in the world of shadows
for the true self. Metaphor of tree,
green and brown against a whisper
of sky and cloud, glides in this ephemera
like a perfect mirror. The exquisite rye
seedhead leans to the dark
with feathery fingers, spider webs
shimmer as if imminently real, as if

>   the world, a thousand reasons for being,
>   held the whole immense truth
>   in one glistening body.
>
>   —Diane LaRae Bodach

"It's interesting," Jane reflected, about the time in her life when she was very sick, but moving toward wholeness:

> Most things in my life at that time felt like a metaphor. The quilt [I was making] was one metaphor, and the piano playing, this garden, and lots of imagery of sprouts. I constantly felt like I was making roots. I have this one picture that has a sprout that's about half an inch long. These roots go for most of the page.
>
> This time was about finally getting myself really grounded where my life, before the crash, had all the trappings of a flower, but the flower didn't have any roots. And it withered and died. And somehow, I had to not be invested in plans and appearances in all the things that I had. I had to totally, just finally, grow some roots. And I feel like that was something really conscious in me [that happened] when I would be gardening.

Through my illness, I am learning to navigate the sometimes treacherous waters between these two worlds—the world of the physical and the world of the spiritual realms. When I was going through chemotherapy for breast cancer, I was terribly sick. I felt so constricted and stuck in a miserable body, but I was very much alive in that in-between world and had learned to let it teach me. I wrote in my journal:

> I slip down the rabbit hole into something. Something that encloses me—touches my form in every spot, like a suit of skintight clothes. At first I think it's too tight, that it binds me and presses on me and makes me uncomfortable when I move. But then I realize that it exactly fits my form. It allows me to feel, to experience exactly what I am. I begin to move with more freedom, to discover exactly where I begin and where I end, who I am, where I'm constricted, and where I'm free.

I thought of Hubert Benoit's description of the "hard and icy couch" in his book, *The Supreme Doctrine*—his vision of what his life felt like in the midst of despair—and how if he somehow was able to simply rest on that couch, the couch of his despair, it fit his form perfectly and supported him completely.

"There were some points," Ken said,

> not many, but there were some points where I actually fell into the experience which I called surrender or grace, where I really willingly allowed my physical symptoms to be there, and there's no way that anyone can say that it's not of great benefit. And in fact, probably more than anything in my life, I experienced more positive depth of appreciation for life, when I was sick, than at any other time.

Father John, an Orthodox priest who has counseled hundreds of individuals and families in times of crisis, observed that many in the throes of severe hardship or loss have had remarkable openings in their spiritual life. Yet one cannot ignore the danger inherent in this situation. There is a very thin line between true spiritual opening and craziness. Getting lost in the jungle of our own darkness is a real hazard. I particularly related to Jane's description of her fear that she would be caught, because of her own inadequacy, in some hell–like place, which to me, is probably what craziness is.

> I always felt a certain sense of inadequacy, like something was being asked of me and I knew that it just had to happen, but I didn't think I'd ever be able to ... the fear was so huge that I couldn't get beyond it. There was a despondence. [I thought] "I'm never going to be able to get beyond the fear, and yet this calling is always going to be calling me." There was also this fear—it wasn't a fear about death—death sounded great, although I never would have the courage to commit suicide—that was at least quiet and peaceful. What I feared was this force calling me out, but my fear wouldn't let me fully go and so I'd be stuck in. I imagined it as this space, this kind of void limbo place ... the imagery was of me scratching at a glass or something, trying to get back into my body but being too far out ... and not being willing to go all the way.

The Dark Night of the Soul

In the Christian tradition this crisis point, or period (it can go on for a long time), is often called the dark night of the soul. It seems, somehow, the law of the way things work, that we cannot have the one without the other. We cannot have the chance at true happiness, everlasting life, Nirvana, union with God, peace, freedom, or whatever name we give to the unnameable essence of the Divine, the joy inherent in existence, without going through the fire, descending into some dark place, or falling into the icy water. Why? Because the darkness or what we think is darkness—the pain, the unpleasantness and discomfort that we have been resisting, pushing away all of our lives—that pea under the mattress—is part of the whole picture.

We have wanted to think we could have happiness and pleasure all the time, but this is not possible. Happiness is gauged by the sorrow we have known. We can have Joy all the time—the deep Joy that arises out of being truly present to our lives as they are, but the happiness we normally think of as happiness is a relative thing known only by comparison to something else. Gangaji, speaking of the story of the Princess and the Pea, says, get rid of the mattresses. *Feel* that pea. The pea, that gnawing discomfort, she says, *is* God. What a revolutionary idea! That which we have been avoiding, that which we want to be rid of, is that which we seek!

So your road to wholeness may begin with your loss—with your grief. It may not feel like wholeness. It may not feel like a road to any place you want to go—you may feel more broken than you have ever felt in your life. Yet the fact that this is happening to you means that, somehow, you are ready for this lesson.

Midnight's Garden

As out of compost does the lily grow,
so from the refuse of our lives, beauty
can be born. The seed does not spurn the low
earth, excrement of worms, but completely

gives itself, is buried in it, fortified
and transformed, taking refuge in that which
the world casts off. Therefore lay not aside
your griefs, but like the good gardener, gather rich

green weeds of mind, dung of low and mean intent,
dry bones of despair, ashes of burnt out desire,
twisted thorned prunings, which your heart rent.
Water with tears, while the alchemical fire

Burns and purifies until, you are not weed,
but humus; rich, black, and sweet, ready for seed.

—Diane LaRae Bodach

CHAPTER 3

Alien

When she said, "I have to stop talking for a while, because I just get too tired from talking," I was flabbergasted. It was like she was from outer space.

—a new friend

I STOPPED ONE DAY to look at a whistling teakettle I had been admiring for several months in the housewares section of my local health food store. "These are very nice," piped an employee. "I have one at home and I love it. I'm glad they've remade the whistles, though, because I have an older model and it's a little hard to get in and out."

I hadn't noticed this feature before and tested one of the whistles. "This may be a problem for me," I said. "I have a chronic illness, and when I'm really weak I think this will be too hard for me to get in and out every time I make tea."

"Oh no," she answered. "If this were the older model, I would agree with you, but these new ones are quite easy." I looked at her blankly, dumbfounded that she was telling me, in essence, that I was wrong about my assessment of my own strength. In her world the idea that someone could be so weak that they could not pull out this new *really easy* whistle was not a possibility.

Another time, I was getting a ride home from my ex-husband's house with a friend of his. I was carrying two gallons of water, thinking her car was just outside the door. When I realized the car was parked in the street about fifteen feet away from the house, I called to her and said I wasn't going to be able to carry the water that far, so I would just leave one in the apartment and get it another time. Then, as I was walking out with the one gallon, I realized I couldn't carry it either, and I said so. I didn't want to ask her to carry the water, but I kind of assumed she would offer. Instead, she said, "Yes, you can." I was shocked and said, "No, I can't." Then she said again, "Yes, you can," or some other similar statement. Again, I was dumbfounded and hurt but I tried not to show it and just started to walk back inside. Then she said she would carry it. I try very hard not to let people's judgments of me as weak or just pretending to be weak (being a hypochondriac) get to me, but this one really did. Whenever I saw this person afterward, I tried to hide my weakness.

One friend was honest enough to say, when recounting her first meeting with me to a mutual friend, "When she said, 'I have to stop talking for a while, because I just get too tired from talking,' I was flabbergasted. It was like she was from outer space. I've never met anyone who said they had to stop talking for a while to rest." Some people simply can't conceive of a person who walks and talks perfectly normally sometimes, not being able at other times to do tasks that seem like nothing to most people. It just doesn't compute. And unless someone is on their deathbed, not having enough energy to talk is simply beyond some people's ability or willingness to comprehend.

My own sister and, in fact, a large part of my extended family didn't accept my illness for years and thought it was all in my head. They thought that, if I really wanted to, I could do things, or if I just went ahead and did things, I would be okay. I have another sister whose chronic illness has also been met with a lot of skepticism. Not until the reality of severe debilitation was brought closer to home by a chronic illness in one of their immediate families did my extended family begin to realize that perhaps my sister and I really were sick after all.

Fifteen Words for Snow

This is not an unusual attitude for well people to have. It is natural to extrapolate from one's own experience of being tired. You just push through it—right? Wrong! Those of us who have experienced the kind of tiredness that comes with chronic fatigue or other kinds of chronic illnesses have repeatedly reaped the bitter harvest of pushing through our tiredness. But those who haven't experienced it cannot be expected to understand. It is just too far out—like my friend said, it's "from outer space." I often feel that way—like I'm from another planet—because my experience of life is so far removed from what "normal" people experience. I often feel like a freak, but my freakishness doesn't show physically, so I guess it's natural for people to think it's mental.

I say I'm tired, and the person I'm talking to says, "I know what you mean; I've been really exhausted lately myself." The person means well and is trying to commiserate, but they are so far off the mark, it causes only frustration. The Eskimos have fifteen words for snow, and the Greeks have four words for love. We have only one word for tired, but after I got sick, I experienced realms of tiredness so far beyond what I had ever known, it might *as well* have been from another planet. If I had made a drawing of a scale of tiredness when I was well, it would have gone from energetic, to tired, to very tired, to exhausted. Exhausted was at the far end of the scale for me when I was healthy, as it is for the normal well person. This exhausted state is as tired as a normal person gets. So when someone says they are tired, the "tired" section of this scale is the experience in the brain that lights up. It's completely understandable.

After I became chronically ill, however, the scale was extended to twice its length. In this scale exhausted was at the middle, and the new part of the scale went into negative territory that is so far beyond tired, beyond exhaustion, that it seemed a different reality. I named these parts utter exhaustion, desperation, and black hole—the black hole state being one that seemed nearly catatonic, in which I could not utter a sound or move even one toe or lift one finger.

These were *new* experiences—experiences I could not have imagined if someone had told me about them before I experienced them in my own body. Finally, I realized that saying I was tired was misleading, and saying I was desperately tired or entering a black hole was too dramatic or unclear. So I took to saying I felt sick when I got to the desperate stage, which, though not entirely truthful, was a lot closer to the truth than tired, and easier for people to understand than any of the other choices.

Planet Scleroderma

If there's one statement that is like a mantra in our chronic illness support group, I guess it is, "People don't get it." We had fun one day talking about feeling like aliens. We named our planet Zicon and ourselves Ziconites, finally getting some comic relief around the things that more often make us cry.

Kim Tusch of Santa Rosa, who has Scleroderma, wrote,

> I am disabled. It sounds funny to me even though I've had over ten years to get used to it. It's not who I am, really. Yet new people I encounter judge and define me instantly when they see me gaunt and somewhat frail, a bit hunched over my cane, having some difficulty breathing. To most, that is who I am now. No longer are the wild and wooly stories from my life the stuff of party chatter. No one asks about the past much, or thinks I have a life now outside the disease. It's like every experience that accumulated and formed me was on another planet. And I'm (here) on Planet Scleroderma now and the atmosphere is life-threatening and I've been modified to make the Sclerodermans feel at ease with me.

John Merrick, the 19th-century man whose body was so deformed and twisted he was known as the Elephant Man and relegated to sub-human status, was actually treated as a freak. The only way he could make a living was to allow himself to be put on display in freak shows and circuses, where people paid money to look at him. Because his vocal apparatus was so deformed, his speech was largely unintelligible. People mostly assumed he was an imbecile and treated him like an animal until a kindly doctor took interest in him and discovered that, not only could he think and communicate, but was indeed a highly intelligent and elegant man, with a romantic imagination.

The Wish to Be Understood

For those of us with conditions that don't show from the outside it's a little different—like the mirrored opposite of what Kim Tusch and John Merrick experienced. What is the same is that people do not understand. People expect them to be different because of the way they look and people expect me and others like me to be "normal" because of the way we look. I don't really blame people for not getting it because I know it is virtually impossible for someone to really understand these things if they haven't experienced them.

I myself don't know which planet I may be inhabiting or necessarily understand the rules under which I will need to be operating on any particular day. When I start doing a little better and/or if I stay home for a few days and can just do things at my own pace, I start to think of myself as a "normal person." Then I am shocked when I go out and see myself juxtaposed against a "real normal person" or experience one of my waves of weakness and bump up against my limitations again. Sometimes I simply forget my limitations in the natural up and down waves I have throughout the day and, when I come up against them, I am astonished at how little I can do. Since I am still befuddled after twenty-two years of experience with this illness, I no longer expect others to understand.

Yet, it is a natural human longing to be understood (especially for us "4's" on the Enneagram), or at least to be met in the place where we are, even though that place where we are *is* like a foreign country for those who have not yet experienced a life-changing illness or loss. What I long for and appreciate so deeply when they appear are friends and lovers who are willing to journey into that country; to learn the customs, the language (twenty words for tired?), the terrain, the weather—to live with the natives for a while.

Jean-Dominique Bauby was editor-in-chief of the French fashion magazine *Elle* and immersed in Parisian society at the time he suffered a stroke in 1995 that left him completely paralyzed except for the ability to blink his left eye. This rare condition is sometimes called, "locked-in-syndrome." Jean-Dominique called it his "diving bell." Once a social butterfly with a keen sense of humor, Bauby found himself in a situation where the only thing that could fly was his mind and he found solace in flights of fantasy.

But his inert body was a source of grief. Lost in his lonely world except for sometimes difficult and painful visits from family and a few close friends, Bauby felt imprisoned in his own body and cut off from society until some painful news from a friend instigated a surprising opening that was to change his "locked-in" life considerably. His friend overheard and shared a bit of gossip being floated in the more snobbish circles of Parisian society that he was now nothing more than a vegetable. Bauby wrote,

> The tone of voice [of the overheard gossipers] left no doubt that henceforth I belonged on a vegetable stall and not to the human race. France was at peace; one couldn't shoot the bearers of bad news. Instead I would have to rely on myself if I wanted to prove that my IQ was still higher than a turnip's.
> Thus was born a collective correspondence that keeps me in touch with those I love. And my hubris has had gratifying results. Apart from an irrecoverable few who maintain a stubborn silence, everybody now understands that he can join me in my diving bell, even if it sometimes takes me into unexplored territory. (pp. 82–83)

The means of this communication consisted of a tedious process in which the letters of the alphabet, which were arranged according to the frequency of use in the French language, were read off by a helper or by someone with whom he wanted to communicate. Bauby waited, poised to blink his working eye, as the letters of the words he had in mind drifted past, at which time the letters would be recorded. In this way Bauby and this relatee would make their way painstakingly through the alphabet hit and miss until, if they were lucky, a sentence emerged. A nurse at the hospital where he lived became his main translator, helping him compose letters to family and friends, and eventually helping him write his book, which was published two days before his death in 1996.

The Language of Disability

My situation is a piece of cake compared to those of Jean-Dominique Bauby and John Merrick, but still causes suffering when I long to carry on a normal conversation free from the fear of having to stop in midstream or sometimes of not being able to carry on a conversation at all. I had prepared one new acquaintance, a possible romantic interest, for the eventuality that I would have to stop talking during a conversation or go long periods of time without talking, and he assured me that this was not a problem for him as he was very comfortable with silence. When we spent time together, however, the actual experience of me not talking to him for an extended period of time was translated by him into "self-absorption" and rudeness on my part.

I began to see that even if people express understanding and willingness to accommodate my physical limitations, their unconscious being does not always go along with the program. We may think communication is about what we say, and that we are in control of what we think and feel, but the body has its own system of transmitting and processing information.

"Body language" goes both ways. Sometimes we can see that what a person says does not match up with what their body language is telling us. Other times we may be telling ourselves what would be the reasonable thing to be feeling, but our bodies are not listening—or at least not following directions. In this case my new friend's history of feeling ignored and abused by his mother and former wife pre-empted his conscious decision not to be offended by my silence.

In any case, it is hard not to feel rejection in the body when someone you are talking to doesn't express attention and interest with verbal or other cues, and sometimes my body is too tired to even say "uh huh" or to nod in acknowledgment. I have checked this out with friends, and those who are willing to be honest have admitted it is true.

A friend with Parkinson's disease shared that people often have a difficult time because, as a result of his disease, he doesn't have much facial expression—the disease has frozen his facial features into a kind of mask. People, he said, are put off by that, and my friend is saddened by his inability to use the kinds of facial expressions that most of us take for granted to communicate subtleties of emotion. After he shared this with me, I realized that I, too, had been put off by his lack of facial expression, but it was such a subtle and unconscious thing that I hadn't been aware of the reasons for my feelings.

I was shocked to realize that I, who have had such intensive training in the language of disability and loss of function, and have prided myself on being able to transcend the barriers to communication that are sometimes presented, had fallen prey to this misunderstanding. That it had affected me on an emotional level without my conscious participation was disturbing, but it helped me to remember what it feels like from the other side and to feel compassion for all those well people who just "don't get it." It was also an eye-opener to realize how subtle communication can be, and what a huge portion of it goes on beneath our conscious awareness.

One can override these bodily reactions and eventually retrain the emotional self not to feel rejection in these kinds of circumstances, but it takes time and willingness. Though it is difficult, there are people (may they be blessed) with the flexibility, compassion, awareness, and adventurousness of spirit to be willing to stretch into another way of seeing or being in order to spend time with those whose physical bodies prevent business as usual. One of my friends knows me so well that she sees the signs when I am wearing down and, without skipping a beat, reminds me that it's okay to not respond to what she is saying with words or nods, and goes right on talking. Or she suggests that we do a meditation together. She knows that when I come over to her house, I may be too tired to interact for a while, and we do our parallel activities, just being in each other's presence, or I lie on the couch until I am recovered enough to interact. But when I meet new people or spend time with those who don't know me intimately, it can be difficult, awkward, or embarrassing.

The Push–Pull of Shame

How can I tell someone that there have been times when I was too exhausted to take off my sweater or roll down my window in a sweltering hot car, or that if I wanted to go somewhere, I had to go dirty and with the torn or unstylish clothes I had on—because if I changed or bathed, I wouldn't have the energy to go?—that if I *were* able to shower, I would try to save energy by washing only the most important parts and anything overtly dirty?

How can I explain that sometimes when driving my car, I have to plan my route very carefully so that I turn the fewest corners possible and even try to make each curve in the road wider than it is, because every corner I turn or curve I go around uses up valuable energy and stresses my muscles, bringing me closer to that dreaded black hole? How can I explain that I really do find my companion's comment funny and would love to laugh if only I had the energy; that the laugh and the retort are right there, but the energy to execute them are not?

How can I admit that I trained my children from a very young age to steer and shift from the passenger seat, because if they hadn't helped with the driving, we would have been virtually housebound?

How can I recount the numberless times I have found myself at a social gathering suddenly marooned in a sea of faces, as lost and helpless as if I had run adrift on an island a thousand miles from anywhere—suddenly at the end of my energy with no lifeboat to get me out of my present conversation, past the hostess and the faces, to the door, into my car, home, and into bed? That there have been many nights I have gone to bed with my clothes, and sometimes even my shoes, on, because I was too exhausted to take them off? And finally, how can I say that I live in shame and horror at the thought of anyone finding out about all these things and at the same time wanting desperately for them to know and understand?

This is such a complicated, but extremely important, topic that I think it warrants exploration. For many ill people, or those that have been emotionally or psychologically debilitated from trauma or loss, the push-pull of shame—not wanting people to know, and the seemingly opposite intense desire to be seen, understood, and accepted as they are—is complex and multifaceted.

Part of not wanting people to know is the shame that arises from the belief that we are failures because we have gotten sick and haven't been able to heal ourselves. The other part, I think, is fear—fear that people will not want to be around us because of our neediness and because it is not fun. So there is the fear of abandonment—the fear of being alone and unloved. Some of this fear arises out of unhealed parts of the psyche and is thus valuable raw material for working with negative emotions as discussed in Chapters Nine, Ten, and Eleven. But there is, in fact, some basis for this fear in the reality of living with illness or disability of any kind, and thus a more practical problem is presented to us, as well, that needs to be addressed in everyday life.

Acquaintances may not say it outright or even think it consciously, but when it comes time to invite someone to go somewhere, it might just be easier to invite someone else. They might think, "Well, she can't do that, anyway. We will be walking too far. She doesn't have the stamina." And, either consciously or unconsciously, they may not want the extra burden of being with someone who will need to be dropped off at the door, have her paraphernalia carried, be pushed in a wheelchair, or be unable to keep up with whatever activity is being enjoyed, and thus be a drag on the group or individual. This, in my mind, is completely understandable. I understand that when people are going somewhere to have fun, they want to be free of burdens. They want to be able to simply enjoy themselves without having to worry about taking care of someone. I often put on that I am doing better than I really am when I go places with people, because I don't want to be a drag on my companions (and I want to be invited again!).

But there is another reason for not wanting people to know how bad things can get sometimes, which is my feeling the need to be protective of my friends and family, those who continue to include me because they love me, in spite of my disability. If they really knew what was going on sometimes, especially when we go out together, their kindness and concern would make them take on more than I would want them to, and more than they are actually prepared to give.

The Difficulty of Partnering

When it comes to partnering, the situation is even more tenuous. Deep soul connection is possible between people on many levels of physical ability but the desire for companionship and sharing mutually enjoyable activities is also an important part of relationship, and cannot be ignored. People rarely acknowledge the truth of the situation. It's very refreshing when someone is willing to say to me, "I don't want to be with you, because you're sick." The truth is, I sense that from people already, but when they are not willing to admit it, and they make it into something else—some other reason—it makes me feel worse than if I know the truth. A few men have told me outright that this was the reason they wouldn't consider being with me. I was very grateful to be told the truth, and felt a very close connection through that simple act of honesty. I have also experienced a partner leaving relationship with me because of my illness. This was much more painful, but I was still grateful to be told the truth.

We who are sick or disabled have come to this situation by fate. We have not been offered a choice. Our mates and friends, when they hang out with us, must take on some of our limitations. In all fairness,

I think we must ask ourselves if we would have chosen these limitations had we been given the choice beforehand. The answer for most of us, I think, would be a resounding no. The spiritual benefits that may have modulated that answer for some of us came much further down the road.

The fact that our loved ones can also share in the spiritual benefits is a saving grace but does not take away the pain of loss that must be faced by everyone concerned. That this loss is illusory can only be discovered by the willingness to enter into it. My honest belief is that the deep emotional and soul healing that has been made possible for me and others on this path through the losses we have encountered more than makes up for our continuing physical limitations. And this healing and emotional maturity is, to some extent I believe, passed on to those who hang out with us, which seems to be borne out by the wonderful friends with whom I share deep loving relationships.

The other side of this coin, of course, is that there are countless ways in which people can be disabled that are not physical. A person may be incapable of giving and receiving love because of childhood trauma or abuse, or live in a state of denial, never having the courage to access deep emotions for fear of uncovering deeply buried pain and, consequently, never touching the center of the true self where joy and real connection can be experienced. A person can get stuck in a belief system that says the world and all the people in it are untrustworthy, making it extremely difficult for him to be in relationships, where trust is an important factor.

To me, the pain of living with a chronic physical illness is not nearly as debilitating as was the pain of living a life defined by a sense of brokenness, incompleteness and the devastating feeling that there was a hole at the bottom of my being that would never be filled, that I sometimes experienced as a well person. In my opinion, these are much more debilitating maladies than any physically limiting condition can ever be.

Prejudice in the workplace is another huge subject I won't go into, except to mention that, as difficult as it may seem in the United States, it is far worse in some other countries. A friend visiting Cambodia wrote about an American there who is helping to maintain a small NGO. He said the man

... employs only disabled Cambodians since it is very hard for them to find work; it's actually illegal for disabled people to be hired by the government, and very few other workplaces will hire them either. Given the number of landmines still in this country, I find this attitude towards amputees, in particular, quite unnerving, but I believe it stems from a need to distance oneself from other people's misfortunes; the disabled are stigmatized in most countries and have only made the progress they have in the US and Europe through long years of political activism.

Though Our Bodies Have Changed, Our Souls Have Not

Even in the more progressive countries where progress has been made politically, it is, I think, an unseen and unacknowledged truth that ill or disabled people are often automatically excluded from many social activities, especially those that involve walking, climbing, dancing, manual labor, or other physical activities. From the standpoint of those who deal with chronic disability, this is very sad, because it cuts us out of a huge part of life. And those of us who were very active in our life as a well person may find it difficult to be relegated to couch-potato status.

Though our bodies have changed, our souls and inclinations have not. I still long to spend time in the wilderness, away from cars and noise. I still long to dance and sing. I still yearn to be included in events that are multifaceted from which I am usually excluded because one of the facets involves physical activity. A hike may culminate in lunch at the beach or under the redwoods. Long river rafting trips include generous amounts of time camping and laying about. So this is a huge loss and one that I think is not completely necessary.

I try to find ways to keep the things and activities that I love in my life. I prefer to think of it as an intriguing puzzle or enigma, which, if approached creatively, can be solved at least partially in many different ways. My friend Jon, who has been in a wheelchair for most of his adult life, still goes dancing with his friends. He gets out on the dance floor and moves his wheelchair around to the music. When I go to dances, I have to sit most of them out but enjoy being there and dancing as much as I am able. There's one dance called "Sweat Your Prayers" (Five Rhythms) where people come and just move their bodies with the music any way they feel like moving.

I have gone to many of these dances when I have been pretty much nonfunctional. I dance maybe one or two dances and am so exhausted I have to sit out for a long time. Sometimes I can still move, but I just can't stand, so I do floor dancing. I can get down on the floor and "dance" with my body and I don't feel like an idiot! (Other people do it too.) Actually many people have gotten on the floor and danced with me there and these floor dances have been some of the most highly charged, creatively infused dances I have participated in at the Sweat Your Prayers dances.

Still there are many activities I have to miss because it just isn't possible or because people don't invite me because *they think* it's not possible. This is hard, but, as it is with all social change, it seems, we, the ones who are disabled and left out, probably have to be the ones who push to expand well persons' (the ones who do the leaving out—sometimes very unintentionally) horizons a bit. For example: one could suggest to a friend or group of friends that you come along on one of those outings that has a more sedentary component in it, or call the Sierra Club and see if someone might consider taking you as a passenger on a canoe ride.

I have to lie down a lot, or I have to be in a *really* comfortable chair in order to make it through events that last longer than an hour. My ex-husband used to be embarrassed by this. He felt that I should go to a back room if I needed to lie down and that I shouldn't lie down in public. I complied for a while, because I didn't want to embarrass him or myself. I guess I took on his assessment that lying down at a social gathering or in public was an inappropriate thing to do. I would then spend half my time warehoused in someone's bedroom listening to people in the other rooms laughing and having a good time, or simply staying home instead of going to an outing that included a long time in public places.

It was very sad for me to want to be out there amidst the laughter while I was shut away like an invalid. I decided at a certain point that I wasn't going to do that any more. I didn't care if it was inappropriate. I just wasn't willing to spend half my life shut away from society because of social dictates. I figured if people were uncomfortable with me and what I had to do for myself, they would have to deal with it.

Now, I often lie down at social gatherings. It is still uncomfortable for me sometimes, depending on the situation, but I am committed to not letting my embarrassment keep me from doing things that I want to do. When I go to a performance, I almost always bring my own chair so I will have head and leg support and a reclinable back, which often makes it possible for me to make it through an event or to come home feeling simply tired, instead of utterly miserable. Mostly, I find, people don't even notice, don't care, or they wish they had thought to bring a chair like mine.

Hidden Prejudice

Sometimes the puzzle of making things work for those of us with limitations requires a little bit of accommodation from companions or passersby. As a Ziconite, not only do I appreciate those who are willing to come to my planet and learn the customs, but also the earthlings who welcome us Ziconites into their world. After all, we are technically earthlings, too. Okay, maybe this is getting silly, but don't we all just long to belong? To be accepted? To feel like we are part of things?

The truth is that many people in our world are very uncomfortable with differences and fear the unknown. This is the ground out of which prejudice grows. The root of the word is "pre-judge"—to judge a person or a group of people before you really know them. And prejudice is a long continuum. Some people are at the extreme. They just don't want "those foreigners" around—or those who talk funny, or those who have a different ideology or look different—and that often includes those who have physical deformities or limitations. But there is blatant prejudice and there is also subtle prejudice. I think we are all guilty of subtle prejudice. When I went to a singles gathering recently, there was not one person there in a wheelchair or who had even the slightest bit of anything unusual (looking) about them physically. I know this is not because there are no disabled singles around.

When I was still pretty bald after the chemo for my breast cancer, I went to a singles event, but couldn't get anybody to talk to me for more than a minute. A number of months later I saw one of the men

I had seen at the singles event at another party. He was shocked when he realized I was the same person he had run into at several gatherings when I didn't have hair. "You're very attractive," he said, somewhat bewildered, and was very interested in talking with me since I then had hair.

I have also noticed that when I use the "riding cart" that some stores provide for disabled customers, I might as well forget about trying to flirt with any men. Though many people are especially kind when it comes to reaching something for me or getting out of my way, I find it nearly impossible to engage a single man in conversation or even to get one to look me in the eye.

The work I have done in opening to my own emotions and learning to offer loving kindness to myself, as well as my experience with my own prejudices, has helped me not to be too judgmental in these kinds of situations. I think sometimes people are afraid. Other times they may simply be so focused on their own needs that bending a little bit to open to or include someone that might be slightly different does not occur to them.

I think this is at least as sad for the "normal" people as it is for those who are challenged, or perhaps more so. For those who are excluded, it may be just another physical challenge, but those who could do something to help and don't, or who actively exclude someone from an activity or decide that he/she is not dating or friendship material on the basis of looks or physical ability, are actually shutting the door to their own hearts and cutting themselves off from a potentially rich experience.

A Small Gesture Goes a Long Way

Some, however, welcome diversity, and relish the richness of life in all its forms. Having done enough of their own inner work to develop an understanding of the web of life and how each part is inextricably bound to the others, they are willing to go a little out of their way to help physically limited people be included. I can't begin to say how much this means to those of us who still long to be a part of this world in ways that are often no longer available to us. A small gesture goes a long way.

Once I was at a Sufi dance, a kind of spiritual dance circle where the participants do what are called Universal Dances of Love and Peace. After a few dances I had to sit down, so I just sat cross-legged a little way outside the circle. I was feeling that old familiar sadness of being on the outside of another activity looking in. To my surprise and delight, the leader of the circle led the dancers single file around me, so that I was sitting on the inside of the circle with the musicians, instead of on the outside. A wave of gratitude and warmth welled up in me at this simple gesture of inclusion. Though I still felt sad about not being able to dance, I felt part of the circle again, and it made a huge difference to me.

A friend once shared this story of a difficult time in her life:

> When I left San Francisco seven years ago, my arms were *not* working—I had a repetitive motion injury from too much keyboarding (while holding tension, anger and codependency with my boss). Injured, I wanted to *get out* of the city, but I couldn't drive myself up here to look at places, because the steering wheel vibrations were too much for me. A chance comment to an acquaintance led to his driving me up here and around to all the bulletin boards in West County. I hadn't known him that well, but he didn't have a car, and for him it was a treat to drive around this beautiful, unexplored area. Sometimes you just never know which way the gifts are flowing.
>
> When I got here, the only people I knew in Sonoma County were people I'd met at a permaculture course at the Occidental Arts and Ecology Center. I really, really wanted to go to the OAEC volunteer garden days on Wednesdays, but there wasn't much I could do—couldn't grip tools for long. But the head gardener came up with some silly easy tasks that I could do near the beds where others were digging and weeding. It was so sweet! ... it still brings tears to my eyes to remember the way he included me.

I think these kinds of actions can be mutually beneficial. Those who are physically challenged get to be included, and the well people not only have an opportunity to touch into their own open hearts, but also sometimes to avail themselves of the rich inner life and experience that may have sprung up in those who journey with such difficulties.

The Loneliness of Living with a Chronic Illness

The loneliness of living with a chronic illness can be intense. There is not only the isolation of being different—being the odd man out—but the very real physical isolation that comes as a result of the physical barriers of exhaustion and disability. You may yearn to be among people but are too exhausted to make the effort to go out or physically cannot get to the places where people gather because of your physical limitations. And if you do get there, you often can't participate. I can't count the number of times I have gotten myself cleaned up and dressed and have driven myself part way to a social event I wanted to attend, and then have had to turn around and go home because the effort of getting that far had simply worn me out.

As a Ziconite living among earthlings, I want to fit in, and I try very hard. Sometimes when I'm at a party or other social situation, I have the feeling that I am pulling a fast one by passing myself off as "normal." But, of course, when I leave the party, it is like Cinderella coming home from the ball. I often collapse onto my bed and cry because my body is hurting so badly from the efforts I have made.

I wrote this in my journal one day:

> Today I'm going to go out and pretend to be a person. I feel a bit sheepish about it, and I wonder if I can pull it off. Of course, I mean a "normal person." The censor in the back of my mind is nagging me. "Take your vitamins. Drink your juice. Give your shot. Get your meds ready to take with you." Maybe I'll just ignore all these voices. If I do all those things before I go, I quite likely won't have the energy left to go out. But if I don't do them, I'll increase the chances that I'll be more weakened afterwards and more susceptible to relapse. More voices chime in: "You can't do this. You're too weak, too sick, you'll do yourself in. You're too greedy. You can't accept your life as it is," and blah blah blah. Will I need to turn around half way there, already too exhausted to drive the rest of the way, like all those other times?

The reason that I put myself in these situations that are so incredibly hard for me is not because I am a masochist (although I feel sometimes that I must be), and it is not about needing to appear normal to others, though, of course, I am not above that and do still struggle with it at times. For the most part, it is because I want, in spite of illness and limitation, to live life to the fullest extent possible, to experience all its richness, and to be part of the human family.

The Paradox of Living with Illness

Here again is another paradox—another kind of push-pull. I see, when I look closely and honestly, that there *is* a small self, little Diane, who *does* cling desperately to life—who wants so desperately to be a person, to have a life—that she will go to ridiculous extremes to do that. And there is the shame that goes along with the awareness of that desperation. Within that small person, however, and mixed up with her, is a being who is not clinging, not desperate, but simply wants to experience life and is willing to risk embarrassment, pain, discomfort and relapse to be truly alive. This is a being, I think, worthy of compassion and even admiration.

Having dealt with severe physical limitation for over twenty years, I have become so accustomed to the situation, I often don't see the barriers that keep me from participating in the most banal of everyday activities. But, occasionally, the poignancy of viewing some very commonplace event will strike straight to my heart. Once, driving home, I saw a group of friends standing on the sidewalk downtown, joking and talking. As I looked, a wave of sorrow swept over me, because I realized that this simple human activity was beyond my reach. I can't stand very long while talking—can't talk very long while standing—can't stand or talk very long, at all.

I got a card from my friend in LA yesterday. She wrote about skiing trips and hiking in the mountains and a plan to travel to Tibet next year. I realized how far her world was from mine. I felt like I lived in my own little third world country in the midst of a land of plenty. Even watching TV or reading a magazine can be excruciating when I tune into the reality of the number of things that are truly out of reach for me—like something from another world.

Everyone is busy and overwhelmed, but while my friend organizes her Tibetan odyssey and a neighbor makes plans to go to Tahoe with her family, arranging for food, lodging, ski rental, pets, etc., many chronically or terminally ill people must plan meticulously how they will make it through the day or the week; must ask themselves, "How can I get the most out of the four hours of help I have from a high school aide?" One man described how he spent almost all of his time and energy arranging, getting ready for, and coming to our once-a-week meetings of The Attitudinal Healing Center. That was his one outing of the week.

Many people don't believe that I really couldn't roll down the window or do some of those other things I described, or think I'm exaggerating. They think that it was my choice—that I was being hypochondriac or just lazy. So be it. Let them think what they must. Again, I emphasize that I don't blame people for these kinds of thoughts and feelings. When I get to feeling a little better, I can hardly believe it myself.

We Are All Aliens

At times, I seem alien even to myself. I can't count the many times I have hit one of my walls and, while my body is screaming "stop," a small quiet voice inside is saying, "but that's unreasonable," and prodding my body to do more because of the total illogicality of it all. It is just too far out and entirely unreasonable not to be able to take off your sweater when you are hot or your shoes before you go to bed, not to be able to send a card to your mother for Easter or return a call from a friend, and most of all, it's extremely unreasonable not to be able to talk or even push out one more word in response when in the midst of a conversation—even the tiny words, "I know," "yes," or "no," or even to nod in acknowledgment.

This idea of feeling like an alien may be useful and descriptive for a time but it is really just another division—another barrier we put between ourselves and others—more of the "us" and "them" mentality that keeps the world at war, the races separated by fear, and men and women struggling for power over each other. Mostly though, it keeps us from touching into our own true heart, where there are no divisions.

Truly we are all aliens. We have come from a world of formlessness, of limitless light and love, and have been born into bodies with physical limitations that will someday die—bodies that trick us sometimes into thinking we are separate from that source and from each other.

The Reed Flute's Song

I think all persons at some time in their lives have felt the sorrow of this "alienation" from our basic wholeness. Rumi, in his poem, "The Reed Flute's Song," talks about the reed flute that sings such a sad song because it has been pulled from the reed bed—the mud that was its source. He says, "Anyone pulled from a source/longs to go back." But adds, "At any gathering I am there, mingling in the laughing and grieving…" (p. 18)

I realized at some point that I needed to move *beyond* needing people, or even myself, to understand. I write this to help well people understand the inner world of the Ziconites and Sclerodermans, but even more to encourage ill people and all who are debilitated by loss or injury—those of us who feel like aliens in our own community, our own homes, even our own bodies—to make lives for ourselves, regardless of what people think and regardless of the fact that our bodies will not let us do many of the things we want to do. We must speak our truth. We must learn to ask for help. But if others don't believe us or refuse to help, we must continue to love and to live and to celebrate life to the extent that we are able. To become bitter is only to invite hardness and hatred into our hearts.

This is much more easily said than done. To forgive a clerk in a store is fairly easy, but to forgive a sister or close friend is harder. Forgiveness is the antidote to the poison of hatred that we often take into our hearts in response to pain. Forgiveness must be an ongoing practice. We think forgiveness is for the person we are forgiving, but again, as with many other ideas, we have it backwards. Forgiving others is what we must do *for ourselves* if we want freedom and true happiness. We are the ones who suffer when we hold onto hatred or resentment. It burns and scars our own hearts more than those of the unforgiven.

Forgiveness Begins at Home

And, as with love, forgiveness begins at home. The first person we may need to forgive is ourselves. We must forgive ourselves for not being the person we expected ourselves to be, and, ultimately, we must forgive ourselves for being ill, because, when it comes down to it, many of us blame ourselves for our illness. But, as with my realization after reading Stephen Levine that healing must go deeper than the physical body, so it is with forgiveness. There are much deeper things for which we need to forgive ourselves than being sick. Our sickness or loss can help lead us to those things.

Many of us have gone through phases of blaming ourselves for our illnesses. Usually, I think of this as a nonproductive path, but sometimes it can be useful to explore these feelings if it can be entered into in a nonjudgmental way, looking compassionately at how we blame ourselves, noticing all our thoughts and judgments about ourselves. If we can sit with this for a while, we may notice some deeper layers behind the judgments.

Sara, a woman in my wellness group, has had arthritis since she was ten years old. In trying to go deeper into her inner self she realized that as a child she always felt she wasn't good enough, that she couldn't do enough. She began to sense that maybe she *did* make herself sick, but it wasn't to punish herself—it was to let herself off the hook. "You don't have to be that good," the compassionate heart was saying to the tender inner child. "You can be sick and you won't have to do that much." As she saw these things, her heart opened in compassion for the child who never felt good enough *and* for the part of herself that tried in the very best way it knew to help the child. Realizing this and beginning a forgiveness practice was a huge step for Sara's inner healing—for the larger healing of her whole being.

Sara was lucky in one sense. She was old enough when she got sick to still have memories of the time before her illness—to be able to sense how and why, in some way, she might have actually chosen to be sick out of compassion for her inner child. Much of the time, these major events are hidden or lost from memory in the preverbal, preconceptual years of infancy.

Once we forgive ourselves, it becomes easier to forgive others. After I began my opening to true healing, I realized at a certain point that I was carrying a lot of resentment for a lot of people in my life. I spent a full year concentrating on a forgiveness practice. I used Stephen Levine's forgiveness meditation (see Appendix) every day to help myself soften my hard stance toward myself and others in my life for whom I had resentments. I found this very useful in opening my heart and moving toward my goal of love.

What Helps and What Doesn't

Sometimes I think it is hard for people to know how to relate to people who have chronic or terminal illnesses. To caregivers, friends, relatives, and loved ones of the chronically ill or disabled, my advice is: ask them what it is like for them, and believe them. Let them describe the pain of loss of many normal functions and the pain of being misunderstood. Try to imagine what it would be like for you to give up everything that they have had to give up.

One friend, who eventually developed a chronic illness himself, shared with me that this was true for him before he got sick. It was a vicious cycle. The longer he stayed away, the harder it was for him to go to visit because he felt guilty for not going. When I asked my friend what was the most helpful thing anyone had done for him in regard to his own illness, he said,

> I think just being with another person, just acknowledging them and just appreciating them where they are at is probably the most helpful thing. Once when I was having a bad relapse, I was feeling very isolated and I just didn't want to burden anybody else. I called my teacher and I asked her and she said, "You have to let other people know. You can tell your wife and your friends, because they're strong enough to take it. You don't have to hold it inside."
>
> I remember that night, I just told my friend all the things that were happening and my fears around it, and she just looked at me, and she looked at me with understanding and she said just a couple of words, just acknowledging that it was happening. And I felt so relieved that someone actually just heard. She didn't have to do anything.
>
> And my wife's stance is basically that I'm totally okay when I'm sick. That I'm better sick than most people are well anyway. She has no problem with me being disabled or sick and she's totally willing to be with me. And that trust that she really feels that way reinforces the notion that there is really nothing wrong with me. Because I think that what most people give you when you're sick is that there's really something wrong with you with all of their efforts to try to help you get better, even if they're well intentioned.

This is something, I think, that many of us who are experiencing long-term illness or loss can relate to. We may not have been able to put our fingers on what exactly was happening at the time except to realize that, even though the person seemed to be offering support with all their suggestions, we didn't feel supported.

Following is another example of something *not* to do to help someone who is or has been sick: Jane recalls something her friend said to her one day:

> Out of the blue—I was talking about how something was hard, and she said, "Yeah, but look at how far you've come." And this is all from someone who does this fairly often ... compares me to my very worst, and is always reminding me of when I was at my bottom and look how far I've come. I hate it. There's something about it that just makes my stomach turn.
>
> I always acknowledge, "yes it's true," but I guess I'm somehow more oriented toward imagining where I want to go. That just feels like another reinforcement or activation of who I was, as if who I was, was this more essential me. And so to always compare to that—it's like a gracious complimentary kind of thing, "Well, good for you!" [But it doesn't feel like that to me...] It feels like you still see me as a sick person and you're amazed that I'm living a normal life. I never put it in words quite like that, but I think that's what it feels like to me.
>
> ... Like I'll never be able to get out from that perspective because no matter what, it'll always be, "well, look how good the sick person's doing."

Some of the things that come up quite often, when I have asked people who are sick or hurting what kinds of responses or behaviors from others have been most helpful or comforting to them, have been to simply be with them, listen to them and believe them.

Jane remembers a therapist who gave her an amazing gift.

> The one thing I remember about her was she was really the first person I had ever known that when I looked her in the eyes, I could see she had one hundred percent confidence that this was a phase, that this was a process. I was on my way out... a hundred percent. Not even a sliver of a doubt. It wasn't even what she said to me. I could just feel it from her. And it did more for me than [anything anyone has ever done].

Offers of physical help are also often very welcome. Usually it is most helpful to make a specific suggestion when you are offering to help. Many people are shy or too proud to accept offers of help, so it is better to make a specific offer, especially the first time you are offering, such as, "Could I bring you a meal or do your grocery shopping next week?" than to say something more general like, "Is there any way I can help you?" or "Call me if you need anything." The specific suggestion makes it easier to say yes, because the person who is being offered the help in this case does not have to take the initiative and she is more likely to think that the person offering help really wants to do it. I do *greatly* appreciate people who say they'll do anything I want, but it's more difficult to accept, at least at first, because I'm afraid they might be offering out of politeness or a sense of obligation.

One of the most poignant memories I have is of a time I came home utterly exhausted and hurting from a fun night out, knowing I had gone way past my limits, feeling that I wanted to simply crawl into bed and curl up in a fetal position. My daughter was there. Without a word she started undressing me. She tenderly took off all my clothes and shoes, put on my pajamas and helped me into bed. She could have left me to my own devices. She could have berated me for doing too much. But she didn't. She simply helped me. This is one of the most beautiful gifts anyone has ever given me. I will always remember and treasure it.

The Hard and Icy Couch

A friend of mine wrote this letter out of pain and desperation to her lover who was having trouble understanding some of the needs of her disability:

> I feel misunderstood. I guess I'm sorry that you/others don't know how what it's like to live with pain your whole f ... life. Do you know what it's like to have to give up everything you ever dreamed, little by little, have your life taken away from you, holding onto your husband because he's the only continuity in my life, only to see him leave? Do you know what it's like to sell your bicycle because it's easier not to see it every day and be reminded? Do you know what it's like to sell your

guitar and know that you will probably never play again? Do you know what it's like to want to ride a horse? Do you know what it's like to want to dance? Do you know what it's like to have two friends with chronic pain kill themselves and try to hold on to your life in the midst of it all? Do you know what it's like to have a plan to kill yourself day after day because it's the only thing that would get you out of a body racked with pain? Do you know what it's like to live with only darkness and holding onto the hope that some way, some day, there will be more light? Hope. Hope. Hope. Do you know what it's like to want to live again but know that the medications that are helping pitifully, but helping, will shorten your life? Do you know what it's like to have wanted to be a mother and know that that is not an option for you? Neither is running, hiking, swimming, traveling? I pay royally for our love-making sessions. I pay for days afterwards. I wouldn't want it any other way because they are so dear to me it, but I do pay.

I feel misunderstood by your words. I know they are just words, but they have the power to hurt. I may pull in some to take care of myself around this.

I love you so dearly, sweetheart. I think you're wonderful and I wouldn't want to change anything about you.

I hope this welling inside me will subside.

Ultimately it comes back to the hard and icy couch. Life is not giving us what we want, and no matter how we manipulate and arrange things, we will not have it—that is the "it" of our material wants. But the truth is that no one really gets what they want in this world. I shared something like this with my friend, John, when we were talking about the difficulties and losses he had experienced as a result of dealing with chronic pain. He responded,

> You know, that's a fundamental truth even without any kind of ailments when you get right down to it. That's one of the lessons that comes from having to meet that head-on, while you still have the belief that you can have what you want. That's where [the hardships of life] become useful. They become spiritual teachers then.

The Epic of Gilgamesh, one of the earliest myths of mankind from ancient Sumer, is a teaching story that uses the timeless archetypes of mankind's spiritual journey to portray this truth. In the myth, Gilgamesh the King is a self-serving and emotionally undeveloped person who misuses his power to conquer and amass wealth, and to have his way with every young woman in his kingdom before her marriage to another is consummated. Only after his egocentric strivings to brand his name upon the earth and gain eternal life in his worldly body lead him to utter failure and despair does he finally accept his limitations, move beyond his selfish drives, and mature into a compassionate human being and a beloved King.

The Eye with Which I See God

Even those who have healthy bodies and get their wishes on the material plane usually remain unsatisfied, because the wanting at bottom is not really about a material or physical thing. It is about wanting to be loved unconditionally and, as Rilke says, "... to belong to something, to be contained in an all-embracing mind that sees me/ as a single thing" (p.98). It is about the longing to return to the reed bed. We want to have love, but what we don't realize is that we can't *have* it because we *are* it. It's like the eye trying to see itself. Meister Eckhart says, "The eye with which I see God is the eye with which God sees me."

Ironically, the conditions that can help us discover this truth are often found in the very same conditions that cause us such pain—the material world of separation from our true self—the condition of our unfulfilled desires. By getting what we want on the material plane and finding out over and over again that that wasn't it (the way to happiness) after all, or by continually not getting what we want and discovering slowly and painstakingly that joy is possible in spite of, or maybe *because* of, not getting what we want on the material plane, we are led back to the truth of who we really are beyond getting or not getting any particular desire fulfilled. And so the separation, the alienation we imagined we felt, was an illusion after all. There is really no way, we find, to actually *be* separate.

CHAPTER 4

Opportunity

...even the stones sing silent arias of being.
—John Sherman, from prison after his realization

ANTHONY DE MELLO, Jesuit priest and author of *Awareness*, talks about how we don't want to be happy. He makes the point that if someone told us we could be happy, we wouldn't trade the various things that we think we need—our degree, our money, our job, our fancy house, our reputation—for that happiness. And I will add another one to that list—our health. The trap we get drawn into is thinking we need to be healthy in order to be happy—that we need to feel good in order to be happy. How many times have you heard people say, "As long as I have my health, that is the only important thing?" Or the other side of that idea—that "life wouldn't be worth living if I'm sick and unable to do the things that I love to do."

When we are sick, the body can feel like a prison, these fleshy walls keeping us from the experiences we long for; keeping us from accomplishing the important work we think we were meant to do, from being the person we feel we have inside that we could be *if only* things were different, even from doing the menial duties that seemingly "must" be done, and finally keeping us from doing the loving things we long to do for our dear ones or for mankind.

Our Obsession with Freedom

We Americans seem to have an obsession with freedom. But freedom, like happiness, is a tricky concept. John Sherman was in prison when he met Gangaji. A cynical bank robber who had given up on life and God, he was the liaison, strangely enough, between various

Eastern spiritual groups and the prison administration dealing with events at the prison chapel. Having arranged the meeting with Gangaji for the inmates, he proceeded to tell everyone he knew not to bother going, and he himself intended not to go. But when he met Gangaji and looked into her eyes, something shifted inside him and his life was never to be the same. Through her teaching and presence, the opening he experienced led him to realize that he had been in prison his whole life, even when he had been out in the so-called "free" world robbing banks and taking what he wanted.

In an interview after he was released from prison, John Sherman said,

> Truly, truly, there's no such thing as imprisonment.... When I was in prison for that first year after meeting Gangaji, I discovered that the same circumstance that I had called prison was paradise. That there was absolutely no difference in the appearance of it—the walls were just as cold and hard, the bars were just as made of steel as they always had been, the fences and the electric wires and the gun towers were all just as they had been, the day-to-day routine was just as it had been, the deprivation that is the lot of people who are in prison remained the same. I still could get none of the luxuries that we think we want so desperately when we're not in prison—we want them desperately in prison too. Still all of that was denied to me. The company and comfort of friends was denied to me.
>
> So nothing, nothing whatsoever about the external circumstances changed at all. And yet that same set of circumstances was seen clearly to be paradise. I wrote to her once during that period and told her the truth, which was that even the stones sing silent arias of being. So whatever prison is, it has nothing to do with the look of it. It has nothing to do with whether I'm locked in a steel cage or out here where I can go wherever I want to go to my heart's content. There was no difference whatsoever between the imprisonment when I was out robbing banks, seemingly free—how could you be any more free than to be out robbing banks—and the prison when I was in the hole in Marion, in the worst prison in the country. Same prison—same exact prison:
>
> *I need something I don't have. I want something I can't get. I don't like things the way they are. I wish they were other. I wish they were something different. I wish I could find what I want.* That's the prison.

From our narrow perspective, it may seem that certain things are bad or wrong. It is bad to be in prison; it is bad to be sick—everyone knows that. But is it true? Of all the people I have met (and I have met many) who are chronically ill, or who have suffered a severe loss in their life, I can't remember a single being who hasn't spoken of the spiritual gifts he or she received as a result of this loss. Many call it grace, and most are awed by the mystery of it. As John Sherman said about the belief that being in prison was keeping him from all the things he thought he wanted and needed,

> And finally that's seen to be a lie. The most fundamental lie of all. Finally it's seen that everything you have ever wanted, everything you have ever searched for, everything you have ever thought to be lacking is permanently everlastingly present as yourself—the last place you would think to look—at yourself. It has nothing to do with anything external to you. And in seeing that, all ideas of imprisonment vanish. All ideas that circumstance has anything to do with you vanish.

The Hindrance Will Become the Lens
with gratitude to STEVEN LEVINE

I heard a story about a woman who sat in her room day after day praying and never went anywhere. Someone asked her why she never went anywhere and she said, "Oh, I do. I go to faraway places." And this has been my experience with loss of bodily function. In the little room of my body I sit and go to the most amazing places. What better time to look into the inner world—the one we always put off for another day—than when we are ill or disabled? It's astounding what you can make of a little bit of life. You take the life that you have and look into it through the lens of your illness, like looking into a microscope at a drop of pond water. When you begin your journey into the heart, it's like going into a microcosm; you discover a huge world within your tiny one. So these deep wounds offer us the opportunity for deep healing and for opening up to our true nature, which is love and joy.

After Jane recovered and became a successful professor at a prominent university, she interviewed a lot of people with agoraphobia for her postgraduate thesis. She wanted to help others understand the debilitating illness that had actually helped transform her own life in a positive way. She found to her own surprise that many others had actually come to see their illness as a tool. "At a certain point they realized that's what it was and that's how they wanted to relate to it. And for that, the amount of gratitude they had toward it was unbelievable."

And even on the level of everyday life, in hundreds of little ways, illness and hardship have rewards to offer us. We fill our lives with the trivia of the modern era, but there's only so much time and energy in the world. So when we're deprived of something, it gives us room to do something else. Everyone has probably had some experience that illustrates this. The "TV turn-offs," sponsored by schools, and other organizations, have been big eye-openers to many people, who found that when they turned off their TVs for a week or a month, members of their family actually began to interact with one another, and to do things that were fun or creative. Others rediscovered the enjoyment of reading or music. Any restriction we put ourselves under, or under which the world puts us, carries with it a certain corresponding freedom.

The Usefulness of Restriction

Most, if not all, of the world religions and spiritual traditions have periods during which the practitioners put themselves under some kind of restriction, either gathered together at a retreat, or during set periods of time such as Lent in the Christian tradition or "practice period" in some of the Eastern traditions, when people forego certain kinds of pleasures and distractions in order to concentrate on the inner life. If you go to meditation retreats, you know that the restrictions are severe: movement, food, even thoughts, are all restricted. But the freedoms are also plentiful: freedom from worrying about what you will eat, what you will do next, even what you will think.

Marc, another ex-con, who had been a part of Gangaji's prison program, received a letter from Gangaji while he was in prison. She said, "While you're inside, I hope you're looking inside."

"That always stuck with me," he said. He realized that being in prison turned out to be the perfect time for him to delve into his own inner self and see what resided there. He had time. He had no distractions. His food was provided. What a perfect opportunity. "This is my personal monastery now," he said. "This is my time now to find out who I am—who I truly am and what I want. Not what I thought I wanted." And it was no longer prison for him, he reflected. "It was a time for me. It was time to find myself. And all the other stuff I felt about being in prison dissolved—all the people I worried about—all dissolved."

If we do a practice period and we say we're not going to eat a certain kind of food, or we're not going to watch TV, or we're not going to listen to any kind of music except classical music—this gives us an opportunity to experience things that we don't normally experience. The enjoyment we can get out of doing the things that we never do because we always do the same things is quite surprising.

Illness and Restriction as Agents of Change

We humans are creatures of habit. We get into a rut. It is usually only when our habitual path is blocked that we are moved to try something new. When I go for a walk, I usually go to the same place. There was a wonderful little oak-lined creek I used to follow on my daily walk, that wound down through a field filled with wildflowers in the spring. One day an electric fence went up around the field, and cows began to graze in my special place. I was so sad and thought I would never find another place to compare to that one. But I did— right down the road another creek and another place even more special than the old one has become the place where I go to walk, dream, meditate, and just be.

When Jim Dreaver had a stroke, he was pushed into making a transition he had wanted to make for a long time:

> Well, I had rheumatoid arthritis for two-and-a-half years, and was taking prednasone for the last year-and-a-half. I was a chiropractor for 25 years, and for many years I wanted to make the transition out of it. I thought the arthritis would do this, and then I had the stroke, and lo and behold I am out of it now. And I was always, well maybe this year I'll leave, but I couldn't quite make the transition, and then it was forced upon me. ... (laughs)
>
> And I'm making a transition to full-time writing and teaching, and that'll happen in time. It's been an interesting journey. I have a manuscript which my publisher was interested in, [but] he wanted a much

shorter book. And I was doing that, but writing of course was extremely difficult when one-handed, and I had to search for the letters, whereas I used to be a touch typist. It was definitely hard to think, but probably good in the sense of my writing because it slowed me down and I really had to focus.

I am deeply grateful to my illnesses, both chronic and life-threatening, for helping to lead me to poetry. I'm a person with a strong creative drive which had taken various forms throughout my life: art, music, crafts, cooking, raising my children, singing etc. When chronic illness had pretty much shut down most of these avenues, I lay in bed barely able to move or talk, and I yearned for some venue, some means of creative expression. Finally I hit upon poetry as a way that might work for me. I thought I could spend much of my creative energies composing in my head, with a minimum of actual writing.

I had written poetry in my youth and dabbled in it throughout the years, but it had mostly fallen by the wayside, partly because I didn't have confidence in myself as a poet, and partly because I was busy with my life doing other things. I began slowly. It was more difficult physically than I had thought, but I found that I could actually do it, if I put off many other things in my life (such as housecleaning!). But it was my brush with death through cancer that really opened me to my inner power and gave my work force. It also gave me the courage to take risks both in my writing and in my willingness to put myself out there as a poet. If you avail yourself to the powerful energies that are attempting to open you, I believe there's no limit to what you can do or be. So when we get sick, we're presented with the opportunity to do something different.

When I'm sick, my body slows down in a way that it never does when I am well. A long meditation retreat comes close, but chronic illness and disability have a different quality to them due to the choicelessness and the indefiniteness or, in the case of incurable illness and permanent disability or injury, the far-reaching *definiteness* of the situation. A meditation retreat has a beginning and an end. But chronic illness or disability has no set ending time. As far as we know, it could go on for the rest of our lives. So we're looking here at a way of life, not a weekend of let's just "tough-it-out-and-get-through-it." We may freak out for a while. One can handle most hardships if they seem to have an end. But if there's no end in sight, one must approach with a different quality of being.

Grief is a given. If we do not grieve the life we have lost, we're not likely to open to a new one. But this is the subject of another chapter. When we have moved through our grief, and we begin to settle in and look around, we see all kinds of things not visible to us before. I never experience the sky or a tree in the same way when I am more well as when I am very ill. I just don't. When I'm ill, I tend to focus on more important things like beauty and truth. I tend to look at the sky and the trees and the hills more, and to hear the songs of birds. I am more likely to attend to things of the heart and of the spirit—to become aware of the feelings beneath the surface that become exposed when the crusty surface layers are peeled back. And when it takes just too much energy to even *have* a personality, I am left with the raw unformed material of my own essence, the very thing meditators and seekers of authenticity try so hard to achieve.

Being Lucky

I have always loved nature. Since tramping the woods and lakeshores of northern Wisconsin as a young child, I have loved the wilderness and have felt most alive and connected at the times when I'm in it. Yet as an adult there were long periods of time when I forgot to even look at the sky or the trees—not so after developing a chronic illness. One of the first things I noticed after being sick for a few months was the great love and appreciation I felt for the natural world. Being outside became sacred to me, and it seemed I could not drink in enough of the sight of blue skies, clouds, grass and trees. When I was too sick to be outside, just to sit by a window and gaze outside was my sustenance.

At some point—I don't know when it was—perhaps two years, maybe five years into my illness, the strangest thing began to occur. I began to see myself as lucky. Who in this fast-paced, busy world has the time to lie out under the sky and just drink in the beauty of the clouds drifting by or the birds swooping overhead? I did, but without the illness, I would never have done it. When I was well, I was too busy.

In addition, the compassion and love I felt for others seemed to be deepening every day. All my life I had secretly looked on myself as self-centered—even selfish. Gradually, through no effort of my own, it seemed, my heart was softening. I felt a kinship with all who suffered and even found compassion for the ostensibly hard-hearted ones—those who seem to cause suffering, the supposed oppressors—knowing that their oppression arises out of their own fear, fear of the loss of many of the things that had already been taken from me by my illness. I saw how these losses were molding me into something soft—someone with more gentleness and compassion—someone I liked a whole lot more than the person I had been when I was well.

The Gift of Choicelessness

I was lying in bed one morning feeling sorry for myself. Perhaps I wasn't so much feeling sorry for myself as having compassion for myself for not being able to take care of things in this life. I was also having an inner dialogue with my sister and with other people who have a lot of judgments about me not keeping my house tidy, and not being able to do this or that. And I said to them silently in my mind, "You try, you just try to do a life, to live a life, with only one-fourth of a body. It's impossible to keep up what one might consider to be a normal life with the amount of energy and strength that I have. That's just a fact." Or is it?

Some small voice began to question. What *is* a "normal life" anyway? I have begun to see that there's no such thing.

And suddenly I realized that what I have with this "one-fourth of a body" is something other people don't—which is time—time in which I can't *do*. Time that is just shut-down time, where there's no choice. There's no question during these times that I will make this body do *anything*. It's choiceless. And so I have this time that other people don't, in which to do things that other people can't.

I can lie and watch the sky and clouds, and listen to the birds. I can tend to matters of the heart. I can't sort my stacks of papers, or clean my house, but I *can* do an internal cleaning. I can begin to look at all the baggage, all the stacks and stacks—the internal stacks, things that I've put into the boxes and closets of my mind and heart throughout the years. I can take them out and look at them. I can do the internal house-cleaning that's been put off for so long. I can get straight with myself and with all the people in my life for whom I hold grudges, or have blockages in the heart—things in the way of love.

What an amazing opportunity. What a gift. How lucky. Yes, there's that word again—"lucky" is the word I would use. And I can reverse that sentence I had earlier about my sister. I can have some compassion for this being who rushes here and rushes there, with never a moment for the interior life, or to lie still and look at the clouds. Mercy. Mercy. Have Mercy on both of us for the things we cannot do, and deep appreciation for the things we can.

John Sherman said in an interview: "The guy who is responsible for me having met Gangaji was talking to me at my house not too long ago and he said, 'You know the difference in you is so astounding. When I knew you in Englewood, you were like dead'."

"So what was this change?" he was asked by the interviewer.

John answered, "He said that I was radiant."

So it is when we begin to open to the truth of who we really are through the auger of our earthly suffering, be it illness, loss, hardship, poverty, pain or deprivation. It is only in retrospect, through the contrast of comparing the way we experience life after our opening to the way we experienced it before, that we realize how constricted we were by our need to have our lives be a certain way.

Our Main Job: To Be

Illness, loss, or deprivation helps us to focus on our main job: to be. It helps us to appreciate the wonderful things life offers us at each moment: the full moon in a deep blue velvet sky; the clouds moving and changing, providing the show of a lifetime for us right before our eyes; a butterfly, the most evanescent of all creatures; the essence of a tree—so sturdy, strong, and grounded. It also gives us the opportunity to work toward healing the emotional or psychic pain we have carried around with us for our whole lives. Jane, speaking about her intense agoraphobic period said,

I think that, one, it gave me a time out. I literally just wanted to check out and in a certain way I did. I was definitely still working hard, but it was like the world really did just stop. Time stopped in some ways to give me a chance to learn things that I just sort of bypassed—or it felt like a going back, and there was obviously, through therapy and everything, so much revisiting the past. So it gave me a rest, which from twenty years of pulling it together, I needed.

I remember at some point I basically had my house, my mom, my grandma—that was the extent of my life. And a few phone calls from people. I realized that this was as blank as you can get and still be alive. And then the first time I added something—I was able to add a regular piece to the week—I was really conscious of the fact that I was adding it.

There was this feeling, once I got down to totally blank, then whatever came on top of that was really, really a conscious decision about the life I'm creating—and I think, up until the crash, I was so unaware and so not reflective of what it was that I really wanted, or what was this thing called my life. And it [had been] about whatever expectations there were of me, the image I was trying to create. [So] I was just really aware that I had had the opportunity to get down to nothing, and that what I was building was my very own.

When I am more well, I tend to focus on things that in the larger scheme of the universe have very little importance, like getting my bills paid, fixing my car or painting the house. I begin to feel the urgency to get things done. As things pile up on the "to do" list, I start to "lean forward" metaphysically speaking. I am not really grounded in now, but leaning into some future time, and thus miss the most precious opportunity to experience this life now—which is the only time it can possibly be experienced. I become more and more enmeshed in the frenetic pace of modern life, rushing here and there, trying to fit it all in and never stopping to ask myself what it is that I need to fit in, what is so important that I can't seem to find the time to watch a sunset or visit a friend?

Kathy, the facilitator of our chronic illness support group, who does not have a chronic illness, went through a long period of being very sick. When she started to get better, she shared with us that she actually missed the slow pace life had taken when she was sick. She saw how she was pulled back into frenetic activity as soon as she began to recuperate. She shared about how, in recovering, the quality of her life actually got worse than when she was ill.

If we can let go of our belief that life should be a certain way, we can see that life is just as it should be at any point in time. Or more accurately, life just is. I have learned that if I think I know what's best for my life or someone else's life, I am misguided and arrogant beyond belief. The lessons are endless, as are the rewards. But we must let life lead.

One night I was sitting, meditating, and about halfway through the session I began fidgeting and getting bored, wishing the time was over, day-dreaming about the snack I would eat and the TV program I would watch when I was done. Then I realized that this time I was meditating, this next fifteen minutes of my life was an opportunity to make contact with the deepest part of myself, to encounter the mysteries of the universe, to touch love, to feel the presence of God. I also realized that I probably would not do any of these things but the fact that the opportunity existed, that I had even the most remote chance of doing that made me see that wishing those fifteen minutes away was ludicrous. For what? Some frozen yogurt and ER? Nothing I could do with the rest of my evening could even come close to comparing with the opportunity I was being given to sit quietly with myself in those precious fifteen minutes. And the minutes, hours, days, weeks we spend in our beds or on our chairs in choiceless inactivity when we are ill are also opportunities—opportunities to heal in a way that doesn't have anything to do with the physical body, opportunities to truly open to the deep joy inherent in each moment of life.

LOVE DOGS

One night a man was crying,
        Allah! Allah!
His lips grew sweet with the praising,
until a cynic said,
        "So! I have heard you
calling out, but have you ever
gotten any response?

The man had no answer to that.
He quit praying and fell into a confused sleep.

He dreamed he saw Khidr, the guide of souls,
in a thick, green foliage.
        "Why did you stop praising?"
"Because I've never heard anything back."
        "This longing
you express is the return message."

The grief you cry out from
draws you toward union.

Your pure sadness
that wants help
is the secret cup.

Listen to the moan of a dog for its master.
That whining is the connection.

There are love dogs
no one knows the names of.

Give your life
to be one of them.

        –Rumi
   (Coleman & Mayne, 1995)

CHAPTER 5

Sickness As Path— Getting to Yes

> *I discovered where my wings were through losing the use of my legs.*[3]
>
> —Laurel Burch

FOR THOSE OF US who consider ourselves to be on a spiritual path, there are often times when we feel we just can't do inner work right now because of this or that. We are sick, or we just lost our job, or our mind just doesn't seem to be functioning clearly, or our child is in trouble and we just can't focus on anything but that, or our partner just left us, or a loved one is dying and we are overcome by grief, or the roof is leaking, or we are simply overwhelmed with all those practical things that just must be attended to—or perhaps life itself is just a little too much to handle right now. For those of us with a chronic illness this is especially persistent, because feeling not well and being overwhelmed is almost a way of life for us.

We say, "When I'm better, I'll practice." "When I get through this crisis, I'll be able to concentrate on my spiritual life." "When I get my life more together, I'll go and talk to a spiritual teacher." Or maybe we just think that when we finally get it together or get through this crisis, peace will come on its own.

Don Juan taught Carlos Castaneda that among the obstacles to a man of knowledge are sickness, old age and death. No matter how together we might be or how much organization we are able to attain in our lives, there will come a time when our lives in this worldly plane will begin to unravel. We will all get old. We will all die. There will come a time when we just can't take care of things any more.

The house that needs painting, the leaves on the front lawn, the tattered couch in the living room—they just will have to remain as they are—undone, unfixed, unattended to—or someone else will have to attend to them. The energy will just not be there.

Eventually this will extend to the physical body. Standing in the shower will be too hard. We will get a chair. Finally even that will become impossible and the unthinkable will happen. Someone else will have to bathe us, or even that most dreaded event, as Morrie (of *Tuesdays with Morrie*) announced to the world in an interview with Ted Koppel, "Someone's gonna have to wipe my ass." (1997, 22). And not just temporarily—for the rest of our lives.

Since we know that this is inevitable, why do we spend so much of our energy trying to run away from this truth? More importantly, why do we think that our spiritual practice depends on our being well, and having it together?

What if these aspects of life—sickness, old age, and death—were not really obstacles at all, but rather opportunities? When we examine our lives honestly, we see that the real growth we have experienced almost always came as a result of painful experiences. When we truly see this, we can sometimes begin to have some appreciation or even gratitude for the pain in our lives and perhaps even for the people who have caused us pain. When we learn to tap into our suffering as a resource, we find a vast store of wealth to enrich our lives.

My first guru (before I was sick) told me about an old Sufi saying, "If you don't have any troubles, get a goat." Well, anyone who has ever had goats knows that, as endearing as they may be, they *are* trouble. So I guess he was saying we can't really do this path—this awakening thing—without hardships of some kind.

Many of the great spiritual teachers seem to agree. When one sees the edge to which illness or loss pushes us, and the extra nudge it often provides to put us over that proverbial edge, we begin to understand why. We can finally acknowledge that, given our proclivities for comfort, pleasure or safety, we would never have taken the plunge without our dark angel. Perhaps, there is something about the friction, the fire that is created in the struggle with our problems, that transforms pain into joy or peace. Of course, we don't really need to get a goat. We all have plenty of troubles, but sometimes we're not aware of them or we're not willing to look at them, so we pretend they're not there, and we need to manufacture something: get a goat, go to a meditation retreat, give something up for Lent.

Until we realize that all these seeming obstacles not only do not get in the way of our spiritual practice but actually *are* our path, we will find ourselves stuck on a side road of our spiritual journey with an empty tank of gas. Metropolitan Anthony, of the Russian Orthodox Church, says in *Courage to Pray*, "How often we think it would be so easy to pray if there was nothing to prevent us and how often this very tumult helps us to pray." (1984, 28) We want our life to be different. We want all these hardships, all these trials, all these difficult situations to go away—we think—then we will be happy. We remember a happy time and we think—if things could be like that again, I would be happy. But we don't realize that these difficulties *are* our path to happiness. By wishing them away we are wishing away our chance to be *truly* happy—to have joy, to have true freedom.

These hard things remind us who we *really* are. They're like the lover's call to home. And home is not some faraway place that we need to travel to. Home is this place, right here, right now, where we find ourselves. The Sufi poet, Hafiz, says, "The place where you are right now God has circled on a map for you." Home is where the heart is. In the deep heart, which is God's Heart, all these things that seem like trouble, that seem like hardship, are just another expression of the love of the existing One—a voice reminding us that we are so much more than just this body: that we are, in fact, Love.

Shondeya, a woman in my support group, saw love open in her life as a result of her struggle with severe migraine headaches that impacted her life in a huge way. She said, "I had to be dragged there kicking and screaming. I wouldn't go there on my own. It's too hard."

Loss of Identity

There are many ways in which illness or loss can help us on our spiritual path. One of the very painful aspects of illness is the loss of some or many of our most treasured identities. Mostly we identify ourselves and others through action. When people meet one another, one of the most common initial questions is, "What do you do?" and by this is usually meant, "What is your job? What do you do for gainful employment?" But further questions may be about what you like "to do" in your free time? Ski? Travel? Play basketball? Write poetry? Hike? Nobody sits down with a new acquaintance and asks, "Who *are* you?" But in our spiritual quest—in the life of the soul, this is the essential question, and the only one, truly, that we need to answer.

Of course, we have ideas of who we are: therapist, executive, artist, homemaker, musician, mountain climber, social or environmental activist, farmer, mother, father, sister, brother, friend. But when we are incapacitated by long-term illness or accident, many of these identities are instantly gone or severely damaged. If they remain, as they must with a mother, father, sister, and brother, our ability to fulfill them may not fit our picture of what that identity "should" be. These are usually devastating transitions—ones most people don't make very gracefully.

When I got sick, almost all my cherished identities, who I imagined myself to be, were shattered or grievously threatened: artist, musician, gardener, hiker, homesteader, homemaker. I could no longer paint or draw, play my guitar, work in the garden, or hike. I couldn't sing or ride my bike. I couldn't cook or bake bread. We had to sell the goats and the chickens. There was a long period of time I couldn't even walk to the back of the property to look at the hills or the garden. But the worst of all was the anguish I felt when I could not take care of my own children, or even read them a story before bed.

I remember lying in bed trying to muffle my crying as I listened to our teenage baby sitter help our four-year old with her bath. Being the best mother I knew how to be had been my most cherished identity. Seeing my darling children set adrift to mostly fend for themselves or be cared for sporadically by near strangers was almost more than I could bear.

Another cherished identity—that of deep spiritual seeker—was also severely challenged. I couldn't attend any kind of meditation group or spiritual teaching. I couldn't sit up to meditate, and mostly, because of the mind fog that seemed to be an integral part of my illness, I could barely even meditate lying down.

And other people put labels on us that are also identities of sorts: genius, bully, saint, freak. Some of these coincide with our own image of ourselves and others may be wildly disparate. These names and labels all point to or are based on something that we or others do. Even closer to home are all those intangible qualities, good and bad, that make up our personalities and are part of our identities as well—kindness, compassion, humor, and generosity or their opposites: meanness or dullness, being down-beat or selfish.

We have a picture of ourselves that we hold onto as "who we are." We may want to hold onto the good things and push away or disavow the bad. I used to like to think of myself as bubbly, fun, active, outgoing, intelligent, a doer, a giver, someone who was a good sport, always up for whatever was going on, whether a spontaneous trip to the beach, helping with the dishes, holding a baby, or having a songfest. But in the shadows lurked the flip side of many of these qualities—the shadow—the view of myself as selfish, dull, stupid, incompetent.

In illness, many of the positive aspects of who I saw myself to be were no longer possible. I saw how my spontaneous impulses—to pick up or play with a child or animal, to jump up to help set the table or do the dishes, to join a last-minute excursion or social gathering—were thwarted by my physical limitations. And when my illness has been most severe, there have been times when I have not even had enough energy to *have* a personality. I have found myself without the energy to laugh at someone's joke or funny comment even though the laugh was right there under the surface wanting to come out. Sometimes my "normal" animated way of talking is downgraded to a dull monotone. I simply don't have the energy to do the intonations or put the feeling that I have behind my words. And finally, speech itself grinds to a halt when my energy has become so depleted I am unable to squeeze out a word.

I remember specifically a day at the beach with my young children when I was in one of my hyper-exhausted states. I saw a new friend there and was absolutely not able to be what I would call "friendly." I simply didn't have the energy for it. Neither did I have the energy to go into any kind of explanation of *why* I couldn't be friendly. However she interpreted my actions or lack of actions, that person was never the same with me after that. Our first blossoming connection seemed to falter and there didn't seem to be anything I could do about it.

The Picture Does Not Match

When we have these kinds of experiences, they come as a shock because we are so identified with our personality. It is our deepest held "identity" on this worldly plane. When it goes, we don't know who we are. All our identities—artist, gardener, manager, politician, athlete, etc.—are extremely difficult to give up, but our identity as personality is perhaps the hardest. We keep trying to live that life, to be that person we were. We keep pounding that square peg into the round hole. We say to ourselves, "But this is not me—I am not myself" and try to explain this to others.

While this is true in a way—and it is important for us to tell ourselves and others this truth because it is part of the knowing adult taking care of the inner child—at a certain point we must acknowledge that this is only a half truth. The other half is, "This *is* me. Circumstances have changed—*I* have changed. The picture does not match. I used to be bubbly, et cetera, but now I am more quiet. I keep to myself more. I don't do that much. But I have a rich inner life. I am more centered, more compassionate." These new descriptions are simply descriptions of what is occurring now. They need not limit us. Change is the truth of existence. At each moment we must ask deeply, "What is true for me here and now?"

With this acknowledgment, this new knowing, comes a new understanding of who we are and are not; that we are not our worldly identities—even the most prized, such as our personality, or the changing labels based on what we do. We are something deeper, something that rides beneath the tides of our personal and professional identities and even our personas, something open and free of doing and not doing. We also begin to develop a new compassion for others because we understand on a deep level that at least part of people's personalities, as well as the things they choose to do, are formed by circumstances and are not necessarily how they would be or what they would choose were circumstances different. Thus we are not so quick to judge.

Jane managed to turn her life around after being virtually homebound for years through opening to her own pain with awareness, loving kindness and the willingness to take one step at a time, allowing herself to feel the horror with each step. Her illness did not go away, but she came into new relationship with it. She continues to deal with extremely difficult situations always with courage and honesty. Once she lost her voice and her response to me was,

> I'm learning how much energy I have used to explain myself, to justify who I am. Now I can't do that and I need to trust that who I am is enough—that I don't need to justify my existence or what I do. If people misunderstand, that is all part of the path—theirs and mine.

Kathy, our support group facilitator, shared with us more about her long and very difficult struggle with a downward health spiral. She described how she saw her identities dropping away painfully one by one: Kathy, the nature trek leader, Kathy, the counselor, Kathy, the active, vital exerciser. But with these losses, she began to see who she really was and what was important in her life. She realized that in spite of these losses, or even *because* of them, she saw herself as a being of light, full and complete as she was, and that this was untouched by the fact that she could no longer do many of the things she used to do, even the things she did to help others or "for health and spiritual well-being."

These identities, to which we are so attached and by which we define who we are in the world, make up what we consider to be our "self" and can actually get in the way of seeing who we *really* are—pure awareness—Light and Love—our true self. There is a Buddhist teaching which says that to lose the self is to find the self. Jesus told us that we must lose our life in order to find it. So these "tough love" teachers, illness and loss, help us to understand who we are by taking away our false identities and reminding us of our true identity.

The Shadow

And what of the shadow identity—the identity we don't want to be, but are so afraid that we are? As the false ego disintegrates, these identities may seem, at first, to get bigger or to be all that remains. Jane remembers the crumbling of her long cherished self-image soon after her breakdown into severe agoraphobia when she left college in the middle of the night to go back home and live with her mom.

> My whole life I had always tried to be so perfect and not be the troublemaker and be helpful and there for [my mom] and ... I remember that first week I was home, one of the feelings was, oh my God, all those years of trying to build up this image and it basically all came crashing down. It was all a total waste, because I can't be anything but a sick dependent person now. It was just a hundred percent opposite of what I had tried to build up.

The selfishness, the anger, the ineptitude—whatever it is that we are hiding, or hiding *from*—may loom larger than ever as our false selves are stripped away and we are able to see beneath the veneer we have created to present to the world. Yet even these, in their turn, are stripped away, at least in the case of intense chronic illness or progressive disease, as the relentless weakness in the body leaves energy for nothing but being.

Phantom Feelings

I remember times when things were not going well in my marriage and my husband would do something or say something that in prior times would have infuriated me. But at the time I couldn't get it up to be angry—I simply didn't have the energy. Sometimes I didn't even have the energy to be hurt or to cry. I wondered what would become of these "almost" feelings, and what would become of me for not having them. I knew, psychologically speaking, it was not healthy to "stuff" feelings, but I wasn't stuffing them—they had not actually even formed themselves. I didn't really have enough energy to even *have* them. So they were in a sense like phantom feelings.

It was an odd thing. I realized that in the big picture it didn't matter at all. It was a bit like the realization I had had on a smaller scale when I first saw that I don't actually have to scratch an itch during meditation. That drive to scratch, as well as the itch itself, that seems so important at the time, will simply pass and it will be as if I never had them. In the end, we will come to this. When we're on our deathbed, it won't matter who wronged us or how. All that will matter is whether or not our hearts are open.

It was very interesting to watch, and I have the sense that I suffered no ill effects from not having these feelings and neither expressing nor suppressing them. So the "shadow" identities, it seemed, had slipped away along with the others, for the time being at least. Later, when more energy became available to me, the feelings returned, and had to be dealt with of course, but what I learned from my experiences was not to take them so seriously—that these feelings are not the solid things we imagine them to be.

To wrest all (or at least many) of our identities from us in one fell swoop without our having to die is perhaps a clever tactic of the divine to bring us up to speed spiritually, or perhaps it's just our good luck. Though it is hard to lose these identities, it is better than getting to the end of our lives and realizing that none of these things ever belonged to us in the first place, that none of these "identities" is who we really are after all, that we have built our lives on sand, that there is nothing solid to stand on, and that we have no time to integrate or realize the enormity of these realizations.

When you become so small that you are about to disappear, you suddenly realize that you are part of something so much bigger, something huge. Illness helps us with this. Illness drove me outside. Cancer even more. When I was so sick—all I could do was lie in bed or sit in my recliner night and day—I got so tired of looking at the walls in my house. I felt like I was in prison. I yearned to be outside beneath the vast open sky. I yearned to lie on the earth beneath the trees.

So I took to sleeping outside under the stars most nights when I could. There is a tree in the field near my house that befriended me. When I slept beneath it, its branches seemed to reach out and enfold me, and I felt the strength of its roots going deep into the earth. The great stars turning on the axis of the heavens and the heavens themselves seemed to hold me, to rock me. I felt a part of all this. I felt huge. John the Baptist said, "He must increase, but I must decrease!." (John 3:30) When you become part of this hugeness, you wonder how you ever thought that little life you had was so important.

Once a woman came to Ekhart Tolle and began to tell him her troubles, which were many. He didn't say a word but simply listened and gave her his full attention. She was very wound up and talked a long time. She had all her papers with her to prove how people had wronged her. She had attorneys' papers strewn around her, and at some point she stopped and looked at him and at the mounds of papers. She said, "None of this has any importance does it?" He answered, "No." And she simply picked up her papers and went home. He said the woman came back to him the next day and asked, "What did you do to me?" She thought he was some kind of wizard. But Ekhart said it was not because he was *there* that she had her awakening. It was because he was *not* there.

"The Bus Hit"

Suzanne Siegel was waiting for a bus one day, and as she watched the bus approach, something extraordinary happened which was to change her life forever: her "self" disappeared. She spent the next ten years in various levels of fear, terror, and despair, going from therapist to therapist trying to restore her lost sense of self. Then one day she met a man, a Zen teacher, who said, "Wow! What you have is what I and many spiritual seekers have been trying to achieve for years." So she began to look at her state in a new way, and as she settled into this new mode of perception, she began to realize that what had seemed like hell for ten years was actually a state of grace. This incident, her loss of self, which she later called her "bus hit," was a defining moment of her life.

Suzanne, it turns out, had a brain tumor and years later died of her condition. Some people were disappointed. The spontaneous loss of self, the miraculous "enlightenment" that Suzanne had experienced was, according to some who had begun to see her as an enlightened being, "phony." It was not some act of grace, but a sickness, which ate away her brain and eventually killed her.

These people are missing the point. The point is not what her condition was or what caused it or what happened to her, but that in opening to her life exactly as it was, she experienced a state of grace in the same exact condition that had formerly seemed like hell. And the condition itself pushed her to an edge where she was so scared and miserable that she made the leap into freedom and grace—a leap she never would have made without the condition of her illness.

Similarly, many of us, whose "bus hit" is an illness, accident, loss of loved one or some other seeming tragedy, may spend years wandering in the desert of despair, floundering in self-pity, seeking revenge, or chasing every snake-oil salesmen that promises a cure in the hope of changing or escaping our current situation. We may think of ourselves as "damaged goods" and see our lives as flawed or lacking or even as basically "over," until one day it hits us. This life—this very life we have tried so desperately to change—feels more precious than it ever has.

This is the crucial point. We think we need *something* or we think we need to *do something* in order to *achieve* Heaven or Nirvana—to *see* or *be* God, or to have true happiness, or whatever our belief system calls that illusive state of pure being which we seek. According to the Dalai Lama, the purpose of life is happiness. But what does it really mean to be happy? Is happiness some pleasant feeling? Freedom from pain? Pleasurable sensations? There is the idea that we have to go somewhere other than where we are, do something different from what we are doing, see some magnificent scenery, accomplish something important or have something: a house, money, or that one and only relationship—or that we need to feel a certain way in order to be happy. Our illness teaches us that there's nowhere to go, because we cannot move. There's nothing to do, because we have no strength to do it. We must make our happiness here, now, with nothing but the wind in our faces and the grass beneath our bodies.

Breaking Through Attachment

The Biblical verse, "It is easier for a camel to pass through the eye of a needle than for a rich man to enter the kingdom of heaven," (Matthew 19:24) might very well be rewritten to read, "It is easier for a camel to pass through the eye of a needle than for a *well person or a carefree person* to enter the kingdom of heaven." And what, one might ask, could be so dangerous spiritually about having money or an easy life? I think that wealth or comfort is not actually the problem. It is our attachment to these things that puts us in spiritual peril and keeps us from freedom. In this verse, money is a metaphor for greed. And greed can take many forms. It can be greed for things, which money can buy, or it can be greed for action, to get things done. It can also be greed for experiences. Most people have a mental list of experiences they want to have, places they want to see, things they want to do.

High on many people's lists are falling in love or having a family, but it could be sky diving, seeing the rain forest (or *saving* the rain forest), going to Paris, climbing Mount Everest, or fishing in the lake one fished in as a child. Some may be wedded to their work and the accumulation of wealth or empire building and power. Others may be into saving the world. We go down our lists, checking things off and filing them away in mental filing cabinets like booty in a treasure chest. The only problem is that somehow we never seem to have enough booty, and we never seem to come to the end of our list. Like the biblical loaves and fishes, it just gets bigger and bigger even as we whittle it away.

The List Dragon

When illness comes, our hopes of attaining or experiencing the things on our list and thus, in our own minds, of attaining happiness, are often dashed because the obstacles created by our ill health seem insurmountable. At these times our lists are likely to turn into "bargains." "You do this for me Lord, and I'll do that for you." A bargain is sometimes simply a prettied-up list that pretends to be spiritual.

I thought I was through with lists. But the list dragon keeps appearing with seven new heads. The human self does not cooperate. It is its nature to want more. Always more. I see with a start as I write about lists that I am still doing it. I have had many wish lists in my life—fewer bargains. The last very serious bargain I remember proposing, before this stark reminder, was when I first became chronically ill and I didn't know whether I was going to live or die. My children were very young, four and seven, and I asked God, I begged, "Please let me raise these children—so they can at least be independent before I must leave them—so they can at least have their mother there for them during their formative years. Then I will willingly go."

When the cancer came twenty years later—Big Surprise—I made my bargain with God—my "last" list—conveniently forgetting that I had already made a "last" bargain with the Divine. "Please God," I prayed, "just let me have three things before I die: A hug from my oldest daughter, love, and to finish and publish my book." This is the list I suddenly remember as I am writing—the list that I still hold in my heart of hearts. And after a moment of true humility—an "aha" moment, I begin to berate myself, to have shame. The false "spiritual" self, catching a whiff of "list," straightens its shoulders and shakes its finger proclaiming, "Thou shalt not have lists!" And off they go, the list maker and the false spiritual judging self, round and round. That is what these "selves" do—fight with each other, judge, and claim to be right. Let them wrangle. Let this simply be. List or no list—it is the same. Leave off trying to reform the human selves. Let them do their human thing and rest in that which you are. That is my mantra to myself, the inner teaching that arises out of my humbling moment.

The Buddha said that the root of suffering is desire. But it seems to me that desire itself is not what causes suffering. Rumi, the Sufi mystic poet, tells us, "This longing...*is* the return message." He says that we must give our lives to be one of those "Love Dogs" that moan and whine for their masters. I think that the Buddha is talking about the negative aspects of desire. Desire, if pure, will burn through our delusions. However, if our desire is for worldly things and if our happiness is attached to their attainment, we are doomed to unhappiness and suffering. Of course, we cannot simply decide to not be attached to the objects of our desire. Through the sometimes seemingly relentless losses in our lives, however, we learn slowly that life goes on and sometimes the losses themselves open us to a peace or joy not previously available.

I learn this over and over again. Each time I go into relapse, I re-experience the loss. I cry. I grieve. One night as I realized I was going into another one of my relapses, I wept bitterly for, again, I had become attached to the gains I had made, the selves that had been resurrected. But each time it becomes a little easier. I am a little less attached. Each time I open a little sooner to the grace that is present in the loss—in the miracle of each moment of life. I dive into the deep heart place opened by the grief and am transformed again. Sometimes these days, a relapse causes no more than a little blip on my radar screen. I seem to be no longer so defined by these passing phenomena and experiences. That feels good.

My teacher used to talk about chains of lead and chains of gold. There are different kinds of attachment. There are the attachments that seem obviously bad, the chains of lead: all of our addictions—drinking coffee, smoking, alcohol, drugs, sex, relationships (if they are addictions), our attachments to negative emotions—anger, hatred, greed, resentment—negative thinking, bad habits etc. These are the kinds of attachments we usually think of as getting in the way of peace or happiness. And the focus of most therapy is to be free of these kinds of attachments. Even meditation and many spiritual paths seem to focus on "letting go" of negativity, anger, etc. and being blissful, peaceful.

There can, however, be a price to pay for these seemingly "good" experiences. If we cling to them and think our lives should always be like that, they become chains of gold. Meditation, chanting, going to church, doing "good works," such as volunteering or community service, and even high states such as blissfulness or peacefulness are all things that can lead to spiritual openings and seem like "progress" on our spiritual path. But in truth, anything we are attached to, anything we cling to, can be a hindrance to our ultimate freedom and joy, even that very bliss and peace that may arise from deep spiritual work.

Spiritual Poverty

I used to hear the word spiritual poverty and wonder what it meant. I had some idea but didn't quite understand. Going through what I call the "black hole" phases of my illness have taught me what spiritual poverty means. When I get so sick and weak that I feel like an inert mass, when I come to the place where nothing can come out—not even light—I begin to truly understand what spiritual poverty really is. I see the futility of all things, or as the Bible tells us, "All is vanity." (Ecclesiastes 1:2)

When an ill or injured person becomes too weak to even feel spiritual (or inspirational), he must rely on grace alone. In those times, I see that the only way love or salvation can come to me is through grace—if I'm willing to surrender to that. I don't get the kind of highs that people can get through working really hard at something, making big efforts, long meditation retreats or giving to others etc.—sometimes that is just the reality of it. There's no way to put a pretty face on it. The door is closed to those things—period. So it seems a loss that is a real loss—no silver lining, no door opening where another closes, just plain loss.

Yet there is something beyond or beneath that. Something beyond those lost deep experiences which are so thrilling, beyond those unreachable satisfactions—something that comes out of this inner earthlike quality of almost catatonia: a humility, a receptivity that is like the earth itself—accepting whatever comes—a communion with all things—not being higher than anything—no way to be proud.

Then we must cut to the chase—go to the bottom line—love. We must extend our begging bowl and ask for mercy because we ourselves cannot do that which is necessary for salvation or enlightenment. If one can accept this state and truly enter it, there is a deep peace in the realization that there's no way to get anything or do anything that could lead to these greater experiences or epiphanies, or nirvana, that you think are possible and that you think you need. And further, that there's no *need* to do or get *anything* or experience *anything*. The ground of being lies beneath those things.

So here's the paradox: with the realization that you simply cannot have those things—those good things, those amazing wonderful things—comes also the realization that it is not necessary to have those things, that what you really truly seek is beyond, or beneath those things. You cannot hold onto them at any rate. Phenomena and experiences come and go. The ground of being is what does not come and go. When you realize this, all striving becomes useless. And the further paradox is that you *do* have those amazing and wonderful experiences, the openings *do* come—through grace. They are simply gifts that come and go, but to try to hold onto them is futile.

Death as Teacher

The great virtues—patience, unconditional love, mercy, kindness, generosity—are not things that come easily. Pema Chödrön reminds us in her book, *The Places That Scare Us,* that those people who annoy us present an opportunity to practice patience and unconditional love. Jesus pointed out that anyone can be loving and kind to people who love us and are loving and kind to us. But to love our enemies? This is hard. Yet it is what we are called to do.

So it is with illness and loss. Anyone can be happy and peaceful when everything is going their way. But to be at peace when your world is falling apart, when you are faced with the loss of everything you hold dear, when death is staring you in the face—that is the path of a warrior—a peace warrior. Death will come—that is a given. We are all called to the table of that divine banquet. We live our lives mostly trying to avoid the awareness of this fact. But in closing off to our dying we are closing off to our living as well. Joseph Sharp talks about living his dying—really opening to and being with dying moment by moment in his life.

> I've come to find that if I don't live my dying, I'm not honestly living my life's wholeness. There's a separation—a compartmentalization, an incompleteness—to my present life experience if I close myself off from my dying.... Dying is inseparable from living. Two sides of one whole coin. (XVII–XVIII)

Our illnesses, whether they be chronic or life-threatening, bring us closer to death, to the reality of our own dying, and consequently open a window for us into life. They present an invitation and an opportunity to truly begin to live our lives fully.

One day I sat in my oncologist's office waiting for the results of a blood test to see if my white blood cell count had recovered enough to begin my third round of chemotherapy for breast cancer. I wondered anew at the strangeness of what I considered to be the inordinate, cheerfulness all around me. "What's wrong with these people?" I wondered, "or what's wrong with *me*? All I feel when I come here is a deep sadness or an anxious quiver in the pit of my stomach."

My eyes fell on the cover of a magazine which read, "Walks on the Wild Side/The Best of America's National Parks/Wildlife Adventures, and Weekend Wildernesses/Hike the Secret Smokies, Herd Wild Horses, Climb Mount St. Helens, Kayak with the Orcas, Find Florida's Wild Orchids, Collar a Black Bear, Track Wolves, Canoe the Adirondacks, Escape from LA." As I read the words, tears began streaming down my face and deep involuntary sobs from the depths erupted past barriers of impropriety.

A flood of emotions and thoughts rushed through my body. First, outrage—how could they put such a magazine in an oncologist's office for people to read who are facing death or are so debilitated from chemotherapy they can barely walk? Then fear—what if the chemo doesn't work? What if the cancer is at this moment growing in my liver or muscles, spreading through my body? Then incredulity—how could all these people, in various stages of cancer, be smiling, as if they were coming in for a pap smear or allergy shots? And finally, deep sadness and a feeling of kinship with all. In the midst of all the brave smiling faces soldiering through their adversity, I sat in my pool of grief, past caring how I looked.

So, as I sat sobbing in the oncologist's office, my heart cracked open once again from the pain of loss with the huge crushing realization that I will die—I saw the finality of that. Whether now or later, this world that I so love will be lost to me. These things that I so long to do—the kinds of things listed on the cover of the magazine, which in reality had been lost to me for over twenty years because of my chronic illness—were still, I realized, on some distant inner wish-list, in spite of the absurdity of it.

At that moment I saw that not only these things, not only the athletic activities and distant mountains, but all things—the soft trails near my home that I walk in the mornings, the birds which still sing to me even when I can't walk, the blue sky and clouds over me always—will be lost to me when death comes. So here again was death teaching the ultimate lesson in nonattachment. Yet somehow this grief—this pure sadness—did not keep me from joy. On the contrary, the cracking open again exposed my deep heart and left me feeling more alive than ever, even in the midst of my pain and my incredible weakness. And more—it left me with a deeper appreciation than ever of the life that I have, however long it might last.

We think we can change outcomes by our choices and we agonize over them. But the only true choice we ever have is to say yes or to say no—to open or to close to what is being presented to us in any particular moment. The circumstances of our lives will change. We will be given things that seem to make us happy for a time, and then they will be gone. We will have experiences that seem to cause us great sorrow and hardship—then they will be gone. We think we have some control over the circumstances of our lives, but illness and loss teach us otherwise. A person could be in Heaven and be miserable; could be in the presence of God and experience it as Hell; or be in a hellish situation and experience great peace. God is all that exists. All else is illusion. For those who open, who say yes, this is heaven. For those who are closed, those who say no—those who chose instead some phenomenal object or experience as happiness—this is Hell because nothing phenomenal can last.

Getting to Yes

This very body and mind we have in this moment, this very life as it is—even this state of mind—are all that we need for happiness, for enlightenment. When we are sick or experiencing great loss, there is, I believe, a certain grace being extended to us. My friend, a very spiritually oriented man, shared with me one day, "It is very hard to meditate when I am sick." I replied without a moment's hesitation from the deep knowing place I had learned to trust, "When you are sick, meditation does you."

We almost don't have to do anything. I guess one could call it the lazy person's way to enlightenment. All we need to do is wake up in the morning and say yes—no making ourselves sit through interminable meditation retreats wondering if we're crazy to be putting ourselves through this. It's all been taken care of for us. Our path is there straight as an arrow before us, and we are in a one-way chute heading straight toward grace. We could resist the ride, and we usually do, but what a miserable struggle we make for ourselves fighting the current and trying to make our way back up the slide.

It may sound glib to say, "all we need to do is say yes." Getting to yes is no easy matter. Opening to the relentlessness of chronic illness or the massive assault of some personal tragedies is exponentially harder than any other practice we would ever visit upon ourselves intentionally. Yes, life is suffering, as the Buddha said. It is the forge that smelts us. Yet, suffering itself is not enough. Jesus calls upon us to pick up our cross and follow him. We must offer ourselves to that suffering. We must allow ourselves to be put into the furnace.

Opening to the extraordinary pain, loss, or hardship that appears in some human lives seems almost too much to ask. Yet we are called upon to bring some intention to our suffering. P.D. Ouspensky, a student of G. Gurdjieff, talked about the merits of "intentional suffering."

Meditation retreats and fasting can be forms of intentional suffering. But acts of nature can also be made into a form of intentional suffering. There is something about the *willingness* to experience pain and loss that is transformative.

About ten years into my chronic illness, I lay in bed one night sobbing and in despair over the relentlessness of my illness. Though I knew my illness—and all the obstacles it had presented to me—were my path, and that many wonderful openings and much grace had come my way because of them, the longing for my lost life was particularly strong that night. The pain and sadness was so deep, I cried out loud to God, "I don't want this. If it be possible, please, please take this away from me." I just didn't want it any more.

A picture of Christ at Gethsemane arose before my eyes. I saw the sweat pouring from him like blood and the gesture from the depths of his soul, "not my will, but Thine be done." And there arose in me, right next to the desperate pleading to have this taken away, a willingness to have it be true, if that, in the Divine will, was what was to be. I said, "Yes," and in that yes I experienced a deep opening, a transformation, and a powerful sense of peace and strength emerged.

I felt like a mountain and was filled with deep gratitude. "Thank you," were the words that came, and that "thank you" was not just for the opening and the peace that had emerged, but for the whole package: peace, joy, and for the illness and pain from which these had issued. Yet, I had no illusions about my path being any easier. And it has not been. But there has been joy and lots of love, right there next to the terror and the pain and the loss that goes on and on.

Mindfulness

My ex-husband said he needed to be hit on the head by several two-by-fours (chronic illness, divorce) before he began to open to his own pain and ultimately to his true heart. Some of us may feel more like a giant redwood is falling on us. But learning and opening doesn't always have to be precipitated by such huge losses. One man in my chronic illness support group shared that he was on disability now because his knee was bad. He had ignored it for a long time because unconsciously he didn't feel justified in catering to his knee since there was no "reason" for it to be bad. Nothing happened to cause it to go out. In retrospect he realized he was basically saying to his knee, "Nothing happened to you. You have no reason to be bad, so just shut up."

He was ignoring his body's signals. When he went deeper, he saw that he was ignoring much more than just the signals from his knee. He had been unhappy in his job for a long time. His inner voice was telling him long before his knee went out that this was not a good thing for him, but he ignored it. Now that he was unable to work, he saw what was going on and gave notice at his job, even though the ego-mind was issuing dire warnings that people would think he was lazy, etc.

In Vipassana Buddhism there is a practice called mindfulness. Mindfulness means to be aware, "mindful" of what is happening in each moment. If you are washing dishes, the practice is to be aware of the dishes and the rag or sponge moving over the plates and cups. It is hard to stay present long enough to actually remember to be mindful. Usually our mind drifts away in daydreams. If we drop something or bang a dish against the sink and crack or chip it, that is usually a reminder that we have not been mindful—our mind was somewhere else. Otherwise we probably wouldn't have chipped the dish.

If we are open and willing, we can use our illness or loss to help us to be mindful. In the case of chronic illness, not being able to have what we want is so relentless—so in our face—that we cannot long forget. We can use this to remember to be mindful in each moment. Chronic pain is another back-door helper in this regard. Whether your pain and loss is physical or emotional, you can use it to open to life as it is. And "life as it is" is the greatest teacher. It is the path that can lead us to fulfillment, and is itself the fulfillment of the path. When we don't want to be anywhere except where we are, or experiencing anything other than what we are experiencing, we can rest in the peace of just this.

Wouldn't it be nice if we could have pleasant and joyful reminders instead of pain and loss? Yes, and sometimes we get those too. Falling in love can be one of those peak experiences that keeps us present. Bearing children is another. When I was pregnant with my first daughter, I was so enraptured to be pregnant that I was almost constantly aware through the entire nine-month gestation of the new life growing inside me. But, we must use whatever means we have to awaken. And what we have sometimes is pain; what we have sometimes is loss.

Being Present in the Now

Most spiritual paths emphasize being in the present moment. For many of us who experience chronic or life-threatening illness or crushing loss, sometimes the only way to survive is to live in the present moment. The future is terrifying and the past is too painful to remember, because of what we no longer have. One woman in my support group said her aunts are all in their nineties and she is only fifty-two and that it is terrifying to her to think that this longevity is in her genes. Without these stark reminders, it is often too easy to get sidetracked. You know the story: I'll surrender to love tomorrow, after I get my brakes fixed and a new washer for the leaky bathroom faucet, or I'll tune into my body in half an hour, after I eat this piece of chocolate cake left over from last night's party.

But life-threatening illness teaches us we may not have a tomorrow; it reminds us that half an hour, even half a minute, is too long to wait for love, too long to wait to inhabit this precious body given for only a finite period of time, too long to wait to live this precious life, in front of us in this moment—the only one we have.

The way to "now" is sometimes a crooked path, and what it actually means to be present to our life as it is may surprise us, as illness and loss relentlessly force us to abandon our fixed ideas of reality. We may feel at times like we are going backwards, like we are losing spiritual ground, like we know less—even after years of spiritual practice, now that we are faced with death or loss of bodily function—than we did before we started a spiritual practice. I wrote in my journal one day in the midst of chemotherapy for my breast cancer an entry to a loved one who was no longer my lover:

> In the deep dark of the night I tell myself things I couldn't say during the day. If you were here, would I tell you too? It's like, I'm so willing to suspend reality. I see how I just wanted to go on this holiday and pretend that I had love. To say to you, let's just pretend, let's just pretend we have love—but only if there's a reality to it in the moment.

It's like all of creation is pretending, is pretending that there's no tomorrow, that they won't die, that it won't fade, that it won't change. I think of the word "reckless." I feel like I'm just being reckless. What does that word mean? "Reckless"? Reck-less ... without a reck? Careless. To live as if there were no tomorrow, because there is no tomorrow. Tomorrow is an illusion. Tomorrow never comes. There's only a succession of todays.

I wrote this the day after:

Okay, it's litmus test time. Do I really believe all this crap I'm spouting? About Joy being present in every moment? If so, I need to stop searching for my happiness out there, enter this pain and find the Joy buried there.

St. Paul said, "We see now as in a mirror, but then face to face." Things, it seems, are backwards. Sometimes what seems true is not, and what seems like illusion is true. In that willingness to pretend, which my mind saw as a betrayal of truth, was buried a deeper truth—the realization, or the near realization, of what the birds already know: that there is no tomorrow; there is only now. And that now contains the love and joy we seek. Sometimes we have to start with pretend, because the myth of time, the myth of separation is so strongly ingrained. It is the common illusion, the common dream constructed and reinforced over lifetimes by humans who have agreed with each other to accept this myth, and have passed it on to their children.

We hold so tightly to these structures of mind, these artifacts from a lifetime of illusion. And when the difficulties in our lives come along and begin to undermine those structures, to break them down, we're right there with our hammer and nails to fix them up or put them back together again. Sometimes it takes a gale force wind, a hurricane, the kind of life event about which this book is being written, to come through and sweep them all away before we can see the ground of truth and love we have covered over with our structures.

In an interview, my friend Jane spoke of the constructed illusions from the period of her life before her breakdown,

That's true, you know, that's what they are, artifacts. And I think that in the middle of a life you forget that they are just artifacts. They become real structures. Real things. And as I'm talking about this now, I see that it was really easy to lose that perspective once I got a life again.

What we are led to is what all the teachers of all great religions and meditative paths preach to their followers—be present in the moment. When we are, we find there can be peace in this moment and sometimes something so much more—an opening—a laying down of the load—a freedom from fear. Our illness is not the enemy. Our bodies are not our enemies. They are our friends—our teachers. Pema Chödrön says illness is like a Zen master hitting her with a stick when she doesn't listen.

There is a Tibetan Buddhist slogan—a teaching—which says, "Abandon any Hope of Fruition." But who is willing to do this? It seems almost human nature to always want things to be better and think that, if we do the right things, we can make them better. Pema Chödrön says, "One of the deepest habitual patterns we have is to feel that now is not good enough." (1994, 96)

Surrender

Sometimes it seems that we must be so wretched that there appears to be no hope of ever being able to live the life that we long for, or even of ever having any kind of satisfying life at all before we unlock the death grip we have on the picture of how our life was supposed to be. Then even in that low, achy, scared, confused place, we can look deeper and find the beauty and joy that exist in this life. The amazing thing is that it's really not *even*, but *especially* in that place, because it is at those lost, low moments, that our tender heart is exposed and accessible, the part of ourselves that never seems to be available when we "have our life together," the part of us that is essential to access in order to truly experience the essence of our existence.

Just when our lives become unmanageable, we are willing to surrender because there is nothing else to do. And when we do, something marvelous happens. The impossible opens up like a soft yellow rose loosening its petals. The sweetness of the simple joy of being becomes available for us to experience. It is there all the time, but we don't experience it. The more "in our face" our pain is, the harder it is to hide, to run away, to seek diversion. Zen teacher, Joko Beck, speaking about the pain in the body, which inevitably arises during long meditation retreats, says, "It is so valuable that, if it didn't exist, it should."

And the relentlessness of chronic illness? The pain that never goes away when a cherished child dies? The loss so cruel it seems to break us into irretrievable pieces? The specter of death that creeps up suddenly and unexpectedly before we are ready? Should they exist? I would never say that—yet when they do, the grace that can flow from the pain becomes a gift transcending our brokenness in some miraculous way.

We must press the "select all," button once and for all. When we do, we can never be disappointed, for we want all that comes, like the character in *The Little Prince,* who commanded things to happen after they had already happened. But we can go one step further. He chose it after the fact; we can choose before.

CHAPTER 6

Practicing with Loss, Illness and Dying

There was a door being presented to me. I needed to walk through that door; to sit in that room, let myself mold to its shape; to rest in that abominable place.

SOCRATES SAID, "True philosophers make death and dying their profession." Joseph Sharp points out in his book, *Living Our Dying,* that in the Eastern spiritual traditions one of the basic aims of life is to prepare for death. This is also true for many of the more simple or primitive societies where death is not a topic to be avoided at all costs as in many Western societies, but is woven into the fabric of everyday life. In India, the dead and dying are everywhere. Funerals are public processions.

On El Dia de Los Muertos ("Day of the Dead"), the Mexican holiday that is celebrated very close to our Halloween, friends and relatives gather in the graveyards to honor and celebrate the lives of loved ones who have died. These events are not solemn or dark affairs. They are celebrations and joyous affirmations of the whole person, the good and the bad, looked upon with warmth and humor as remembered by friends and family from their shared journey of life. If the loved one was a gambler and a drinker, the altar may contain tiny skeletons sitting around a table playing cards and drinking tequila. This kind of celebration stands in stark contrast to the American way of honoring the dead, which is usually with solemnity, sadness, and a tendency to focus on remembering the "good things" about the deceased while conveniently forgetting or excluding "the bad."

I remember seeing a movie about a family in some mid-century European country where a dying grandmother, the matriarch of the family, had her bed in the living room amid the comings and going of the extended family. Teenage grandchildren kissed her on the way out the door and great-grandchildren proudly presented their paintings and drawings for her praise, or a doll's "owie" for a kiss. She phased in and out of sleep as family life continued around her.

"What a wonderful way to die," I thought, juxtaposing this scenario with others I have seen of elders breathing their last breaths hidden away in the back room of the house or in a hospital bed hooked up to a multitude of tubes and monitors. And how wonderful for the children and young adults coming of age in such a milieu, where death is accepted matter-of-factly and openly as part of life.

But in the West we hide from dying, push it away into the back room of the house or a hospital room. Twice in the last year, after all my work to bring death and dying to consciousness and openness in my life, I have visited family or friends who had suffered the loss of a loved one in the not too distant past and I have failed to bring up the subject of this loss. It's shocking to realize the enormity of our cultural taboo against speaking of death, a taboo that clings to us despite our conscious strivings to the contrary. My mind made excuses, "This isn't the time or the place." "It would make her uncomfortable." While these were partially true, the real reasons were cultural conditioning and fear.

Our society is not satisfied with simply putting death out of sight and out of mind. Anything that reminds us of our mortality is downsized, hidden, changed or ignored. Thus we have seventy-year-old women sacrificing their bodies to the god of eternal youth, going under the scalpel time and time again to maintain an illusion of girlish beauty. Millions of dollars are spent each year on cosmetics and other beauty aids, workout machines, gym memberships, and every conceivable diet plan or pill to attain or maintain a facsimile of our cultural icons, Ken and Barbie.

For many years the chronically ill, disfigured and disabled were also shut away out of sight in their homes or in institutions. Only in recent years has this trend begun to reverse itself, evidenced in such things as mainstreaming in schools, the Americans with Disabilities

Act, and laws requiring access for wheelchairs in public places. But the chronically ill are still mostly an invisible subculture in our society.

Notwithstanding wheelchair access and other advancements, a person who deals with chronic fatigue or other chronic illnesses that may not require a wheelchair at all times is still hard pressed to find a chair to rest on in any store or other public place, such as the post office. I have asked clerks at more checkout counters than I care to remember to please find me a chair as I am unable to stand in line for more than a few minutes. Quite often they have been unable to find one for me, and I end up sitting on the floor or leaving.

We also have a long way to go toward acceptance of disfigurement. Terry Healey was a young man at the top of his game. He had everything going for him. He was a good looking, popular homecoming prince in high school, president of his fraternity at UC Berkeley, with a beautiful girlfriend, good grades and a promising future, when his life was turned upside down by a facial cancer that left him horribly disfigured. Looking in the mirror in the morning became too painful to bear, and the same girls who used to look at him with stars in their eyes, now pointed and stared or turned away in horror. People can be pretty cruel," Healey says.

> Their actions leave a mark on your psyche. Little by little you start thinking, 'I'm a freak,' and that just feeds on itself. You carry yourself differently. You cower. And then, people treat you differently because you act that way. (From *The North Bay Bohemian,* February 7-13, 2002. Copyright Metro Publishing Inc. maintained by Boulevards New Media)

However, it wasn't his horrendously scarred face that lost him his girlfriend—it was his loss of heart and attitude toward himself and his disfigurement, that turned her off.

> After I asked for the millionth time how she felt about my looks, she told me that my problem wasn't physical, it was mental. I was just too insecure, and she couldn't deal with it. So she broke up with me. It was devastating, but also eye-opening and liberating. I thought, 'This is great! It's not my looks that are the problem—it's me!' I mean, there was nothing I could do about my looks. But me—that's something I could work with.

That was the beginning of his transformative journey, shared in his book, *At Face Value* (2006). The disfigurement, he came to realize, was the agent of change that helped him become a wiser, more compassionate person.

Though we have seen how great loss, serious or chronic illness, and encountering the experience of death can and has changed the lives of many in a very positive way, not everyone has the "good fortune" of experiencing one of these masterful teachers before the end of life is actually upon him. "The good news," says Joseph Sharp, "is we all have a life-threatening condition if we open our hearts to life as it really is." (1996, p. 16)

When I was young and healthy, there was a dark shadow over my heart, a hard sheath that kept me from really connecting authentically with others or with myself. It also kept me from truly living my life fully and joyously. This, in my opinion, was more debilitating and "life threatening" than anything I have experienced as a result of illness or cancer. If we really allow ourselves to experience life as it is, we don't need chronic illness or disfigurement or the threat of imminent death to crack us open. There is plenty of pain in every life to accomplish this.

As an adolescent, I used to dream up make-believe scenarios where I and a wonderful, handsome, sensitive man would be marooned together on a desert island or some Anne-Frankian or 1984ish situation. I think that in my simple young mind I already sensed the disappointment and disillusionment that comes when the ardent idealism of youth or the flush of young love has passed. So I constructed a situation where that couldn't happen—a situation where life is precious because it is perilous, where it is lived on the edge fully in the present moment, and each moment is sweet because the future does not exist.

We are always in that perilous situation, but we don't know it. Life is so fragile and short. Illness, loss, or the threat of some fatal disease helps us remember, but the truth is, no one knows when their time will come. If we could live with that awareness in each moment, every breath would be a miracle.

We practice many things. We practice what we want to learn or what we think we need to learn. Some of the things we want to learn are things we love like music, dancing, golf, or tennis. Other things we practice because we think they make our lives easier, such as driving a car or learning computer skills. Sometimes we may practice things like swimming, shooting a gun for self-defense, fire drills, or another activity to help divert some disaster that may never happen.

What we don't practice is loss; what we don't practice is dying, though loss and death are the two things guaranteed to come to us. The gift of illness and death is "no one to be, nothing to do." The gift is in allowing us to stop the striving, stop the constant pressure to be someone.

My friend Joe was riding cross-country on his motorcycle in his twenties when he suffered some kind of mental breakdown. He watched himself descend slowly into a space where he could barely talk or move. He had no friends, no family, no employer nearby to help him or even notice what was happening to him. Luckily some kind and compassionate stranger did notice and offered him a place to stay and some home-cooked meals, as well as an easy kind of friendship that allowed for no, or little, conversation. "My life got so small," he said,

> I'd get up in the morning and try to think—"what do I have to do today?" Then I would remember—"Oh yea—brush your teeth." I remember a problem with staring. I'd go in the bathroom and get stuck there. I'd just stare at the mirror, not being able to remember what I was there for. I saw that I had no control. Whatever comes next, comes next. I have nothing to say about it.

The man allowed Joe to hang around his auto shop and tinker with the cars. Eventually he was employed there.

> I had to learn how to exist without planning. It was a long process, but when I stopped being afraid of being alone and not having anyone, when I finally was able to exist without planning anything and just be—when I was okay with that—that's when I started healing.

We can do this even now—even in the midst of our lives—if we realize the essential truth of emptiness and the irrefutable truth that our bodies will, at some unknown future time, die.

Practicing with Loss

You can take the occasion of near misses to imagine what it would be like if you had really lost your house, your job, a loved one or something dear to you: the plane your son didn't get on that crashed; the day your husband was so late coming home and couldn't reach you to tell you; the time your child almost died from appendicitis; the fire that started in the oven and you managed to put out with a kitchen fire extinguisher. It is not necessarily gruesome to imagine that these things you were afraid might have happened, actually did happen, and to allow yourself to experience the grief that naturally arises. It is important to make a distinction between practicing with loss, illness or death in this way and the morbid obsession some people have with these events, playing them out in their minds over and over again and paralyzing themselves with fear. This practice is not playing out or wallowing in a morbid fantasy—it is bowing to and honoring life as it is.

Loss and illness have all happened to someone and they could happen to anyone. They are a part of life. And when death comes, all these people and things *will* be lost. One of you will die—your beloved or you—eventually both. Your house, all your possessions will go. We think we cannot bear this, but we can. We can because we must.

When my daughter was depressed, she once envisioned a noose rope hanging from her chin-up bar and a bottle of pills in her hand. I must have pictured them a thousand times in my head. And what I saw was what a flimsy membrane my life and happiness rest on. Even though she assured me she would never take her own life, the truth that she experienced wanting to die—that her unconscious summoned up two ways of actually accomplishing this—and the fear I experienced before I got her reassurance, shook my being to such depths that I knew this was something I needed to allow myself to experience.

I saw that it was bigger than just me and her, bigger than the small universe of family and friends in which I lived. Parents lose their precious children to suicide every day. Simply knowing unequivocally that this exists in the world brought up immense grief for me. My own daughter's proximity to this truth helped me access my own experience of that, and with it the tender heart of Bodhicitta (compassion), as well as the realization of my connection with people everywhere who may actually be experiencing such a devastating sorrow.

And of course, notwithstanding my daughter's reassurances, I still needed to continue to work with my own fears, most of which were irrational. I questioned whether a severely depressed person could even *make* such a promise and surmised as well that things could change, i.e. get worse and she'd change her mind. My questioning and my thoughts seemed rational; my anxiety was not rational. It touched the place of my deepest, most out-of-control fear. The rationality or non-rationality, the reality or non-reality of the situation were both irrelevant in one sense. There was a door being presented to me. I needed to walk through that door, to sit in that room, to let myself mold to its shape, to rest in that abominable place.

Practicing with Illness and Death

Now we get down to the illness and death of our own bodies. Though it's easier for those who have actually had an illness or accident which has brought them closer to the real possibility of death to access the reality of their own dying, there are ways to practice with dying in everyday life without having to experience such a traumatic event. Even so, it is probably the rare person who has not been touched directly by death or tragedy in their circle of family and friends. So I think it is not our lack of access but rather our lack of willingness to enter this realm that keeps us distanced from the depth of experience that opening to our own death and dying, as well as to that of others, can provide.

One exercise I have found very useful is the practice of using our pains or small sicknesses to imagine that we are dying, or to imagine that the sickness or condition we are experiencing will not get better, but will stay the same or get worse. If you do this, if you "take the occasion" as Joseph Sharp suggests (1996, 38) you have a tool to help you to access the truth of the fact that you *will* die, and that you could in fact at any time become incapacitated through accident or illness.

I used to think there were certain times when I just couldn't do a spiritual practice, i.e., when I was too sick, too tired, when I overindulged myself, especially in eating too much (or did too much and made myself too exhausted), and that I would just have to wait until the condition passed. I realized at some point that just being with my illness, my tiredness, my miserable fullness, etc. was also a form of practice. And now that I have been practicing with dying, these practices take on a whole new aspect.

When I am sick or in pain or uncomfortable in any way, I can use these situations to practice dying—to practice my willingness to be with my discomfort in a different way—to practice with the reality of what is already happening. I *am* dying, we are all dying, this is simply true. Of course we are living too, but the dying part is the part we rarely acknowledge. The fact of our dying will never go away. It is *not* some imagined thing.

So we practice with it and get closer and closer until we are finally simply present, experiencing our living *and* our dying as they truly are, not morbidly, but joyfully, or perhaps at least with the deep appreciation for the opportunity to be here that often arises when we are fully present to life as it is. When we truly live with the experience of our dying, it is like the grandmother in the living room: our living and our dying, joyfully and compassionately intermingled—not some horrid idea of dying that we keep in the back room which we know in some subconscious area of our psyche will some day have to be faced.

The experience of your own dying or the real possibility of having a long-term chronic illness may be more accessible to you at these times of discomfort or illness than when you are well and strong. Say you have the flu and you feel so sick you actually need to stay in bed, or at least you feel like you can't get out of bed. Usually when we are sick, there is an unspoken belief system that props us up. Even if we are incredibly miserable, something in us believes or "knows" this experience is temporary and looks forward to the time we will be well again.

Just for a moment, see if you can suspend that belief and imagine that whatever condition you are experiencing—pain, discomfort, exhaustion—is permanent. Allow yourself to experience that. Feel the feeling—the pain, the nausea, the fear, the sadness. Let it sink into your bones. Imagine your life. What will you do? Who will cook? Who will clean? Who will pick up the children from school and take them to lessons? Who will pay the bills? Who will you BE if you can't do any of these things?

Then take it a step further and imagine that you are dying: that whatever sickness or discomfort you are experiencing is just one stage in that process. Give yourself over to whatever feelings arise, whether it be sadness or grief, or perhaps a sense of relief or freedom. It may surprise or frighten you if the latter (sense of relief or freedom) is what you feel if you truly give yourself to this process. Steven Levine used to have people at his workshops divide a piece of paper into two columns. On one side participants were instructed to list the reasons they wanted to stay alive; in the other column, the reasons they wanted to, or that it just might be okay to die. Again, here is an opportunity to open yourself to the possibility that death may not always be the worst possible thing, or that you may even have a hidden longing for death that perhaps wants to be explored. If you feel inclined, try these exercises.

Tibetan monks are given a practice of imagining or actually experiencing their own deaths. I tried this practice once when I thought I might be dying from cancer (or perhaps from toxicity of the poisons being pumped into me to kill the cancer). It wasn't a huge stretch. My body was so weak, it felt almost transparent—like I was already entering some other realm of existence. I was lying in my backyard on the grass beneath the mulberry tree and I imagined myself dying: my breath, my heart, slowing to stillness, blood pooling in my arteries.

I watched my body disintegrating—the cells dying, breaking down, the boundaries that separated me from the world around me weakening and blurring. And that which was alive in the earth crossing those boundaries to further the deconstruction. Ants, grubs, beetles, carrion came to feed on my dead body—to take the dead material into their living bodies. I felt myself slowly merging into the soil, into the air, into the creatures—becoming one with the earth I have so loved, feeding the tree that has so graciously watched over me.

I was amazed at the peace I felt during this meditation, the serenity I experienced as my body melted into the earth. I have also, of course, at other times, experienced abject horror at the prospect of losing my life and everything I know and love. I have experienced the terror of becoming nothing. Whatever comes up, whether it be peace, joy or terror, is what we open to. Joe said he got to the point during his breakdown and recovery when he didn't care if he died—he knew, he said, that if he did die, it would be okay—and that experience has transformed his life after his recovery. "It humbles you," he said, "My personality is so proud, it was good for me. I know that I can fall to the bottom of the world at any moment."

What you are trying to imagine is not something that may or may not happen. This is something that *will* inevitably come to pass. You will die. Though you may not have children depending on you, which I acknowledge is (and have experienced as) one of the worst scenarios, you undoubtedly have *someone* depending on you even if it is only yourself. Many people say they are not afraid to die. This is easy enough to say when you are alive and well. Not as easy when death is staring you in the face.

Another way to practice with loss or dying is to use an exercise given to hospice trainees to help them have some taste or glimmer of what their clients will be experiencing as they die. Get a stack of blank cards. On each card write the name of a loved one or a possession, identity or activity you can't imagine being without: your partner's and your children's names, those of your friends and other beloveds; the cherished identities of mother, father, friend, artist, gardener, provider, nurturer, etc.; activities and possessions that bring you great joy, such as singing, hiking, working, skiing etc., a treasured photo album or keepsake.

When you are done, turn the cards over so the blank side is up and choose one at random. Then imagine that you have lost whatever is represented by the word on the card—the person has died, the possession is irretrievably gone, you are no longer capable of doing the activity, or perhaps the card you have drawn is the identity of mother or father, which may also indicate your child has died or left—a double loss. Take your time and allow yourself to experience your life without that person, thing or activity. Feel deeply into it. Open your heart to the feeling of loss. Let yourself be with whatever arises. Stay with the feeling. Try not to go into thinking but simply stay with and follow the raw feelings as they open and change, going deeper and deeper as you allow yourself to experience the loss. One by one, draw the cards until they are all drawn. Sit with each loss until you feel complete with all the feelings that want to come to the surface. Then imagine who you would be without any of those things you have lost.

Life is filled with an abundance and a great variety of experiences and emotions, some of which we judge to be "good" and move toward, some of which we judge "bad" and want to avoid at all costs. Mostly, we want a "fix," we want "happily ever after," we want the ultimate experience that will make us happy and keep us happy—end of story. But do we really want "end of story?" End of story means death—at least in this human form, in this lifetime. Why are we in such a hurry to get to the end of the story? Not that death is a bad thing. Death is a natural part of living. And judging from my experience with facing the possibility of death through severe illness and cancer, I believe that the process of death and dying, if truly opened to, will be very rich and will open new doors of unimaginable beauty and depth of experience.

The point is that by wanting to freeze ourselves into one experience—"happy," "joyful," "peaceful," or whatever we have decided is the ultimate or desirable emotion or experience of life—we are basically denying our human-ness and killing our aliveness. And by pushing away the so-called negative emotions and experiences we paradoxically are shutting ourselves off from desired experiences as well.

Often it's when we think we're not afraid, that we are really the most afraid. Because we're so afraid, we push it away, we deny it. The paradox here is that it is the unacknowledged fear of death we carry, and are in denial of, that causes much of the suffering in the world, both in ourselves and in the terrible things we do to our fellow humans when we are acting out of that unrealized fear. Killing other human beings, whether in war for idealistic notions or murder out of anger or retribution, or ridiculing others for their appearance or disability, all have their roots in this ground of fear.

People are afraid of fear. They think it's a bad thing. But fear is just another emotion, like joy or sorrow. We all remember Franklin D. Roosevelt's quote, "The only thing we have to fear is fear itself," which I think is about right.

The truth is that death from the inside is not nearly as frightening as death from the outside. That is, when you're actually facing death and are able to truly open to it, it's not nearly as frightening as looking at it from the outside. In fact, there's a certain peace in the surrender because there's no longer any need for the desperate striving and struggling that we do in our lives. We've struggled and striven for so long, we have forgotten when it all started and what life was like before all that efforting began. When there's *really* nothing more we can do, we have to come to peace with our lives as they are right now.

But we can do this *before* there's *really* nothing more to do—before death is imminent. When we bring our awareness to life as it is, we see that death is always with us. When we are finally able to open to the reality of death—to experience it, to know it in our bones—we can perhaps begin again to simply BE as we were before all the efforting. We can begin to truly live, and in this living we may see a quality of loving kindness that wasn't there before—that has changed the way we experience ourselves and what we send out into the world.

CHAPTER 7

The Function of Emotions

Wisdom is the accumulation of all our experiences stored as emotion. When you cannot feel what is true, then you cannot utilize your wisdom.

—Erica Chopich and Margaret Paul

WHEN OUR CHILDREN WERE YOUNG, we had a book the kids loved named *Be Nice to Spiders*. It was about a zoo. This was a beautiful zoo. The mayor was coming for a visit, so the zookeeper admonished the grounds keepers to get the place cleaned up, and especially to be sure to clean up all those unsightly cobwebs. They scurried around with their brooms and their mops, swabbing and cleaning until the place was spotless. There was not a cobweb to be seen. The mayor was very impressed and gave the zookeeper a prize for having the cleanest zoo in the county.

After the mayor left, the zookeeper, wanting to keep his high status, made sure that the zoo was always kept shining and clean. But after a while there was a problem. All the animals were getting sick, and no one could figure out why, but there were flies everywhere making the animals miserable. One day one of the grounds keepers noticed one of the animals, an elephant I think, that was thriving. His pen was in an out-of-the-way place and had been missed by the cleaning crew. There were cobwebs everywhere, but there were no flies, and the elephant was very contentedly munching his hay. The grounds keeper went to the main zookeeper and told him about the elephant. He said, "It seems spiders are kind of useful, boss." After that they no longer cleaned up the cobwebs and the mayor gave the zookeeper an award for having the zoo with the healthiest animals.

A Bum Rap

In spiritual circles, emotions, specifically the negative ones, often get a bum rap. In Zen practice they may be seen as *makio* or illusion and ignored. They are sometimes looked upon as that which gets in the way of being in the present moment, experiencing joy, or seeing the truth. Christians may view them as sinful or self-indulgent, things which block our connection to God and keep us from being loving people, and are, thus, things to be struggled against. In therapy, negative emotions are sometimes analyzed, dissected, expressed, and talked about *ad nauseam,* all with the ultimate goal of getting rid of them.

While these outlooks and approaches have some truth in them, and perhaps some therapeutic value, they are only half-truths and the therapeutic value is limited. We cannot just drop our negative feelings or stop the actions that arise out of them, which are often harmful or hurtful to ourselves or to others. Even if we could, the result may be different from what we had hoped, and actually cause more harm than good. We find ourselves time and time again caught in the same web, the same patterns. We want to tidy up our lives—dust away those cobwebs—make our lives shining and clean like the zoo. But beware—the price may be more than we're willing to pay.

In December of 1982, my ex-husband and I, after a year of separation, decided to give our marriage another try. We were determined to make it work. I decided that nothing was more important than harmony in our relationship, and that all those "little things," that used to get me so upset, were simply not worth the heartache. Therefore, I would just "let them go." I also decided I would not let myself get involved in the tempestuous relationship between my husband and our oldest daughter, in which I had often in the past found myself enmeshed.

Several years later, I ended up on a psychologist's couch, being told to read a book on battered women. I was stunned. This was a category in which I would never, in a million years, have imagined myself. I protested her recommendation. I didn't see myself as some weak female incapable of standing up for herself. But when I looked closely at what I was experiencing, I realized it *was* battering. Only *I* was the one—really—who was doing the battering. It was a psychological stance, a state induced by my own decision. Instead of fighting for what I thought was right, which is what I had done for the first ten years of our marriage, I had pushed it all underground; in psychological language, I had suppressed it.

On the surface, things seemed more harmonious, more shiny and clean, but underneath, there was trouble. This wasn't about my husband—it was about me. My husband hadn't suddenly changed into a wife batterer. I was the one who had changed—I had deserted myself for the sake of peace. But peace didn't come. Instead, the end result was a woman on the verge of a mental breakdown. I had painted myself into a corner and I couldn't move in any direction.

Usually these dysfunctional states are brought about by decisions made in early childhood or when we were mere babes. Thus the origins are lost and we come to believe our pain or dysfunction is caused by others, when they do something that momentarily touches on the place of the pain that precipitated our original decision, or perhaps that we are irretrievably flawed. Because this one was brought on by a conscious decision I had made in the not too distant past, I was able to see how it was self-induced—how I had created it.

Though I had surely suppressed feelings all my life, I had never gone to this extreme. It allowed me to see clearly the danger inherent in this activity—how a disconnect from feelings can lead to mental illness. It was quite frightening to be gazing into the abyss of craziness. Luckily, I had caught myself in time, and was able to reverse the effects shortly, chalk the whole thing up to a failed experiment, and go back to my normal old neuroticisms and marital disharmony—a much healthier state of affairs.

I was also able to acknowledge that my approach to life and self, though definitely dysfunctional, was healthier than I had previously thought. In going back to fighting for my truth, I'm not saying that my perceived truths *were* true and it was my job to make things right—though it might have been. The point here is that we cannot change from the outside. We cannot change by imposing moral dictates or rules upon ourselves. I still believed, however, that more harmony in relationships and more peace within my own soul was possible. So there had to be another way. I continued, in the years that followed, to search for that way to peace.

I realized along the way that I had to first make peace with myself. The process of figuring out how to do that spanned many years. I finally admitted defeat in making my marriage work, stopped blaming my husband, and took responsibility for the fact that I just didn't want to try any more. I knew I had a lot of work to do on myself, and had always felt I "should" be able to do it in the marriage.

Accepting the fact that I couldn't, or didn't want to, was a big step for me. Yet, I still wanted healing in this relationship from which I seemed to be fleeing, as well as with others in my life. Though I acknowledged that I couldn't do it then and there within the marriage, I held out a dim hope that somehow with some distance and the work I hoped to be doing on myself, there could be some kind of healing over time between my ex-husband and me.

As it turned out, we, having both done a lot of inner work and maturing, have become very good friends. Many of the issues which were way too hot to handle during our marriage are now being brought out one by one, talked about and worked through in a way that I thought would never be possible with us. We have also been able to acknowledge that we are much better suited for friendship than for marriage.

A New Paradigm of Healing

As I began to be more responsible for my feelings and grope toward a new paradigm of inner healing, I was discouraged by the fact that, though I had been a meditator for twenty years, I still experienced fear, embarrassment, annoyance, judgment, feelings of being unlovable, unworthy, boring or incompetent, and many other unpleasant emotions on a regular basis. Somehow, I had expected this to change as a result of spiritual practice. Not expressing my negative emotions didn't work either, as I learned from my foray into craziness. Yet negative emotions seemed as ubiquitous as grass. And from what I could see, others around me, even the supposedly "spiritual" people, were having no better luck than I was in dealing with them. So what are we to do with these constant companions, these cobwebs of the soul, and what exactly is a negative emotion anyway?

The term, "negative emotion" is, in a sense, an oxymoron. Emotions are simply feelings, a combination of thoughts and bodily sensations. They are simply the body and the mind doing what they do. But we have opinions about these emotions—we judge them to be "positive" or "negative," based on deeply held beliefs. In one sense, all emotions are good. Just as symptoms of physical illness, such as fever, aches and pains, or weakness, are not bad in themselves, though they may feel bad, so the "negative" emotions are often an attempt to make right something in the life of the soul which has gone askew.

Some people take aspirin or ibuprofen to get rid of a fever, but many wise doctors counsel patients not to try to bring a fever down too far. A fever is not some nuisance or punishment that is visited upon us as penance for some misdeed. It is one of the body's important defenses against attack from foreign invaders such as viruses and bacteria. The elevated body temperature provides a hostile environment in which these life forms cannot exist, thus protecting us from harm. Negative emotions are not some evolutionary dead-end to be dispensed with, but a symptom of a deep malaise that our being is attempting to deal with to the best of its ability, and like the symptoms of physical illness, are not just symptoms, but an integral part of the cure.

The Ecology of the Soul

Just like everything else on this planet, emotions have a very important function. In the ecology of the soul, emotions are the compass, the map, and the vehicle by which we can travel, all rolled up into one. They give us direction in our lives. They point the way in which we must go, and enliven our will to go there. Without the energy of our emotions to drive us, we would be little more than automatons. In their book, *Healing Your Aloneness*, Erica Chopich and Margaret Paul speak about emotions,

> Our society has long diminished the importance of feelings, worshipping logic while downgrading the wisdom that comes from feelings, touting the left brain while ignoring the right. This has created a terrible imbalance—the power of logic without the power of wisdom.

Wisdom is the accumulation of all our experiences stored as emotion. When you cannot feel what is true, then you cannot utilize your wisdom. (10–11)

The so-called "negative emotions" are distortions of this basic wisdom. Like a beam of light shining through water is bent, so our basic human wisdom is distorted as it tries to make its way through all the armoring we have constructed around our hearts—the seat of wisdom—to protect ourselves from pain. Though it is distorted, it is still wisdom, and if we begin to open to it, it can still teach us, and take us back to the source. With a child's intuition, Jane, even at age nine, had a sense of this wisdom underlying her own fear. She used to have panic attacks when she felt she was being pulled from her body by some other-worldly force. One day she said to her aunt,

> "I have this feeling that if I wouldn't slap myself to get myself back and just let myself go all the way, I'd go some place amazing." So I always felt it was my fear that was in my way and that my fear was always bringing me back.

Pema Chödrön talks about "poison as medicine." Describing the Tibetan Buddhist practice of *lojong,* she says,

> ... when these poisons arise, the instruction is to drop the story line, which means—instead of acting out or repressing—use the situation as an opportunity to feel your heart, to feel the wound. Use it as an opportunity to touch that soft spot. Underneath all that craving or aversion or jealousy or feeling wretched about yourself, underneath all that hopelessness and despair and depression, there's something extremely soft... (1994, 32)

All the stories we tell ourselves about what we're feeling and why and how and who is to blame, etc., etc., keep us from experiencing that softness.

We Are Programmed for Joy

The human psyche longs to be happy. Like a plant growing in a dark spot will lean toward the light, we humans have something in us that is programmed for joy, and we will strive for it with all the strength of our being. Sometimes this longing and this striving comes out all wrong because of false beliefs we have about ourselves or about what will really make us happy.

On a very basic human level, our negative emotions are often a mistaken attempt to take care of ourselves, to make ourselves happy. How often I have heard people say, "The only way they will listen to me is if I get angry." Parents may feel that way about their kids, bosses about their employees, or teachers about their pupils—even mates about their partners. Tears are often unconsciously used in the same way—to "make them listen." Criticism may be used to cover low self-esteem. Our unconscious rationale is, "If she looks bad, maybe I will look good." Controlling behavior covers over the total helplessness and loss of control we feel when life assaults us on all sides. These strategies are actually cries for attention or help—they say loud and clear, "Please pay attention to me," "Please help me," or "Please don't hurt me." On a deeper level, what they are saying is, "Please love me."

Looked at in this way, perhaps we can begin to have some compassion for ourselves and others, who, in our clumsy ways, are only striving to be happy, to get love, or to protect ourselves from some real or imagined danger. The problem is, trying to bring happiness to ourselves with these strategies does not work. Harville Hendricks in his book, *Getting the Love You Want* (2007), points out that the psyche does not actually distinguish between outer and inner. So when we direct anger or hatred out into the world—onto another person, as in our relationships, or onto a group of people, as in our prejudices—the psyche experiences it as being directed toward our own selves and our own heart reaps the same bitter harvest. Consequently, we suffer. When we see this clearly, our mistaken belief that we can find happiness by attacking others or putting people down will begin to fall away.

Conversely, we cannot extend love to others while hating and doing violence to ourselves. We think our emotions are telling us truths about things and people in our lives, but usually they are pointing instead to the unhealed territory in our own hearts. We think the compass points out, but we have it backwards. The direction is not out, but in. When we finally attend to the suppressed emotions that are calling out to be healed, when we finally allow ourselves to experience our long-held pain, we find that our emotions can then begin to be a true compass in the external world as well. Without the baggage we have carried around most of our lives that befuddles the mind and clutters up the pathway to our hearts, we can begin to truly see and feel what is happening around us, and thus to relate to the world and the people in our lives with more integrity and compassion.

In addition to being our compass, emotions are the interface between the external world and our inner or soul world. They help us process, chew up, digest, and integrate our experiences. We cannot short-circuit emotions with impunity. An experience that has entered our psyche is like food that we have eaten. Once it has entered our system, it must be dealt with, digested, or processed in some way. Sometimes, in our lives, experiences have been so intense or traumatic, and the resultant emotions so overwhelming, that, in order to cope, we have put them aside or erected barriers or false personalities to keep from feeling them. But these experiences have nowhere to go. They sit there, like the leftovers in the back of our fridge, or undigested food in the stomach, until we are ready to do something about them. In the meantime, they can stink up our lives.

Brother Donkey

In the infinite wisdom of the body, these experiences are held for us; they are preserved lovingly and kept safe in the cells of our backs, shoulders, necks, guts, and the deep recesses of our brains until we are ready to finally take them in. Jalaja Bonheim, in *Aphrodite's Daughter,* says:

> Saint Francis called the body "Brother Donkey" for the way it patiently carries the overload of our psychic baggage, our unprocessed pain, and our unfelt emotions. Incorruptibly truthful and innocent, the body is a great spiritual teacher and a powerful catalyst for transformation. (1997, 293)

Like a tumor in the body, this excess baggage we carry with us throughout our lives keeps poking us, prodding us, crowding us, and, generally, making our lives very uncomfortable. It turns up in the most unwelcome places and at the most inopportune times. Manifesting as anger, resentment, neediness, fear, anxiety, greed, or even sometimes as physical illness, it makes our lives miserable until we finally pay attention.

Emotions provide the lifeline that connects us with that original event and our reaction to it, which took us off the path in the first place and is the real block to our happiness. This was the point at which we split ourselves into two or more parts to avoid experiencing something that seemed just too painful or frightening to bear. In order to be whole we must experience everything that comes to us. We cannot pick and choose our curriculum.

All that is needed is simply that we accept and be willing to reside in whatever life presents to us. We must say yes, be willing to take the cup and drink as Christ did at Gesthemane. Because we are imperfect beings we cannot always do this. Sometimes we say no. If not for the body holding our experiences, keeping them for us until we are ready, we would be shut out of the kingdom, blocked from wholeness for eternity. When a negative emotion arises, it is our opportunity to access that place that needs healing. So, as bad as it may seem when our demons come knocking, we should thank our lucky stars that we still have the opportunity to do this work.

CHAPTER 8

Working with Negative Emotions

It's hard to imagine that one would spend one's whole life protecting against something that could easily be done—that is, experiencing our feelings—simply by having the intention to do it.

SUPPOSE WE ACCEPT THE PREMISE that negative emotions, like spiders, are kind of useful. That still leaves the question: how do we work with these things, useful as they may be, that just don't feel good, that lurk in the shadows and scare us, that wreak havoc in our lives, that we would rather ignore?

In the beginning, it is helpful to simply become more aware of what our situation actually is—what we actually do, think and feel—in other words, to know ourselves. Although not absolutely necessary, I believe instituting a meditation and mindfulness practice in your life is extremely helpful in the process of working with negative emotions. I would suggest looking for a Vipassana teacher to help with this beginning step of developing a meditation practice.

In our everyday lives, we get so caught up in our attachments to things, people wealth, power, sickness or hardship etc. that we cannot see the forest for the trees. Meditation helps us to pull back just a bit, to begin to access a deeper part of ourselves, and to develop the witness, which is so essential to our ability to study ourselves. I look at this kind of practice as the container in which the more specific process of working with negative emotions can be held and nurtured.

Over the years, within this container of daily practice, three important steps have emerged from my own work with emotions that I have found to be consistent and indispensable aids in this process:

1. Developing a loving kindness practice
2. Experiencing
3. Exposing and working with false beliefs

These steps can be done in any order. In fact, any one of the steps can be complete in itself and can actually lead to more freedom and a more satisfying and fulfilled life. Starting with loving kindness, however, can help to soften the ground for the sometimes harsh, and often frightening, second step of experiencing. For most people, I believe it to be a necessary step which opens the door to a possibility that was not there before. We humans spend our lives frantically reinforcing the walls we have constructed around our hearts, that keep us from experiencing what we are feeling and thus, also from freedom, and from love. It's hard to imagine that one would spend one's whole life protecting against something that could easily be done—that is, experiencing our feelings—simply by having the intention to do it.

The depth of fear or anxiety which often arises when one begins to open to long-suppressed emotions is hard to fathom, and harder yet to face. This is hard work. By instituting a daily loving kindness practice, the frightened inner self or child can begin to experience the unconditional love that allows us to open to the painful inner holdings that have constricted us for so many years. I have done the loving kindness meditation daily for years. It has been an indispensable aid and support for me in dealing with the very difficult path I've had to walk with my illnesses as well as with the psychological baggage I carried with me from childhood.

The second step, that of experiencing, is actually the essential one. It is the alchemist's pot, in which the transformational cooking occurs. This is the process of actually being with and "experiencing" our emotions in a very intimate way.

The third step, exposing and working with false beliefs, deals with the domain of the inner adult in relation to the inner child and can help us understand why it is so important to do the step of experiencing. This step leads us to a clearer understanding of how we are keeping ourselves stuck by continuing to subscribe to mistaken beliefs that we have taken on throughout our lives, beginning perhaps as early as the gestation period when we still lived in our mothers' wombs.

Step one and step three may help supply the *segue* and support the possibility of experiencing, or actually lead to an epiphany that includes it. Conversely, as we develop our ability to experience our emotions, loving kindness as well as the understanding and/or the transformation of false beliefs about ourselves and about life will flow out of that experiencing as a natural consequence.

As we come to understand that emotions, and specifically negative emotions, are not an impediment in our spiritual journey, but can be our guides and helpers, we can begin to open to and work with these almost universally despised pariahs in a new and more constructive way.

CHAPTER 9

Loving Kindness

The way of love is not a subtle argument.
The door there is devastation.
Birds make great sky-circles of their freedom.
How do they learn it?
They fall, and falling, they're given wings.

—Rumi

THIS BEING HUMAN IS A HARD PATH. It is hard to face the crushing losses that each human being must inevitably face at some point in his or her life. And if we have an aspiration to wake up, to actually know the truth, the full truth, Big Truth, it is even harder to face and open to the totality of one's own self. All those petty, selfish, fearful selves, our brokenness, the deep flaws we see in ourselves which may seem, at times, irredeemable—all those parts of ourselves that we have hidden in the shadows and refused to look at for most of our lives—loom larger than ever when illness or loss threatens to dismantle our life, our psyche, and, it seems, our very souls as we have known them up to that point. This is a hero's journey. To see and to open to all of this pain requires incredible courage, the kind of courage that we just may not think we have. This kind of journey cannot be undertaken without the support of the gentle arms of love.

What do we really want? Go deep and ask yourself this question. For me, I know the answer is love. I want love. I want to be held and cared for like a precious being in the arms of love. There is also desire for safety, and yet the desire for love supercedes that. I see in my own life how the risks I have taken at times totally disregarded my own safety in order to have even the possibility of love. Love is the prize—the deepest yearning of our souls.

A friend of mine who gives me a ride to doctors' appointments in a nearby city has coexisted with cancer and thus the threat of imminent death for upward of six years. She has active tumors growing in the site of her mastectomy which several times have been removed but always grow back. She also deals with a lifelong disease that has required many operations and makes her life very difficult. One day when I got into the car and asked her how she was doing she said, "I knew you would ask me that and I've been thinking for days how I would respond (pause). I am in the midst of the most difficult and tumultuous period I have ever experienced."

I was shocked but braced myself for the bad news. I figured the cancer must have spread. But she went on to tell me that her lover of fifteen years was leaving her and how this was the hardest thing she had ever faced. I immediately understood because of my own experiences with facing death and loss of love—how I had realized that the loss of love was worse than the thought that I could die. I marveled again at this human condition. We value love, it seems, above life itself—because what is life without love?

Illness or loss can be an asset in this journey of the soul. Illness brings me to stillness, because I cannot move. Illness brings me to silence, because I cannot talk. Illness brings me to simplicity, because I have so little energy. And illness brings me finally to love, because love is what remains when everything external has been stripped away.

The Alpha and the Omega

Love is the Alpha and the Omega—the beginning and the end. We must start there and we will end there. We must start there, though it is impossible to start there. We will end there when our long circuitous journey is over and realize that we had love all along. But the journey is long and may lead us first through perilous territories of bitterness, disillusionment, fear and self-hatred.

Violence is rampant in our world today. It is the topic on everyone's lips and in every headline. It is difficult to find a movie that does not pander to the seemingly endless public appetite for it. The violence we see in society is a reflection of the violence we visit upon ourselves and each other both emotionally and physically on a very personal level. We feed ourselves food that cannot sustain life, read books and watch movies that help to perpetuate the cycle of violence by feeding our minds and hearts the equivalent of junk food, put ourselves in the company of people who abuse us, and drive our bodies relentlessly until they are about to break. When they do, we berate ourselves endlessly for driving ourselves into illness and continue on to blame ourselves for not being able to heal. It is time to stop this cycle of violence. If there were one thing I had to choose as the most important first step in spiritual healing as well as in healing the world, I believe it would be to develop an attitude of loving kindness toward ourselves.

There's a lot of emphasis in our world on being a kind person. We look up to and admire those who give themselves in service to others. Likewise, we don't like people we consider to be very critical, unkind or mean. We usually think of them as selfish, as thinking more of themselves than they do of others. Yet while it may be true that these "unkind" people are most certainly thinking about themselves a considerable amount of the time, it does not follow, as we might suppose, that they think highly of themselves, or that they like who they are. These are the people who often secretly think of themselves as the worst of the worst. The violence they do to others is often a pittance compared to what they inflict upon themselves. But the "selfish" have no monopoly on self-inflicted violence. This is an open shop, an equal opportunity employer. We all have a critic who stands on our shoulder spouting some version of unworthiness.

The Shadow

Most of us go through our lives with a picture of who we think we are. We have a picture that we present to the world, and often to ourselves as well. But there is another picture that we keep hidden, one that contains the attributes, actions and emotions that we find unacceptable or "bad." This picture we push underground, label "not me," or distance ourselves from in some way. Secretly, though, we may fear, or actually believe, that this picture is who we really are, that if people really knew us, they would see that we are fake or flawed or unlovable.

This aspect of ourselves is called the "shadow." Sometimes the shadow is pushed so far underground that we don't even know it is there. This rejection of parts of ourselves has a huge price. We have become fragmented. We are not whole, and because we are a microcosm of the universe, we cannot then accept the parts of others that we have rejected in ourselves. Thus we feel isolated and cut off from others and from life.

The things we don't like in others are the disowned aspects of ourselves. When we were babies, we had no clear boundaries separating ourselves from others. We saw ourselves reflected in the eyes of our caregivers. When they were displeased or angry, we saw ourselves as defective. Our fear that they would leave us was the fear of dying, which was the same as being non-existent, because our existence depended on them. We split off from the behavior that was displeasing to them—made it "not me." The problem with this approach is the old "throwing the baby out with the bath water" difficulty. As Pema Chödrön says,

> Our wisdom is all mixed up with what we call our neurosis. Our brilliance, our juiciness, is all mixed up with our craziness and our confusion and therefore it doesn't do any good to try to get rid of our so-called negative aspects, because in that process we also get rid of our basic wonderfulness. (1991, 6–7)

We enter adulthood as disembodied beings, walking around wondering where our zing went, wondering what is wrong with us, wondering why we feel so disconnected, wondering why we can't feel love for those around us. Having never reclaimed our lost selves, we are only half-alive. Seeing this can be useful to our spiritual development or it can become just another excuse for bashing ourselves and perpetuating our negative core beliefs about ourselves. We may ask ourselves, "How could I be so stupid, so inept, so fearful as to damage myself, and to carry the wound with me through my whole adult life?" And we conclude, "I must be inherently flawed."

The truth of the matter, however, is that at the time of making such decisions, the child was acting in its own best interests, and in the only possible way it saw of protecting itself under the circumstances. These decisions arose out of our inner nature, which is always loving and kind, always acting out of love to take care of us and protect us, and thus were, at the time, sound decisions. Our existence did depend on those adults caring for us and our only power lay in our ability to modify ourselves to be more acceptable to them or in some cases to be so annoying that they would have to notice us and perhaps do something to make us stop crying. So, in adulthood, because we have forgotten who we really are (Light and Love), we perpetuate the patterns and the strategies that served us as children, even though they no longer apply. Even though we're no longer dependent on another for survival, we act as if we are.

Being chronically ill, in pain, or experiencing great loss exacerbates our false beliefs about ourselves. If we have felt worthless, we feel more worthless. If we have felt incompetent, we feel more incompetent. If we felt helpless before, now we really feel helpless, or actually are. If we consider ourselves unlovable, our illness or pain, and the loneliness we experience as a result of it, verifies that unlovableness in our minds.

In a sense, especially if we are ill, we have become like little children again. Many of the attributes of the child are there. We are weak. We need to depend on others for help. We have no power, or at least we feel that we have none. We may even feel that we deserve what we have gotten, because we are bad, wrong, or selfish. "I remember one time," my friend Jane said,

> [My mom] was doing yard work and—oh, I just remember looking through the window at her and just sobbing in my room, angry that—doesn't she know?—I'm nothing without her, and then also just feeling horrible that I feel this way and horrible that I'm in my twenties and really like an infant, totally dependent on my mom. So that would come out in bitterness sometimes and sometimes she'd had enough; she had to get away, you know. So it was just such a mix of appreciation, guilt and resentment all at the same time.

This Is No Accident and No Dirty Trick

Our illness or loss dredges up all the unhealed pain in our lives and drops it squarely onto our plate. As I mentioned in the first chapter, this puts us precisely in the right position to begin our work of true healing—that is, healing on a being level, which may or may not include the healing of the physical body.

We may think the gods have played some nasty trick on us, bringing all of our woundedness out of cold storage just when it seems we are least able to deal with it—when our energy is at its lowest ebb, and our world is crumbling around us. But this is no accident and no dirty trick. It is precisely *because* we have so little energy that these wounds are able to rise to the surface. To suppress feelings requires huge amounts of energy. So the grace of illness and loss is that we are less able to suppress, and therefore more able to access, that which has hitherto been inaccessible. To heal, we must first open to the pain we are experiencing in the present. If we really do that, we will be opening ourselves up to deeper pain, the grief of a lifetime, which began the first time we saw reflected in our caregivers' eyes that somehow we weren't enough.

In order to open to that pain, it is helpful to first lay the groundwork of loving kindness. When we think of a loving kindness practice, we naturally think of trying to be kind to others. We have all been taught it is unseemly to love ourselves. We have been taught to put others before ourselves, and the needs of others before our own. But this is backwards. We cannot be kind to others until we can be kind to ourselves.

Trying to be kind and loving to others first is not a bad practice. It just doesn't work. It can be very useful, however, in showing us where we're stuck. Either we will end up not really being kind, or we will do something that appears to be kind, but inside will be telling ourselves how that was really a selfish act or we're just trying to make ourselves look good. For a long time, I tried to be a kind person with mixed success. Sometimes I would actually do something that appeared to be kind, but usually it rang false for me in some essential but still unfathomable way.

Most of us carry a belief deep inside that we are unlovable or unloving, which to the psyche is one and the same. This belief has been with us for so long that we often don't even realize it is there. It just seems like the natural order of things, the way things are, the way *we* are. When we first formed that belief, the rejection and aloneness we felt must have been immense, which is why we walled it off. That place of desolation feels too big, too bleak, too hopeless, too joyless, too fearsome to bear. The only way it can be borne is within the context of love. We will not be able to heal ourselves until we can attend to our own healing in the way a mother attends to her child. And we can never attend to our healing in this way unless we're moved to do so by love—because love is the only force strong enough to enable us to do what we need to do, to make the necessary sacrifices.

The "Catch–22" of Spiritual Practice

Sometimes when I get into a very narrow spot, I become lost in it. The world closes down on me or everything seems to be spinning so fast and out of control, I just want to get off. I recognize that I'm not centered, not in my heart, not residing in love, but seem to be helpless to do anything about it. What is happening here? A lot, but what it boils down to is this: I'm not in my heart, and because I'm not in my heart, I'm incredibly judgmental toward myself. This is the crux of the problem. It is the "Catch-22" of spiritual practice. You cannot enter that place of love without love. And because we have walled off our hearts to keep from feeling the pain, we have walled off love as well.

The alchemists said, "You must have gold to make gold." And the Bible tells us, "For whoever has, to him more shall be given, and he will have an abundance; but whoever does not have, even what he has shall be taken away from him" (Matthew 13:12). This is the abyss that all persons who embark upon a spiritual quest will eventually encounter—the impassable divide between the blocked, closed down human heart and the Divine. Is there then any hope?

When I first read Jerry Jampolsky's book, *Love Is Letting Go of Fear*, in the '80s, I was very excited, and at the same time I was very sad. He said that, if we make love our only goal, we will be happy. The concept was tantalizing and inspiring, yet I knew in my heart that this kind of happiness was not for me. I saw how far I was from having love as my only goal. Not only did the distance seem far, but there was someone in me who saw myself as incapable of ever doing that. The gulf between me and God seemed an impassable abyss. I was just too flawed. This was something for saints and gurus, and for people with basic goodness and kindness and depth—not me.

Yet there was something in this simple exhortation that was so appealing, and the freedom of it was so tantalizing, that a tiny part of me held it out as a distant hope. Lama Kunga (who was not a Lama at the time but my teacher in another tradition) once said to me, "Man can do nothing, but if we try, something may happen." And so a seed had been planted. By surrendering to the moment, making a start, and putting one foot in front of the other, things began to open up for me.

A Saving Nightmare

A few years later I had a dream—really a nightmare, but a saving nightmare. I was driving a car following another car. There was something sinister about this situation. I suspected that someone in the car in front of me was up to no good. Then a bundle or package fell out of the back of the car, or maybe somebody threw it out. It was too close and I ran over it. Then I realized with horror that it was a baby and that baby was me. I saw with startling clarity how I was deserting myself over and over again—and not only deserting myself, but doing actual violence to myself, all under the guise of being a "good and kind" and even a "spiritual" person. That was part of a series of events and realizations leading me in a whole new direction in my spiritual journey.

Fast-forward seven or eight more years: I was visiting my family in my hometown. I sat with my sister at a wake for a distant relative as she told me that she and my two brothers and all their spouses were going out for dinner and dancing later that evening. It dawned on me that she was saying without saying it that mom and I were not invited. I had overheard them talking about the evening earlier and assumed we would all be going, yet it seemed odd that no one had actually said anything directly to us about it.

She made some excuse about me being tired and was a little more direct about not wanting mom with them because it would spoil their fun. But I knew they didn't want me either for similar reasons. They wanted a carefree evening of dining and dancing. They didn't want to be saddled with an oldie and a sickie, both without mates. I could tell that my sister was uncomfortable. I think she knew inside that what she was doing was an unkind thing.

For a few brief moments I was stunned and devastated, but the work I had done opening my heart over the previous ten years had changed me dramatically. The knife I felt twisting in my heart could have become a wound that festered for years forming a wall of scar tissue between me and my siblings. Yet I knew that the main person who would be hurting during all that time would be me. My heart didn't want that pain. My heart wanted love. I realized with a shock that at that moment my only goal was love. I hugged my sister and told her to have a good time. And I meant it.

Having an Intention Is the First Step

How can we learn to love ourselves? This is a difficult question, for, like letting go of fear, we cannot simply do it by willing it. Having an intention is the first step. Intention is a very powerful force. The second step is seeing: setting the witness the task of observing what we do to ourselves over and over again; observing our strengths and our joy as well as our weaknesses; observing our intentions. We may have an intention to have love as our only goal one minute, and the next all we want is to get even with our husband, sister or co-worker for hurting us. And so we learn that not only can we not will ourselves to love, we cannot even, it seems, have an intention to love. Intention can never be pure in the beginning. We must *ask* for pure intention. Julian of Norwich said, "All shall be well, and all manner of thing shall be well with the purification of the intention in the ground of our beseeching."

It is the function of the witness to watch, not to try to change anything, but simply to notice without judgment what we do, what we think and say, under all the circumstances of our lives. If we have been diligent in our observations, we will see that not only do we have lots of inappropriate judgments and do many unkind things, but we also have moments of real kindness and generosity. If we make a map of ourselves, we will know the terrain with which we are dealing. We will see that we are not the mean ogre we at times think ourselves to be—and neither are we the kind, gentle, loving person we hold up at other times to the world (and to ourselves) as who we are.

And when we fall into the same hole or swampy territory for the umpteenth time, we can say with Stephen Levine (and hopefully with the same loving kindness one would have for a child who fell and scraped his or her knee), "Big surprise." We might set one day aside each week to concentrate solely on observing the judgments we make on ourselves and others throughout the day—not just the big judgments, but even the tiny ones, like when we call ourselves stupid for forgetting where we put the keys. But noticing can lead to bashing, and so we are led back to the need for love. How do we hold this witnessing, this new and painful awareness of what we really do in our lives, with tenderness and mercy?

One must first examine one's notion of what love is, and most likely get rid of it. Love is probably one of the most misunderstood words in the English language. Most of what passes for love in our society is simply self-serving tit for tat. You do this for me, and I'll do that for you. Or sometimes, I'll do this for you, and you love me. Mostly when we do things out of what we think is love, we're actually trying to get something, to fulfill some need that we think we have, perhaps for security, to make ourselves feel important, to feel needed, to get what we want, or to fill up that hole in the center of our existence. We rarely do things out of real love. Try the acid test some time: do something kind for someone close to you. Really put yourself out, but do it in such a way that the person will never know it was you who did it. When you see how hard this is, you will realize how self-serving most of our actions are.

Somewhere in Us We Know Love

Yet even in the most wretched soul, there is some shred of real love. If you have children, you can usually find it there, though even with our children, much of the love we offer is self-serving. However, we can find moments when we amaze ourselves with true selfless love for these beings who have been entrusted to our care. And this, the love of a parent for their child, is perhaps the best model of love that we have.

When my first child was born, she got jaundiced after the first day and had to go back into the hospital. I couldn't stay in the nursery with my baby, so I came every three hours to nurse her. Once I came in and found that the headband that had been put around her head to protect her eyes from the fluorescent lights that were treating her jaundice had been put on so tightly it caused a bruise around her tender little head. I had no doubt that the woman watching over my baby was a good person, but I realized that my child was a job to her.

Even if she was very conscientious and tried to do the very best job she could possibly do, she would never be a mother to my child nor do the things a mother would do. That would not be possible, because a mother would sit up day and night and watch her sick child. She would attend to every detail with the love that only a mother can have—would give her own life for her child if that were necessary to save her. There is a Zen story about a mother whose son was a robber and a murderer. He cut off his mother's head and was carrying it down a rocky road. The mother called out to him, "Son, please be careful not to trip and hurt yourself." So this is the kind of devotion we must ultimately have for healing our own inner child.

If you have never had children, perhaps you had a dog or friend that opened that place of unconditional love for you, if only for a moment. And of course most of us are children of someone who had moments of real love for us, and in those moments, we felt and knew love. Finally, there is the Love we came out of—the Primordial Love—God, evoked by the Buddhist koan, "Show me your parent's face before you were born." Somewhere in us then, though it may be hidden, we know love. So, like the drummer boy, we offer whatever we have to the tiny frightened soul in us struggling to be. Meister Eckhart, the Christian mystic, said we must sail across the sea (the abyss) on a ship of love. But, if we only have half a sail, he urges us not to despair and to set out with what we have.

If you still believe you have no real love in you at all, try to set aside, at least for the moment, the notion that this is the eternal and immutable truth about you. The facilitator of a chronic illness support group I attended for many years used to say, "What if..." followed by some statement of belief that was different from the one we were discussing about ourselves, or had a different slant or interpretation. In this case it might be skillful to ask yourself, "What if this notion, this idea I have that there is no real love in me, is just a deeply held belief, and is not necessarily the deepest truth about me?" Or "What if I'm simply refusing to acknowledge the truth of love that lies within me?" Or "What if there is love in me, but I just can't feel it, because there are things blocking it?" "What if the true essence of my own being is love?" One or more of these questions may be palatable to you, and may allow you to imagine for a moment that what has been proposed in them might possibly have some truth in it, or at least open the door a crack to that possibility.

The Truth Is, We Are Love

The truth is that we *are* Love, and the deepest urging of our soul is to reconnect with that Love. When we have invited those long banished parts of ourselves back into our hearts and are whole again, when we can look with a smile of mercy on the beaten-down child in us who lashes out at others under the mistaken assumption that by putting others down, we will be made bigger, when we can extend a warm embrace of kindness to that most crushed and devastated part of ourselves that thinks itself unlovable and thus distances itself from those who would love us, then loving kindness will flow naturally to others, for we will see in them the same sad efforts to boost themselves up that we have made in our vain effort to cover up the hole in the center of our being.

I have learned from experience that as I began to acknowledge, open to, accept, and even love (not as something to be desired, but as something deserving of compassion) these undesirable parts of myself, I began to be more accepting and loving of others as well.

If you have tried all these things and still feel you are the one hopeless case, you are not alone. One night in my meditation group we were talking about core beliefs. One man spent ten minutes describing all the negative qualities about himself. Actually he wasn't describing real negative qualities about himself; he was describing himself as he saw himself. Our teacher said something about these being false beliefs, and that his true nature was love. The man asked, "Why isn't it true that I am what I think I am?"

I Met Myself Face to Face and Didn't Like What I Saw

I remembered asking myself that question thirty years ago. I had come to a crisis on an acid trip. I met myself face-to-face and didn't like what I saw. In fact it was so frightening I couldn't face it at all. The man guiding me in my trip said, " Suppose this really is the truth about you? What could be so terrible about the truth?" It stopped me in my tracks. It was show-down time, the moment of reckoning. I had spent my life trying to avoid seeing that I might possibly actually be the person I feared I was. This put me in a terrible bind, because I also saw myself as a person seeking truth. And the deepest part of me wanted the truth. But this fear—actually terror—that I was bad, even evil, at my very core, was too horrifying to allow into full consciousness. But there it was, no longer avoidable. I had to look, or know forevermore that I had come to the truth and turned away.

At the point of decision-making, I contemplated turning away. After all, if what I feared was true, I was (as I believed then) doomed to eternal fire hell anyway. Wasn't it preferable to live in denial, and have the illusion of love, enjoyment, fun, even joy, at times during this sojourn on earth? But I guess the seeker in me was too strong. I decided against that option and considered the possibility that I might finally stop turning away from fear and start down a path of truthful inquiry into my true nature, wherever that might lead me. That was the beginning of a loving kindness practice toward myself, though I didn't know it at the time. When nothing else is possible, to allow the truth as we see it to just be is the kindest thing we can do.

So, we begin with gentleness, and a basic friendliness toward ourselves, or perhaps a willingness to open to the possibility of loving kindness. And, if none of these are possible, may we bring simply a willingness to open to the truth.

Practicing a daily loving kindness meditation may be helpful in this opening. I have practiced the Loving Kindness meditation from Stephen Levine's book *Healing into Life and Death* for many years and will probably continue to practice it until I die (see Appendix).

CHAPTER 10

Practicing with Negative Emotions

*Let no place in me hold itself closed,
for where I am closed, I am false.*

—Rainer Maria Rilke

How We Avoid Experiencing

WE MODERN HUMANS, generally speaking, are emotionally constipated. Usually when we have a bad feeling, instead of processing the feeling, that is, letting ourselves experience it, we hang onto it. We stick it into a little dark corner and try to forget about it. Consequently, it can never move through us, and we will not be free of it. Unexperienced emotions held in the body can cause blockages, leading to loss of flexibility and spontaneity, or sometimes even to physical illness. The only way to clear these blockages is to experience the emotion that has been repressed. It may take years, but we can eventually pare down these blockages to allow much more freedom in our lives. And if we allow ourselves to experience emotions as they arise in our lives, we will spare ourselves the hardship of dealing with yet more pain down the road caused by more blockages.

Normally, there are two ways we respond to a negative emotion: we either suppress it or express it (act out). Many consider the second response a healthy way of dealing with emotions, but in actuality, both of these responses can be ways of avoiding feeling our emotions, that is—experiencing. Even acting out in private by hitting a pillow or other object, as some therapists recommend, though preferable to saying or doing something hurtful to another, may still be a way of avoiding truly experiencing what one is feeling. In some instances, these techniques may actually help us *access* deeply held emotions. Generally speaking, however, when strong feelings are already presenting themselves, journaling, talking things out with a friend or therapist and otherwise expressing feelings, though all important and valuable tools, are best kept for *after* you have had a chance to *feel* your feelings, and process them on an experiential level.

The Shadow "I" and the Impartial Observer

When we are experiencing a negative emotion, things are usually moving very fast. Our thoughts are swirling around us, and we're basically caught in reaction mode. Our standard patterns of behavior are reeling out like an old-time movie, and the director is out to lunch. All we want to do is blame the other person or get the hell out of Dodge, or cry, or laugh, or follow whatever strategy we've developed to deal with this emotion.

If we do happen to even think about spiritual practice, we usually don't have the time or the presence of mind to actually see what it would look like, or the willingness and fortitude to implement it even if we did. This is true partly because the "I" who is "up" just then, is not the "I" who practices.

We may notice at this time or later that this "upset I" seems like a totally different being from the one that usually inhabits our bodies. We may say to ourselves or others, "I just wasn't myself," or "That wasn't really me." Yet, when we're in the eye of the cyclone, or sometimes when we're alone, we may feel that *this is* who we really are, and the other "I's" are just a show, a sham to conceal our true self from others and from the world.

Even when you're back to "yourself," that sickening feeling of self-doubt may cling to your being. Floating just beneath the surface, it ruins our peace of mind and makes us feel uncomfortable in our own bodies (as if the boom may fall at any moment). This "I" is the "shadow I," the frightened inner child, the one we label "not me" and ignore to the extent that we can.

The best we can usually hope for, when reaction takes over, is to try very hard to have some kind of impartial observer frantically taking notes, or a mental handicam set up in a corner of our mind to record the whole scene. And, if we can possibly manage it, to have a stand-in available to run interference, to keep us from harming ourselves or others, either physically or emotionally. If we've laid the groundwork of loving kindness, or if the adult has established some connection with the frightened inner child, we may possibly be able to offer some support to this struggling being at this time.

Of course the most desirable scenario would be to allow all emotions to be experienced fully while the unsettling event is actually taking place. In reality, however, especially in the beginning of this work, it is rarely possible to do that. The armoring we have built up over the years is too thick, and it may feel too overwhelming to enter those fearful emotions while the person or event that triggered our fear is present. Later, however, I have found that with practice it is possible to become more comfortable being with these aspects of ourselves, and to do more processing during the actual upset.

No More Important Task

As soon as possible after an upsetting event, try to find a quiet spot where you can be alone, or a public place where you can be anonymous and feel safe enough to explore your feelings. Don't wait until you get home, or put it off until the end of the day, if you can help it. I find the longer I wait to work with a particular situation, the more likely it is that I will have lost touch with the actual feelings I was having, and it becomes a worthless mental exercise.

There is no more important task on God's earth than what you're endeavoring to do in this moment, which is to heal into the pain which has held you prisoner for ten, twenty, thirty or more years. I would recommend, however, that the first time you practice with experiencing that you do it at home or in a place where you are fairly sure you will not be interrupted. *Not* that anything terrible is going to happen—it's not. But until you are familiar with the way your particular body will react, it might be best to be alone, or with someone with whom you feel safe, and who understands experiencing so they can simply be there with you and allow you to go through your process.

I specifically remember the first time I decided to try to actually *do* this "experiencing" thing. It was terribly frightening. I felt the flush of one of those old familiar really "yucky" emotions that I had tried to avoid all my life rising in my chest, in my throat. And I realized I had never allowed myself to get anywhere near actually *feeling* this emotion because it had seemed too scary. I felt myself sinking into what felt like an altered state of consciousness. I think this was because in order to actually experience this emotion, I had to go back in time to the moment I first experienced it, the time I decided that it was just too scary and put it into that little box. So now I was opening the box and there was something warning me not to go there, that something dreadful would happen to me if I allowed myself to explore this feeling. It felt like I was entering forbidden territory and would be punished, perhaps eternally—even that I might die.

But the fear we feel which guards the entrance to our hearts, trying to keep us from going there, trying to keep us from doing this work, is not the demon we suppose it to be. Rainer Maria Rilke, in *Letters to a Young Poet*, tells us fear is the dragon that guards our most precious possessions. So what is this dragon guarding? What *are* those precious possessions?

The Past Is Where We Live

Back when we first encountered this fear, we were probably babies or small children. Someone close to us, perhaps our mother or father, perhaps another close relative or caregver—someone we depended on for the basic necessities of life—may, due to overwork, exhaustion, or stress, have neglected to care for us in the way that we needed. Or worse—they may, out of their own woundedness and pain, have hurt us, either psychologically, by shouting at us or calling us names, or have actually physically or sexually abused us.

To the tiny beings that we were, totally helpless, totally dependent, these events probably would have felt like death, or perhaps made us feel so bad, so wrong, so unlovable, that we thought we would be left alone, which in our baby hearts was worse than death. Being helpless and unable to protect ourselves or help ourselves in any way physically, the only way to protect ourselves was by disassociating ourselves from feeling these experiences. This may have been a necessary and thus loving step taken by the baby ego to protect the delicate developing soul.

Usually we don't remember the step taken out of desperation to save ourselves, but in the case of Naomi, a woman who had been sexually abused by her own father at a very young age, formerly repressed memories began to emerge when she embarked upon a path of healing. Jalaja Bonheim tells Naomi's story in her book of women's sexual stories and the journey of the soul: (1997, 291)

> Like many victims of abuse, Naomi survived only by shattering into pieces. Unable to stay present in the face of such incomprehensible torture, her inner being splintered as the agonized psyche tore herself away from the tortured body. "I recently remembered the moment my personality shattered," she recounted. It happened one nightmarish day when her father took his daughter—just seven years old—to the house of one of his friends to be gang-raped. While this was going on, a kind of guardian presence appeared and said: "Come on, we're leaving. We're not staying in this body." "I was already fragmented into 'we' by then. This guardian took my hand and started pulling me away from my body. I was flooded with incredible grief that I had to leave my body forever and I could never go back because it was too awful to stay. First I cried, 'No, no, I don't want to leave.' But then I looked at the scene around me and was convinced. 'Oh, I see. Yes, I guess I'll come with you. I really can't stay here.' From then on, I just lived somewhere else, dissociated from my body."

And so the tender child soul may become encapsulated in a protective shield to be saved from destruction. Most of us have not had the kind of horrendous circumstances that caused Naomi's drastic splintering, but all of us, I think, have suffered circumstances as children that were just too frightening or felt too unloving to experience and thus to some degree split off from our true heart as a protective measure.

But there is a problem with and a paradox in this necessary shielding or separation that occurred and was perpetuated past the time when it was no longer necessary. The problem is that the heart, which experiences pain, vulnerability, and grief, is also the repository of joy and love. So by protecting ourselves from pain, we have also, inadvertently, shut ourselves off from the possibility of realizing and experiencing our own true nature, which is love. This is the essential human problem, and the work of a lifetime is to reconnect with that original nature of love and joy. This means, of course, that we must also be prepared to experience sorrow and pain.

To do this we must take the lifelines that have been thrown to us through our emotions, which connect us to the primal event, and, at last, surrender to the feeling. *We don't need to remember the event itself.* We are not really *going* anywhere, or re-experiencing something from the past. The past is where we live—we have carried it with us and relate to our life from this ancient place. We don't have to scratch around in our past looking for the original wound, an emotion to heal. It's all included in the emotions we encounter in our everyday life and the sensations in our bodies, if we are willing to open to them.

That original pain, however, may be encoded as something else. We have put quite a bit of protective wrapping around it the way the body builds up a tough callous around a sliver that hasn't been removed. This doesn't imply that we must go to decoding through analysis—looking for meaning in any kind of intellectual way. The way is *always* to stay with experience—stay with the body—with sensation—with "what is this?" So what we experience at first may be just a slight discomfort, or irritation, a pain in the back, an uneasiness or anxiety when a loved one is about to leave, anger when someone criticizes us or leaves us out, resentment when someone keeps taking what we give and never gives anything back, annoyance when someone tells us what to do.

Experiencing

When you have settled down somewhere safe, let whatever is surging in you just be there. In the actual situation, you may have struggled to control it, change it, or hide it. Let yourself feel these feelings without any judgment about them. This includes all feelings—even feelings of self-hatred. There may be some confusion about this point after all the talk about Loving Kindness. But it is loving and kind to allow ourselves to have any feeling without rejecting ourselves for having it. John Ruskin says,

> Self-rejection does not come about because you have negative feelings—self-rejection occurs when you reject the feelings. In other words, feelings are never self-rejecting or accepting, even feelings of

hatred toward yourself. It is the attitude toward the feelings that is accepting or rejecting. (1993, 126)

Have mercy on yourself. If you can bring to bear some loving kindness on this being who suffers, all the better, but if you can't, don't add more suffering by judging yourself for your inability to do so. Give yourself to the process. Let your feelings wash over you. Let them just be there. Feel yourself opening to whatever it is. Be willing, once and for all, to let the truth be—and to accept whatever it may bring.

Tune into your body. What is going on there? Notice where the emotion seems to center. The gut? The heart space? What does it feel like? Is there tightness? Pain? Heat or cold? What about the rest of your body? Check out the whole body, but try not to get into a checklist mode. Maintain a Gestalt awareness of the overall feeling. Go deep. Don't analyze—just experience. It may feel very old. If pictures or memories come into your awareness, pay attention to them (unless they are mundane worries or distractions.) You may feel very frightened. Perhaps a memory is trying to surface that feels too terrifying to allow into consciousness. Remind yourself that you are experiencing a memory. There is nothing you can remember that you haven't already lived through.

You may feel like you are going to throw up. You may feel cold or small. You may even experience sexual feelings. You may feel great discomfort, as if there are too many people in too small a space, or as if someone for whom you have disgust is in the same room with you. You may experience two conflicting things so strongly that it feels unbearable—that you can't stand being in your body—that you have to move, runaway, distract yourself—anything just to get away from the feeling you're having.

Try to stay with it. You won't die or burst. The buffers that you have erected to keep your various selves from seeing each other are dissolving. This is good. It means you are close to actually experiencing something that has been pent up inside you for a long time, and to seeing the truth about your life—that you have been living a half-life, acknowledging only the bright side of the penny, while denying all the parts of yourself that didn't fit the picture of who you thought you needed to be in order to be loved. But the truth is, that you, just as you are, are all that is needed. You *are* love. There will be no better time than now to open to these poor exiled parts of yourself and to begin to welcome them back into your heart, and the circle of life.

As you allow yourself to experience deeper and deeper levels of feeling, your body may begin to do strange and perhaps frightening things. You'll probably cry, but you may also laugh, shake, twitch, gasp for breath, take deep gulps of air, or do a lot of yawning. Don't worry about this. It is simply energy being released. Your body is clearing out blockages that have been held for many years and this is a good thing.

Our minds will play tricks on us, try to get us involved, so we don't have to feel. Maybe it will try to convince us that we have important business to attend to in the world. Perhaps you forgot to call your friend back. She will think you don't care—maybe it was urgent. Maybe she really needs you. Or perhaps you suddenly remember a bill you didn't pay. If you don't get it off today, you will be fined. The mailman is coming in twenty minutes, etc.

If we resist those temptations, the mind will try to draw us off into analyzing and understanding this emotion, producing amazing insights with which it promises to free us. The mind thinks—that's what it does. It's the function of mind. It is not thoughts that are the problem. It is our attachment to our thoughts that is the problem. Stephen Levine said, "The mind is a wonderful tool, but a terrible taskmaster." Often, I think, we confuse thoughts with feelings. But feelings are not the problem either—it is our resistance to our feelings that is the problem. The only way to free ourselves is to let ourselves feel the pain.

Have paper and pencil ready to write down any insights that come to you, but don't get bogged down in ideas. The insights may be valuable, but I have found, writing down ideas can get in the way of, or actually take the place of feeling feelings. You'll have to decide by trial and error, if it's better for you to make the note, so as to get it out of the way in order to feel feelings, or if it is taking the place of feeling feelings, or letting the steam out of your feelings, so they are no longer as powerful.

The main job here is not figuring out what is happening or why, but to experience the "whatness" of what is happening. These ancient emotions have been waiting for us all our lives. The only way out is through, and when these difficult emotions, the ones from which we have been hiding, present themselves, we have another shot at healing. When they do, we can ask ourselves, "Will I finally say yes to them? Or will I take a pass, and put them back on the shelf yet again?" I think we've all seen the truth: they don't go away. They keep coming back in one guise or another until we are finally ready to surrender.

We Need to Unwrap Our Pain Slowly

Sometimes we need to unwrap our pain slowly, layer by layer, allowing ourselves to experience what comes up, letting the wrappings be peeled back one by one to expose the deeper feelings. There may be layers and layers of feeling. The first feeling you encounter is the top, outer layer. You're like an onion with layer upon layer that has been laid down, one after another, over the years, each one putting you farther and farther from your true heart. So you peel the onion, one layer at a time, until you reach the center.

The first emotion you encounter may be embarrassment. Someone says something that makes you think you said something stupid or inappropriate. In reality, the person may or may not have thought that what you said was stupid, and may or may not have said something that could be seen by an objective observer to imply that what you said was stupid. For the purpose of the basic processing of experience that you are doing now, it doesn't matter. Whatever feeling comes up, whether it is "warranted" or not, is what you work with. (Later, when you dialog with the inner child, the truth of the circumstances will be more relevant.)

If you're very aware, you may notice that there was a fleeting feeling of hurt, which came first, but was quickly replaced by embarrassment. This hurt feeling was a primary emotion. All the emotions that follow, except the very last one, are secondary emotions. That is, they are feelings, which cover up or take the place of the primary feeling.

Feelings are composed of thoughts and bodily sensations and will usually be accompanied by an impulse to do something (a strategy). For example, the feeling of embarrassment may include a thought that you have done something inappropriate, as some so-called friend has so obligingly pointed out.

You may feel flushed, and want to run away or hide. Notice this, and stay with the feeling. Second may come anger, with a further rush of heat, and the words you should have said, or the impulse to actually hurt someone. Beneath the embarrassment and the anger, if you can go deeper, may be shame, or the feeling of total unworthiness or unloveableness, and beneath that, the fear of rejection. Finally, you may get to the base fear, the terror of being left totally alone or the fear of death.

It is helpful to remember that this intense emotion is the emotion of a helpless baby or child, who was utterly dependent for life itself on the person who precipitated the original emotion. At that time, we actually could have died or been hurt very badly, but for the care of the other, and had no defense against being hurt by the person who to us was like a God. Now, however, we're no longer babies. We are adults. We have the means to protect ourselves from harm, and to lovingly care for ourselves. Remembering these things may help us to allow ourselves to experience these painful feelings.

If you are a meditator, you may feel that this kind of work is not what meditation is about. I know there's a kind of rule that many of us follow when some strong emotion or thought comes up during meditation: You don't suppress it, but you also don't follow it. You just let it go through. The reasoning is that meditation is about being present to our experience in the moment, and that these "remembered" emotions are from some past time.

The approach I'm suggesting may appear to go against that rule. Looking closely, however, we can see that this doesn't really defy the rule after all, because the kind of situation I'm talking about *is* an experience—it's something that's happening *now*. There are *external* experiences and there are *internal* experiences—so this is an internal experience—an experience that we have perhaps suppressed for a long time or even repressed, so that we have no idea of it even being there. But it exists, nonetheless, and has kept us *out* of our hearts for years.

If we allow ourselves to experience whatever feeling is present in the moment, we may see that what's present came from the past. And if we're holding it in the body, it is present in the body right at this moment. So being with that pain, allowing that pain to be there, experiencing that pain or that sorrow, that terror or that fear *is our work* as meditators, as spiritual aspirants. So with normal thoughts and monkey-mind kind of things—the constant chatter—yes, you just let that be there, and let that go through, let it do what it does, but don't latch on to it and don't follow it. I think, however, when something very juicy comes up, something with a big charge attached to it, it can be extremely helpful in our practice to actually go into it *as an experience.*

Try to stay with the feeling aspect of the experience—the visceral quality of the body/mind. Allow yourself to experience in your cells, in your bones, in your blood, what has been kept so closely guarded for so many years. Feelings are always about *now*—about "what is." Leave the mental constructs and beliefs about what you are experiencing for processing later. These constructs of the mind are *not* the substance of meditation, though they may provide useful insight for later contemplation. They do not concern the present moment or "experiencing." They are not about "what" is. They are usually about the past or the future, or explaining our experience to us.

Deep Inquiry

I want to emphasize that there are two different levels of being with the present moment, i.e. of opening to "what is." One, there is the level that simply stays with awareness of body sensations—the level of noticing—noticing when I get angry that there's tension in the chest—the muscles tighten, the throat tightens. And I can experience those sensations just as sensations, and that's very useful, because there's a little bit of detachment. I can notice the body sensations and know that that's not necessarily me, that it's just phenomena. And I can move back into a more open awareness or deeper meditation.

And two, there's another level of experiencing that goes much deeper which is, in my experience, more transformative. Certain emotions, it seems, catch me up time and time again. And it feels like they have me in their grip. These are the emotions I've carried with me from childhood. So when I feel myself in the grip of one of these emotions, I feel lost. They are such familiar feelings—ancient feelings—like a prison. They ruin my peace and steal my joy. And, in fact, almost all of the emotions that carry a big charge for us involve these old emotions. By "charge" I mean something that causes reactivity in us—when we feel some strong emotion surfacing in reaction to some event.

Getting to this level requires deep inquiry. It's almost like an invocation, a beseeching—and it definitely involves more then simply noticing. It involves entering the experience on a deep emotional level as well as coming to an understanding of the false beliefs we carry that keep us trapped in these old emotions.

These kinds of feelings have receded considerably for me since I began my deep inquiry in the mid-eighties when everything seemed to be falling apart, but still rear their unwanted heads occasionally. One particularly persistent and challenging early emotion was triggered again long after I thought I had seen the last of it by a disconcerting interview with a spiritual teacher whose book I had loved. I was doing a session with her based on the book and her reputation. Yet in my interview with her, I didn't like her. I thought she was wrong in her assessment of something.

But because this teacher had such a good reputation, I began to doubt myself. I began to question my authenticity. I thought, "Well, she's a famous teacher. It can't be her. It must be me." I asked myself, was I just trying to get out of facing the truth about something in myself? Was I lying to myself? Maybe I didn't really want to know the truth after all. I felt myself sinking into an old feeling/belief pattern that said, "You are the one and only person on earth incapable of doing this work and thus doomed to eternal hellfire. Or worse—the person who is false: who pretends to have chosen the path, but really on the deepest level, turns away and refuses to do the work that is really necessary."

This shocked me—I hadn't seen this old ghost in ten or more years. That particular fear had, in the past, been my worst nightmare on a soul level and plagued me at various times and under various circumstances throughout the early part of my spiritual life. It was a place I recognized immediately as being deeply connected to my core beliefs and fears. In this case, I saw that I was dealing more with an old belief pattern (covered more extensively in Chapter Eleven). Because it came up, I wanted to look at it, but I also noticed that it didn't have a huge charge connected to it as it would have in the past and I knew that was because I had done so much work in this area already. Thus the fears and doubts that arose on a feeling level were not that deeply imbedded and passed through fairly quickly.

Whether or not what the teacher said was correct was not as important as the fact that I did not make this experience into a huge fire and brimstone scenario like the ones I used to conjure in my head under similar circumstances, and that I was able to make the decision that this teacher was not the right one for me without a lot of fanfare. My tendency to make high drama out of a situation that did not warrant it was not winning out this time. That was a good thing.

However, I had another encounter with my core wounded self about six months later that unearthed such intense feelings of fear, doubt and shame that I was on my knees begging for mercy. I had a nightmare in which I molested a child—a young boy. When I awoke I felt intense shame. I asked myself, could I somehow be a latent child molester and be hiding it from myself and others? Or worse, could I have actually molested a child and suppressed the memory of it?

I didn't think these things were very likely, but the dream had such reality to it and had touched such a deep part of me that I knew it had to have truth to it on some level. I thought it was more likely to be some kind of rape or molestation by me of some part of myself—my inner child.

But these were thoughts. I knew I needed to open to this on a deeper emotional level. I knew this had to do with a deep core being shame that thoughts or analyzing could not touch. The shame and the fear were overwhelming. But there was desire behind it too, a deep wanting to know, not on an intellectual level, but on a soul level.

So when we come to a place like this in our journey, we will recognize it—the doubt, the fear, the shame of our old familiar swamp. Or something even deeper—unfamiliar territory—something terrifying and new. And when this appears, it is a huge opportunity. Simply being able to see it this way is a huge step. But something more is required. We must pick the lock—open up those closely guarded secrets—take a good look at the self that we thought was absolutely unlovable and unworthy, and finally experience the feelings we thought we couldn't bear.

I wanted freedom, wanted to access the love that I knew was there, the truth, the wisdom, beauty, peace, clarity and joy. But when I was caught up in those emotions, I didn't experience any of those things.

So in this deeper way of experiencing we ask, "What is this?" and go into it. What is this surging? What is the heart of it? "What's happening? What's *really* here?"—questions that come out of the deepest desires of the heart—a real wanting to know on an experiential level what this devastation is about. My experience is that this can be terrifying. It's not some little tight muscle or queasy stomach. This is huge in the life of the soul. It can bring up a feeling that is so intense and terrifying that I'll do anything to get away from it. And yet if my desire is strong enough to be free, I'll go into it and may be willing to experience it.

The Longing Itself IS the Connection We Seek

It may not always be that intense, but when there's a charge, we know *something's* going on. So if there's a charge, go into whatever the charge has brought for you. There's energy in that charge, and you can use the energy of the charge to go deeper. This again goes back to the reason I'm encouraging people to work with experiencing difficult emotions, or any emotions really, as close as possible to the time they actually occur. I find that, if I wait until my day is over or for some pre-designated meditation times, I am very likely to have lost the energy of the charge that can carry me to a place of deeply productive inner work. But also please *do* this during meditation if intense emotions arise during meditation.

We may be inclined not to want to do this if we're meditating with a group because, if we really go deep, something may happen that we think may disturb the other meditators or that may be embarrassing. This is something you can discuss in your own meditation group if members are open to it. It could be fertile ground for deepening and strengthening the group as well as your own personal practice.

We want to be free of that charge in a sense. We want to be free of our anger and our irritation and our anxiety, or reactivity, and yet there's some deep truth buried there. So it's tricky because while we're not saying things should be different, there is that sense, there is some feeling that they should—that things should be different, that *we* should be different. Sometimes it's not other people who push our buttons, but us, with all of our feelings of unworthiness and unlovableness. So just absolutely go into those feelings, whatever they are—with your desire, with your desire to be free. Remember what Rumi said, the longing itself *is the connection we seek.*

Advaida teacher, John Sherman, explained the phenomena to me once in a way that I really got it. And it goes to the depths of the truth that we have heard over and over again from different spiritual teachings, which is basically that "all is one," but of course we can say that and hear that and not understand it. I was asking John about some difficult emotion and he said that there is only one energy. And the energy that's buried in our negative emotions is that same energy. That's why our wanting to throw them away or bury them or get rid of them doesn't work.

Pre-verbal Experience

If you get to a place for which there are no words, you may be in a pre-verbal stage—like a very tiny baby, or even pre-birth. This may feel awful, and be very frightening, but in my own work, I take it as a good sign. It means I am allowing myself to experience ancient blocked emotions. When I was going through chemo, my body felt so bad that I thought it was going to die a couple of times, and during this same period, I was experiencing rejection from someone important in my life. These two intensely difficult experiences happening together had a synchronous effect that was greater than the sum of their parts. It forced me into, or perhaps allowed me to surrender and open to, a very deep part of myself.

At one point I went into my bodily feelings, but it was more than the body I was referring to in the previous section on deep inquiry— even though we are focusing more on bodily sensations, it goes deeper than that. It's hard to describe or grasp because, when we do deep inquiry, we discover that the idea we're merely physical is really an illusion. If we go deeply into the physical, we find that it can be a gateway into another dimension. At that point you're not *just* in the physical— you can't really separate these layers.

So what I experienced was going into a black pit. I was in this thick, yucky mud-like medium where I couldn't move and I just felt terrible. Of course "terrible" is just a word and the experience didn't have a word. It was pure experience. I knew somewhere in me that I was having a pre-verbal experience. I was experiencing something as a baby and it was absolutely terrifying.

My belief is that I hadn't allowed myself to fully have this experience at the time it occurred when I was a child or a baby and it was held somewhere in my body, in my cells. The stimulus of my present situation helped me to go to that place and unlock that experience. Although I didn't have words or even thoughts for this experience, I assumed it must have been a time when, as a baby, I was experiencing some overwhelmingly painful or frightening physical sensations and a sense of rejection, aloneness, or abandonment. After this experience, I felt changed. I felt more free and open. My body still felt sick from the chemo, but I moved through the feeling of rejection with more ease and experienced myself as more "whole" and well then before the processing.

Another time I was working with a psychic and we were going into some areas of my body that were very tight. She asked me to go there and feel my experience. I suddenly realized I was experiencing my mother. She was huge and very frightening. This was a surprise to me because as a teenager I had begun to see my mother as weak and as something of a sad and pathetic figure because of her extreme nervousness. This was also how I saw her as an adult. After this experience however, I realized how frightening her hysteria must have been for me as a baby and small child.

When I am having an intense experience, I try to stay with the feeling as long as I can. If I find myself judging myself or someone else, I don't push it away—I let that be part of the process, but only to the extent that I am experiencing what it feels like to judge and be judged, and to notice what the judge is saying. I try to write these judgments down for reflection and integration at a later time when the intense feelings have passed. That judging being is coming out of the same place, the same fear, that my embarrassment, anger, shame, or whatever feeling I am working with, came out of. Whatever arises, I just let it be there, and enter into it as fully as possible, while still maintaining an awareness of the bigger picture, i.e. that I'm not really small, cold, sick, bad, in danger, etc. and that my adult self (if possible) is there to offer loving kindness.

Allow

It's not that we keep part of ourselves separate. We go into ourselves and our experiences completely—we just *are*. But it is all held within a larger awareness, a benevolent awareness, a soft awareness. This is not a hard driving "push through the pain" type of effort. In fact, this is not really even something we do. It is not really something we *can* do. The key here is to *allow*. To allow whatever is there to be there. To allow ourselves to be whoever we are. We have shut ourselves out of our hearts for too many years. Now is the time for welcome. Now is the time, not for closing doors, but for opening. Now is the time to, finally, just be. You're the one, right here, right now, in this place, at this time, appointed to love yourself.

You may balk at this idea. The words may come, "I'm too little, too small, too selfish, too self-absorbed." That is because you're still identified with the small scared self or selves that are in exile. The ego, the false self, is trying desperately to keep you from knowing the truth, which is that you're much, much more than any of these. You *are* love. If it seems there is no benevolence available—that's okay. Just let these words float in awareness. And let your hardness float in awareness. Let there be space around them—around the feelings that carry them. Imagine just the slightest loosening, softening, around the edges of this tight holding.

For me, this work has been of prime importance in my own healing. One example of peeling the onion for me began with a feeling of uneasiness or discomfort when I realized that I wasn't happy for my friend who was describing an experience that was really great for him. I was feeling kind of left out of that and uncomfortable. Then I went a little deeper and realized I was having a judgment about something that had happened a little earlier in the day—he had made a new connection with a woman and was going off to do something with her that didn't include me. A judgment is not a feeling, but it's part of the process to notice judgments and try to go beneath them to the feeling. So I tried to stay with the feeling, just exploring, asking, "What is this?" and going deeper with it.

Beneath the judgment I found there was hurt, and beneath the hurt, sadness and fear of loss, because I felt there was going to be a certain loss involved with this person, a loss for me. And then even beneath that, another feeling was rising. It was very strong. It was like this big massive thing in the center of my chest which I recognized as anger. I had begun to realize recently that I had more work to do around anger. Anger, I saw, was still somewhat frightening to me and not "okay." I remembered Advaida teacher John Sherman's admonition: "That which we push away is that which we seek." So I let myself experience it.

I put aside all my thoughts and judgments about my friend and the situation that had triggered the anger. I allowed myself to simply feel my body and the various sensations sweeping through it, without the story of my friend doing whatever he had done to "make me mad." I very quickly surrendered to the surging feelings and realized with a start that what I was experiencing was raw power—energy very similar to sexual orgasm in its intensity and force.

Release

It just surged up and down my body and suddenly my body was opened up, and there was some gasping in my breathing and there was some twitching in my muscles.

I find it's almost a trance-like state to really go into these held emotions because I think they have kept us in a sort of prison for many years. So when there's a release of this holding, it's like the body goes a little berserk and suddenly all those pent up emotions are released and become available for more positive purposes.

We generally think of anger as a negative emotion and we have all seen and felt the energy behind anger in its out-of-control destructive force, but in this experiencing without the story, there was nothing negative about it. It was thrilling and vitalizing. It filled my body with the drive and strength to do whatever great thing I decided upon. I was astounded at this secret cache of energy, available to use in whatever way I chose.

This, for me, translated mostly into psychic and creative energy as my physical body was still quite weak from the ravages of chronic illness and chemotherapy. But over time, as I opened to and worked with various emotions, I saw more of this psychic and creative energy spilling over into my physical body and imbuing it with more strength and more vitality. Sometimes it is hard to tell if my physical self is actually improved or not because the psychic energy shines through and permeates my body. But whatever it is, it is a force to be reckoned with and used.

This particular time I got clarity of what I needed to do for myself. I realized that I wasn't taking care of myself and that the anger and my inability to celebrate with my friend was coming out of that. I saw that what I needed to do was make our friendship more clearly friendship and relinquish the aspect of our relationship that still had romantic overtones. Immediately, the distance that I felt between us vanished and I was celebrating with him the joy and the expansion that he was feeling.

So this experience came with an insight, but that's not always the case with experiencing. And of course we may not always be capable of *acting* on the insights that are presented to us. The process of experiencing stands on its own and doesn't necessarily *give* us anything in the way of knowledge or understanding that we can measure by the standards of this world. Sometimes I just go into a state and it's intense and my body does weird things and I may not get any insight at all. But afterward I feel different. Most of the time the problem, or whatever had seemed to be a problem, has disappeared, even though nothing in the external situation has changed. I've found this to be true time and time again.

I have found that doing this kind of work frees up a certain energy in me and I believe it clears something that doesn't come back, that it's doing some kind of work that doesn't need to be repeated. That doesn't mean the emotion won't come up again. It keeps coming up, and we need to keep clearing *what seems* like the same thing over and over again, but I think we're doing pieces of it. In the above example with my friend, I don't think my hurt and anger had entirely to do with the current situation. I believe part of it had to do with ancient holdings, though I didn't become aware of them in my processing of this particular situation. We don't always need to bring old experiences to conscious awareness in order to clear them. If we truly open to our current experiences, our old holdings will automatically be accessed as well. And our backlog of holdings will get smaller.

I know for sure that there comes a point where there's more spaciousness in the heart. More ability to be present. Less reactivity. And I think that if we keep doing the work, we get to a certain point of being fairly clear where we don't have a lot of built up old emotions and our reaction time is a lot shorter. We might have an immediate reaction and if we just allow ourselves to feel it, it moves through us like a storm and is gone. I've found this to be true in my own experience.

Jane knew about "allowing" on a gut level but was completely incapacitated by her extremely intelligent but overactive mind, which would take her tripping on the kinds of things most people take for granted, such as seeing or thinking. This mind-tripping was not at all the pleasant kind. It brought on extreme anxiety and panic attacks. Luckily, she was also very much in touch with the very sound basic wisdom underlying her roof-brain chatter.

> I knew that if I was going to make it, if I was going to stick around here, I had to get to a point where I could have some sort of faith in existence. I knew that the answer wasn't going to be in this mind-tripping. I was always tempted by it. And every time the next mind-trip started, I felt like if I just kept pursuing it, there would be satisfaction, and yet when I finally got to the point where I was paralyzed, I knew it had to stop. And the only way that was going to happen was to develop some guttural faith that had nothing to do with thinking. Talk about letting go—[when everything for me] was about holding on and defining—and to basically saying, "you've got to go all the way!"
>
> There was some recognition about the nature of the mind, that the mind was actually a tool, an organ, just like the digestive organs, that it had a purpose and it was to be used for that. But since the mind can feel like its own entity, its own existence, it feels like it should be able to know everything and understand everything. I realized that's where my trap was, that because the mind was the [tool I had practice using], I would use it just because it was what I knew how to do. Yet somewhere I knew that there was another way of knowing, a completely different way of knowing that required actually getting to the recognition of where the mind's limits are, but I didn't know what that was yet.
>
> So the mind would take me to these places and I would panic when it couldn't take me any further. And that realization, at the edge of where the mind could go, was where I had to step back and learn this other way of knowing.

Because thinking had taken on such a huge presence in her psyche for so long and she had become, one might say, addicted to it, giving it up for even small periods of time was actually terrifying for Jane, as, in fact, I think it *is* for everyone who seriously begins to *do* it. The courage, ingenuity and perseverance with which Jane approached her situation in the face of sometimes terrifying experiences allowed her to move slowly toward true healing and a state of mental health I would say far surpasses what might be called "normal." Her description of her process is long, but I think it's worth including here as another template for people working with frightening situations.

> I made a rule for myself. It was really hard to keep. It took a long time to get to the place where I could, but I would identify some of those trigger thoughts that were going to start me on that freak-out path, and I would say, "I'm only allowed to have them at 5:00 in the evening in this chair." If I started seeing that I was doing it, I'd have to say, "You can do it at 5:00, you can't do it now. Go do something else." And the other thing was that I wasn't ever, ever, and under any circumstances, allowed to have a single one of these kinds of thoughts at night in bed with the lights out.
>
> And so I worked with these techniques or strategies [for] breaking this habit [of] my mind. I was so split. It's like I really, really believed these things, and yet I was so not believing at the same time—if someone wanted to ask me my feelings about human nature, I'd say I believed that kind of faith was a natural state even though I was so, so, so, so far from that. I believed that first I had to stop the habit [of mind-tripping] to allow room for this natural state of faith to just be. There was that feeling that I was getting in the way of the faith, or the mind was getting in the way.

So Jane stumbled upon the truth that we must all answer in our own way: that we have the truth already in us—we only need to find it. Her work was not specifically about "practicing with negative emotions" in the sense of "experiencing," but it was a step in that direction and an inspiring example of someone who, as terrified as she was of life, and as faithless as she thought she was, still, on some deep wordless level, understood or believed that that faith, or basic wisdom, or ability to heal, existed in her, and that if she could just get out of her own way, i.e. clear the path to it, and simply "allow," it would be there.

When I told Jane how courageous I thought she was and how profound it was that she really already had the faith she was looking for, she replied,

> It *is* profound. Wow. It kind of reminds me of that saying that the most courageous people are the ones with the most fear. And my image of myself was of such a fearful, weak person, but from this perspective here's somebody that didn't have the faith to even take a breath.
>
> I think it was a combination of getting comfortable and familiar with that space and a certain degree of quietness. The mental tension, the physical tension, the vigilance, it was all very, very loud inside me, and it took up every bit of space. Any amount of space terrified me, so to say something to myself like, "Here's a thought that you fill up a lot of space with and the thought has to go." Or, "You can only have this thought at 5:00 in that chair. What are you going to do with that space in the meantime?" There had to be this real intentional effort. I knew that was the only way, and I had to get comfortable with that.
>
> So I think it was so incremental to say, "You can have this thought but not that thought," and I would create little periods of time to have to feel that. The analogy is, if I had a stereo on full blast—[or rather] six stereos on full blast—I might turn one of them down a few notches but leave all the other ones blasting. And then when I got comfortable with that, maybe I'd turn two of them down a little bit, and then maybe at some point I'd just turn one stereo off completely, but the other one would still be on high.
>
> It was creating the space really slowly, but I often felt physically nauseous when I had to get comfortable with a new level of space. What also happened, and this had sort of a cumulative effect, was that, as I would have some success (like I knew I was comfortable with stereo six on level two or something, and that it had been uncomfortable), [I knew I could] eventually get comfortable with it. And that started becoming the thing. To this day, I actually still *use* this [technique] when I have to. I just recognize that [uncomfortable feeling] as a sensation, [and say to myself,] "I know this one, here we go, we have to go through that uncomfortable-getting-comfortable-with-the-void thing again. I still don't want to do it, but I know it's possible." So there's a willingness to say, "No, I know I can do this. Okay, it's temporary, let's go for it."
>
> That has ended up being a humongous tool for me. Especially in the work that I'm doing now with the chakras, so often I'm pushing myself or allowing myself to go to the edge of my comfort zone in any number

of ways. It's always that same kind of nauseous [feeling that comes up when] facing that void or discomfort. I guess it's just about change and that it's almost like a natural reaction for me now to just somehow refer back to that agoraphobic time, and say, "Oh yeah, okay, I know this one. I obviously can do this one."

CHAPTER 11

Dialoguing with the Inner Child

The idea is to know yourself as you long to be known, to really see yourself as you long to be seen, which is the child's deepest longing.

AT SOME POINT, if you have gone as far as possible with just experiencing the feeling, or if you're having trouble letting yourself experience it—that is, you're resisting the feeling—you can begin a dialogue with yourself. Imagine that there is an adult and a child. The frightened being that we want to label "not I" is the child—that is, the *wounded* child—and the adult is the one there to offer loving kindness and maintain a larger awareness.

Everyone has within him/herself an adult and a child. The child is the feeling, being part of us. The adult is the thinking, doing part. It is key that these two parts be present and balanced. In a healthy adult, the inner child is exuberant, joyful and playful, and the inner adult makes careful choices about what to do, when and how much, as well as to maintain healthy boundaries. Most of us, however, have not developed in a balanced way. One or another of these parts is usually underdeveloped, leaving the other to compensate, or has developed in an unhealthy way. Most of us have a wounded inner child, and an inner adult who has not experienced good modeling.

It is the adult's job to watch over the welfare and happiness of the child. The inner adult will often parent the inner child in the same way the real physical parent parented the real physical child. If the real parent was controlling and abusive, the inner parent will usually treat the inner child in the same way, perhaps calling her stupid and incompetent or driving her relentlessly to succeed, while at the same time, depriving her of the simple pleasures of life. If the real parent was absent or emotionally unavailable, the inner parent will often simply disappear, leaving the child adrift to fend for herself.

Re-parenting the Inner Child

With awareness, and conscious effort, one can learn to re-parent oneself. This may take a long time, as anyone knows who has ever tried to heal a relationship with their own flesh-and-blood child. The child may not open to you at first, and it may take several sessions before she even feels safe enough to talk at all. I think it is a good idea to have a certain time each day set aside for dialoguing with the inner child, even if nothing seems to be happening. If you show up every day, the child may begin to trust that you actually care.

I know many people have an aversion to the notion of inner child work. There's part of me that also resisted working in this way at first, until I saw the value of it. Dialoguing with the inner child, or whatever else you choose to call this feeling part of yourself, is only a tool, a technique to help you to access deeply buried feelings, and to process them, in order that you can have more freedom in your life. There are many ways to do this. Yet I have found dialoguing, at times, to be an almost miraculous aide for healing and for accessing hidden parts of myself.

Words can be very powerful, especially a kind word at the right time. You have all probably experienced a time when you're in a great deal of pain and it was all bottled up inside. Then perhaps someone came along and noticed your pain—a dear friend, or perhaps even a stranger. This person said a kind word or asked you with tenderness if there was anything they could do for you, or simply hugged you. And suddenly the floodgates opened. There was no stopping the flow of tears that gushed forth, and before you knew it, you were telling this dear one or stranger the story of your sorrow.

One day in church I noticed a young woman come in whom I had seen many times, though I had never met her. When she walked in, I knew immediately something was wrong. The narrow confines which constitute acceptable or normal human behavior were breached and flashed like a glaring neon sign, though not a word had been spoken.

This young woman was obviously in the midst of some kind of mental breakdown. The anxiety of the mother was palpable. She hovered near, trying fruitlessly to buffer her daughter's paranoia.

After the service, I saw the mother standing in the back of the church. My inner knowing told me what to do. I knew this woman only superficially, but we had had enough of a connection to make my impulse feel right. I approached her and hugged her, actually held her. This was not our usual greeting. Normally, we would smile, say hello, how are you and perhaps touch hands or have a short casual hug. This hug was deep and long—I didn't let go until she did. She began to sob—deep, wrenching sobs, dredged up from the depths. When we finally separated, I took her hand, and she, through tears, said, "She's getting better." I nodded and squeezed her hand, and that was that. Nothing more seemed needed or appropriate at that particular moment. Yet, two beings had met in a deep way. She had released some of the deep emotions locked inside, and felt seen and understood, and I knew she was grateful.

Meeting Your Inner Sorrow with Mercy and Kindness

So, too, can we meet our own inner sorrow with tenderness and mercy. If you saw a suffering being, the natural inclination of your heart would be to offer comfort or a sympathetic ear. But with ourselves we are merciless. Practices of loving kindness, along with a growing awareness of the pain of our inner child, can begin to change that. Let us have the same mercy and compassion for the suffering being within that we would offer to our only child, or to a stranger on the street.

If I step outside of myself and look at myself as I would look if I were someone else, I can see that this being deserves compassion. No one else can see that as I can—no one else knows the difficulty and pain of this life as I do. No one else knows the bravery with which this being keeps on plugging, under the most unworkable conditions. That which is great in me can have mercy on that which is mean and small, or weak and sick. All this may sound self-pitying, self-aggrandizing, or downright unchristian. After all, doesn't Christianity tell us to think about love, and care for others? Doesn't it emphasize humility, and the fact that we are all sinners? Well yes, but there's also the part about loving others *as we love ourselves*. This is the model Christ uses to tell us how to love. The second great Commandment is "Love your neighbor as yourself." So if we don't love ourselves, how then will we know how to love others? Likewise if we hate ourselves, this is what we will send out into the world. Pema Chödrön says,

> Compassion for others begins with kindness to ourselves. The reason we're often not there for others—whether for our child or mother or someone who is insulting us or someone who frightens us—is that we're not there for ourselves. There are whole parts of ourselves that are so unwanted that, whenever they begin to come up, we run away.... Only to the degree that we've gotten to know our personal pain, only to the degree that we've related with pain at all, will we be fearless enough, brave enough, and enough of a warrior to be willing to feel the pain of others. To that degree we will be able to take on the pain of others because we will have discovered that their pain and our own pain are not different. (1994 6, 4)

So the idea is, to know yourself as you long to be known, to really see yourself, as you long to be seen, to offer unconditional love to yourself, which is the child's deepest longing. If the idea of adult and child doesn't work for you, don't use it—it is just a model. The main thing is that there is someone there listening, and there is some sense of separateness between the two identities. If the suffering being wants to talk, let him talk. Actually encourage him to talk by asking questions. Then listen wholeheartedly, and with compassion and understanding. It is important that you have the dialogue out loud and not just in your head. You may be amazed at the things that come out of your mouth (out of the mouth of the child or the suffering being).

Tell the child that he is not bad for feeling what he is feeling—that there is a good reason for these feelings. There is always a good reason for feelings, though they may not be the reasons that we think. Tell him that it is okay to experience it and that you will take care of him and make sure he's not hurt or left alone.

The important thing is to really listen and learn from the inner child. We must learn what the inner child really wants and needs, because the adult, as the thinker/doer, is the one who must act in the external world to actualize these wants and needs, and most importantly, to see to the child's joy.

Telling the Child the Truth

The adult always tells the child the truth. The first truth, of course, is what we talked about earlier—there is a good reason for having these feelings. You will need to deal with the feelings on several levels. There is the superficial level of the actual circumstance that is occurring in real life, and there is the deeper level of the original event, probably from early in life, that we resisted feeling because it was too overwhelming at the time.

The real work, and the real gold, is in getting to the original feeling, and realizing that what you are experiencing has little, if anything, to do with your present circumstances. But remember—the child isn't experiencing only in real time. The child is carrying the past with her, and experiencing it through the catalyst of present circumstances. This realization in itself eliminates many of the unpleasant secondary emotions, such as self-judgment or embarrassment that spring up when we feel we're being too sensitive, acting inappropriately to circumstances, or behaving like a child.

When we see the true plight of our inner child, we can begin to have compassion for this suffering being, and gently offer support and love to ease the pain of this very difficult work. This is the layer we attend to first if it is available. We can get to this more easily if we don't jump in immediately to deal with the circumstantial layer, telling the child that the other person's actions came out of their own pain, or some other such thing. Though this is true and the adult always tells the child the truth, there is the deeper truth to deal with first.

Simply focus on the feeling, saying things like "You're feeling really scared/sad/angry right now, aren't you?" Or, "Do you feel lonely/sad/scared?" Or, "That must be really hard." Don't go to conceptual explanation or thoughts. Don't try to take the feeling away. Just stay with offering safety and support at first. "It's all right for you to have these feelings. I'm right here. I'll take care of you," etc.

At some point you can remind the child who she really is. The mind often knows the truth that we are love, but the deeply wounded child cannot feel it. The adult can help the wounded child to feel loved and beautiful by expressing these truths out loud. "You are a beautiful person. The essence of you is love. That is what you are at the very core of your being. Nothing can change or alter that—not what people say or think about you, not what you feel about yourself, not even the fact that, out of your pain, you may at times, do or say unkind things. Have mercy on yourself." Say these words, or words that may be more authentic for you, with as much heart as you can muster. Say them as if you were speaking to your only child—because you are—with love and encouragement—because it is the truth. If the child feels supported and loved, this can lead back into direct experience—the crux of healing.

Lack of Feelings Can Signal Trouble

Sometimes it may be a lack of feelings that may be a sign that your inner child is in trouble. After I went through my third chemotherapy session for breast cancer, I noticed that, though I had been really into baths in the year before the cancer, experiencing them as sensory enjoyment, I suddenly had an aversion, or at least no desire to get into the tub. When I did, it suddenly dawned on me that I wasn't feeling. My body had shut down. My inner child had turned off the sensory input valve. The last chemo had been so traumatic, so intense, so devastating that the inner child, it seemed, had just decided, "No more! If this is what feeling is like, I'll have none of it." I could see that it was going to require considerable nurturing and loving care to bring the child back into the realm of feeling again.

And it was a lesson, a very clear demonstration of what occurs when we are babies and children and have no tools to deal with the traumas that befall us. Here I was, a grown woman with nearly thirty years of meditation experience, as well as years of therapy, loving kindness practice, and working with the inner child—and still I was caught in a downward vortex over which I seemed to have no control. The cancer, on top of twenty years of chronic illness, had made me very vulnerable and childlike. The onslaught of the chemo, it seemed, had been overwhelming to my inner child, leaving me at the same time with no energy, no physical or emotional resources with which to deal with the problem. How much less, then, is a baby or small child able to deal with heavy emotional or physical trauma, having neither physical/emotional resources nor spiritual understanding/practice experience. Thus we carry our wounds with us into adulthood until we gather enough awareness, love and courage to finally open to and heal them.

After you have experienced as deeply as possible, you can go back and address the issue of the actual circumstances that precipitated the child's feelings. Say you're in a social situation, and feel you're being ignored or treated badly. The adult can assess the situation and tell the child what she sees. "So and so was really very busy with her party, and had too many things to think about." Or "She was ignoring you, but it was not because you're unlovable—it was because she has her own inner pain, and was trying to make herself feel important."

In 1980, when I first became ill, chronic fatigue wasn't even a known illness. When all my tests came up normal, many of my doctors, instead of acknowledging they were stumped, jumped immediately to psychosomatic explanations, and told me to look for a therapist. I remember the flush of shame I felt. To be *so* ill, and to have doctors telling you it's all in your head can be devastating. I began questioning myself—could I be making all this up? I knew how sick I felt—how real the physical symptoms were, and yet, I questioned my own mental health, because those in professional positions, those in authority seemed to be telling me it probably wasn't a physical illness at all. Who was I to question them?

Because illness or loss weakens us and makes us so vulnerable and childlike, we are especially susceptible to this kind of abuse. Years later, when I learned the techniques described above, I could tell the inner child that the doctors, as humans, were afraid of not knowing what was wrong with me. It brought up their own feelings of helplessness and incompetence. Naturally they wanted to go to a " known," so they could feel in control again, and not feel afraid. While it is important to be open to the fact that there may be, and probably are, psychological components to any illness, it is also very important to honor the truth that the body is telling us, and not to use our doctor's words as another excuse to beat ourselves up. What the doctor is saying may or may not be true, but the fact that he is saying it doesn't make it true. This is an extremely important inner distinction to make.

Having Our Buttons Pushed

There's also another important distinction to make—the distinction between the outer truth of the words themselves and the inner emotional or psychological truths that the words elicit for us. If the words have a particularly strong sting for us, a "charge," we can be sure there is a truth there. It may not be the literal truth of the situation. But there is a truth that lies hidden in the feelings we are carrying from some past experience which are brought to the surface by the words we hear or perhaps even someone's expression. This is called "having our buttons pushed." These are the feelings held over from a time when we felt judged, misunderstood, abandoned or unloved, or perhaps all of these, in the past, but for one reason or another chose not to or were unable to experience the feelings. So again, the process is always the same—first experience the truth of what you're feeling. Having done that, you can then turn to the circumstances and deal more appropriately with them.

There are so many issues that come up around illness and loss—it is really important for the adult to run interference. Many persons with chronic or even acute illness and those who have suffered great loss look normal. None of the chronic fatigue, fibromyalgia-type illnesses have any external visibility, and someone who has lost a beloved son or daughter or mate to cancer or tragedy may be crumbling on the inside and virtually nonfunctional while having a body that is physically intact.

Since we appear to look normal, others tend to expect us to act normally. When we sit after dinner instead of jumping up to help with the dishes, or other chores, this may be viewed by others as being lazy or inconsiderate. There may be indirect hints or even blatant comments. Or, we may hear about people's uncharitable thoughts through mutual friends or relatives. This can be very hurtful, but it is also another opportunity for us to do the work of a lifetime—to experience whatever hurt or rejection is being held in the body. After you have processed whatever deep feelings of unworthiness or rejection you're holding from the past, you can dialogue with the inner child, helping her to understand that the hurtful comments came out of ignorance.

People cannot possibly know what is going on for you in your body or soul. You are the only one who really knows.

Then you can assure the child that you'll take care of the situation if that is possible. If the child is lonely, you'll look into calling a friend, or if friends are lacking, explore the possibility of joining a support group or book club or something that will provide the possibility of making friends or feeling supported. Again, I want to stress that the main objective in this work and the deepest healing is to access the deep feelings of pain or loss and experience them.

If doing any of these practical things to take care of the inner child is being used to avoid experiencing, it might be better to put them off until the feeling has been processed, or at least to understand that these practical steps will not change us in any fundamental way. We will continue to bump up against those old familiar feelings until we finally stop resisting them and allow ourselves to experience them. However, taking these physical steps to care for and nurture the child, if done within the larger context of the loving kindness we are attempting to extend to ourselves, can facilitate deeper changes in our relationships with ourselves and others as well as our approach to life and spiritual practice.

Also there are several practical steps the inner adult can offer that will serve both the outer and the inner worlds. Those would be things like beginning a meditation practice, forming a practice group, finding a spiritual teacher, doing yoga, or simply finding more time to be alone in nature or with oneself.

CHAPTER 12

Getting to Yes and No— Taking a Stand Against False Beliefs

This is my no and I'm saying yes to it.

Sometimes Getting to Yes Means Accepting That You're Saying No

ONE EVENING, I lay on the couch unable to move, dishes and food splashed around the kitchen, stereo blaring too loud. I had found myself in the middle of a project when my energy just ran out. To make it to the couch was miracle enough—walking ten more feet across the room to turn the stereo down was beyond my strength. I'm used to this, but the frequency with which it had been occurring during the time I was receiving chemotherapy was taking its toll. I felt myself sinking into a black pit.

I tried to do my usual practice of surrender—allowing the moment to be what it was, doing my practice of getting to yes—but my whole being seemed to be rising up with a gigantic NO that completely overshadowed the Yes. The activities I had done were not frivolous. They were part of my cancer therapy—making myself vegetable juice and cooking some healthy vegetables. Of course I should have known better after going to the doctor and making juice that cooking anything would be too much. But it all caved in on me—the tininess of my life—a life that seemed to be getting tinier and tinier every day. Was I about to disappear?

All evening I struggled—crying and crying, trying to come to yes, like I have so many times in the past, and was not able to do so. I was not able to surrender. The NO was too big—too strong. My experience that evening is an example of how the three steps of working with emotions—extending loving kindness to ourselves, experiencing, and uncovering false beliefs—intertwine with one another and feed one another. I thought I was working with experiencing, which I was, when I came to the big NO. The gigantic NO—the resistance again so strong, and not wanting the cup I'd been given, like that night so many years earlier, when I had finally been able to say yes to my chronic illness and it gave me such strength and peace. But this was stronger. It was mammoth, and I couldn't seem to get around it, through it, or into it.

I saw clearly that the only way I would ever come to yes in this grappling was to wrap a yes around the no, more or less—just say yes to the no, to surrender to it and to willingly experience what seemed like a massive wall of resistance. I said to myself, "Okay, if this is what's here—this is the no, this is *my* no and I'm saying yes to it." It wasn't like one of those big cathartic things, where I gasp and shake, but there was more of an inner catharsis, like an understanding—like, "Oh yeah, no is part of life." And so including that no seemed like a really important thing.

Beneath the resistance was anger. I thought it was anger at God. Though my concept of this Being I had called God and continued to do so along with other names, through lack of a better system, had changed considerably through the years. I was amazed and somewhat alarmed at my words and demeanor toward the High Spirit I had revered, honored and worshipped most of my life. But the words welled up in me with great strength and power. They were not disrespectful. I simply stated with a sense of great authority that I did not accept this place given to me—I did not accept this suffering.

So I thought at first that who I was saying no to was God, to the cancer, and to this miserable body I had been given; that I was not going to simply accept this sentence that seemed to be imposed on me. I actually thought at the time that I was going to give the cancer back to God and that my body was going to change; that I would finally heal because I had broken through the barrier of being passive and taking whatever was thrown at me. I realized only later that what I was saying no to were my false beliefs, my drama, my story of who I am.

God Save Me from God

In a sense I *was* saying no to god—but it was the false god of false beliefs—the idol that keeps us enslaved to materialism. I think this is what Meister Eckhart meant when he said, "God save me from God." If there is something "out there" that we seem to need to get, that is not God, because God is inside of us all the while. But even if it's something "in there," something inside of us, that we think we need to get or access or open to, which really means that it is still an object outside of us—that's not it either. My first guru said,

> Throw everything out. Throw out your ideas of what you think you need or don't need. Throw out your ideas of what you think you can't possibly stand to be without or to be with. Throw out your expectations, your shoulds, would haves and could haves, your regrets, your ideas of how your life was supposed to be. Whatever is inside you, good or bad—your worst nightmares and your most treasured or sacred dreams—throw them all out. *And when only emptiness remains, take a good firm hold of that and throw it out too.*

Twenty years of chronic illness got me to YES. That was a big deal. That was tremendously important. But it took cancer to get me to NO. It took 54-3/4 years of living with my false beliefs about myself before I realized I could just say no to them—to those negative dreams—to those descriptions that were simply stories woven out of other people's dreams, dreams that I took on as my own.

The particular picture and belief I was saying no to that night on the couch was the belief that I was "less than" because I had a body that was sick and weak, a body that had grown a cancer, and a body that didn't allow me to do many of the things other people can do. I was saying no to the dream of "damaged goods" and powerlessness. There was an immense freedom that came with the realization that I do not have to accept that dream—that I can say no to that dream. I do not have to take the place assigned to me. I do not have to fulfill those pictures that other people have of me or that I have of myself.

At the same time, I realized that I still do need to say yes—a resounding and complete yes—to the physical and emotional reality that is present in each moment. Feelings, experiences and situations such as pain, aloneness, a body that does not work—perhaps even a body that is dying of cancer—the reality that because this body is limited, certain experiences are simply not available to me, the pain I may cause others with my own words or actions, the fact that loved ones die or suffer, and the resultant feelings that arise from all these events are things that I must continue to say yes to, and open to completely. This is a difficult path to tread.

My "Yes" Religion

I have learned that if I stay with my deep body knowing, it will teach me things that are beyond my comprehension, at least beyond anything I could come to with the conscious mind. I had attended a healing circle a few days earlier led by a Ph.D. therapist, who spoke about how we need to say no sometimes very strongly to certain things. I had disagreed with him, espousing the belief, which seemed to have become my "religion," that we need to say yes to everything. Of course this *was* a religion that had emerged out of deep inner searching, and an authentic inner knowing. Therefore, there was a deep truth in what I was saying. The leader deferred to me, because he saw this truth. And the others in the group recognized the truth in what I said, took it in, and learned from it as well. However, after this experience with the no, I realized that there was also truth in what he had said, and what John Ruskin, in his book, *Emotional Clearing,* had said about affirmations and about the value of saying no to certain beliefs.

So there was that reminder again about not settling down in any one truth. Once again I was humbled. I had used affirmations when I was younger, but developed a disdain for them as I learned the value of experiencing and saw the dangers of covering over painful experiences with Pollyanna statements. Many people, I think, use affirmations in this way, hoping for a kind of "shortcut" or easy way to their desired healing or individuation. While this practice can lead to momentary feelings of release, exhilaration or a sense of power, it ultimately does nothing to heal the deep wounds most of us carry from childhood which can be healed only by opening to the painful blocked experiences. Rusian says,

> Affirmations are used correctly when the intention is to recondition the unconscious mind to be accepting. As with positive attitude, they are used incorrectly when the intention is to avoid what is perceived as unpleasant experience or feelings (1993, 262).

This is where it is vital to be able to distinguish between thoughts and feelings, which are very commonly confused. If you ask someone how they feel about something, their answer will often be a thought rather than a feeling. For example, in answer to the question, "How do you feel about Sarah?" A friend said, "Sarah is stuck up." This answer is a thought. It is a belief or assumption about Sarah. Feelings are never about the other person. They are about the person expressing the feeling. The feeling about Sarah might have been, "I hate Sarah," or "I resent Sarah," or "I'm angry with Sarah for not going out with me." On a deeper level the feeling might be, "I'm hurt," or "I'm sad." And the belief about himself might have been, "I'm a loser," "I don't have what it takes to get a girl," or "I'll never be loved."

Beliefs Are Not Feelings

Beliefs are not feelings, and in most cases feelings must be dealt with before belief systems can be changed. My friend may not be able to change his beliefs about himself by simply affirming, "I am a winner," or "I am lovable." The feelings themselves must be accessed and experienced first. Beliefs are then sometimes changed simply through experiencing the suppressed emotions. In my case, allowing myself to experience my anger led to a realization of how I was keeping myself stuck with my negative false beliefs of "not enoughness."

Sometimes, however, simply becoming aware of a restricting belief and being willing to question, even for a moment, its unremitting truth can lead to an opening for change.

I used to have a pretty well entrenched belief that I needed to be understood. This belief impacted my life and my relationships in a big way and led to a lot of unhappiness. One of the big reasons I thought I couldn't be with my ex-husband was that I didn't feel understood. A few years after we separated, I was dating a man and saw that old familiar frustration of feeling misunderstood arising again ("Big Surprise!"). I remember walking down my road one morning and suddenly being struck by the most bizarre idea: "What if I don't really *need* to be understood?" The fact that it even occurred to me to ask the question, and that I was willing to, meant that something was already changing.

The "no" experience sheds some light on what I see to be the meaning behind a ritual in the Orthodox Christian Church that once stopped me cold from taking the final steps to actually *becoming* orthodox a number of years ago. The ritual is part of the baptism ceremony, where the person to be baptized turns around at the door of the church so they are facing the outside and spits "on the devil." I couldn't bring myself to do that for a number of reasons. For one, I must admit it seemed a little ridiculous. And I didn't really believe in the Devil as an entity. But it did bring me to some serious introspection when I tried to look beneath the words and the forms to what I thought were the real issues they represented.

I felt that the Christian idea of the Devil was the same as what is called Maya, or "illusion," in Eastern practices. I thought that to turn around and "face the Devil" would be to give form and weight to something illusory; and that the result would be exactly the opposite of what it seemed must be the intention behind the ritual: to take a stand against evil and to move toward God. I felt that I needed to keep my eyes on God, that I had already made the irrevocable decision to go forward on the spiritual path and had already metaphorically "turned my back on the Devil" or what he represents, which to me is falsehood.

It seemed that making this formal turning around to face the devil would be spiritually tantamount to the ill-fated turning back of several biblical and mythological characters. Lot's wife, for example, who was warned not to look back but did so anyway, was turned into a pillar of salt; and Orpheus, who was warned not to look back when leading his beloved Eurydice out of Hell, looked back in a moment of doubt at the very doorsill of the underworld to make sure she was following, and consequently lost his love forever.

From the Christian tradition, I thought of Peter when he saw Jesus walking on the water. After Jesus called to Peter to step out of the boat and come to him across the water, Peter began in faith, but halfway to his Lord, he was overcome by fear and doubt and took his eyes off Jesus to look down at the storm-whipped water. At that point he began to sink.

So, in contemplating all this, I reasoned that to turn back around and address the devil in any way would be losing my path. But on this night, my own inner being was teaching me about the value—the necessity, really—of taking another stand against falsehood; of facing it again squarely head on and saying no boldly and firmly; and of the prospect that it would most likely be necessary to continue to do this time and time again into the future. So in one sense I think I was correct in my interpretation of the myths and stories about turning back. The way I see it now is that turning back does represent taking my focus off the divine, which is life as it is. But I must also keep an eye on my false beliefs, which continue to control or interfere with my life in many ways and cause me to doubt and turn away from my true self, my path, and life as it is.

We Usually Have It Backwards

Of course, there is still truth in my "yes" religion. The yes is vital and leads to the transformation of negative emotions and states of mind through the willingness to simply experience them. Many people are so firmly entrenched in the "no" religion that learning the wholehearted "yes" can be life-altering. Even that night, in the larger sense, I *did* need to say yes. I needed to say yes to the great "NO" that rose up like a lion from some deep place of wisdom within to teach me. Learning the "No"—what it meant and how and when to use it—was extremely important to me. It was like a bookend to the yes. Like Gangaji said when I told her about my experiences with the yes and the no, "We usually have it backwards—we usually say yes to our story and no to our experiences." Turning these tendencies back around is part of our work as spiritual warriors.

Learning the inner yes and truly opening to our experiences and emotions is pivotal, but it is only half the equation of deep healing. The other half is saying no to our negative belief system and our endless opinions and judgments about everything imaginable—in other words, to the story line of our personal drama. Our deepest beliefs and opinions—about how life "ought" to be or about who we think we are—are so thoroughly ingrained that we do not even know they are beliefs. They are the unquestioned shadows that hang over our lives like a dense fog that has shrouded our perception of ourselves and our lives for so long that we have come to believe that this is how things really are, that this is the true face of reality.

These beliefs are closely, perhaps inextricably, connected to our suppressed emotions because they were often put into place at a time when we were young children or babies and certain emotions were too overwhelming to experience. Thus many people may have the common negative or restricting beliefs that the world is unsafe or too difficult, that they are too small, too weak, too incompetent to deal with life, or that they are unworthy or unlovable.

Illness Can Begin to Eat Away at Our Self-Esteem

Most of us go through life thinking that we're not quite good enough or that life itself should be some other way than what it is. There is almost no end to the negative false beliefs that we humans have adopted and carry around with us all the time that make our lives much more limited and painful than they actually need to be. When we are sick, these negative beliefs are accentuated, or beliefs may appear that weren't there before. Illness can begin to eat away at our self-esteem. We can begin to see ourselves as no better than a lump of clay lying there—worse in fact, because we depend on others for help. We begin to think of ourselves as impacting our loved ones in a negative way—being a burden to them, a downer in their lives, a liability.

This may be accentuated when important people in our lives collude with us in these negative beliefs. Marie, a woman in my support group, has a debilitating illness that is accompanied by almost constant pain, making it impossible for her to do many physical activities. Her husband never accepted her illness or the limitations it imposed on the kinds of things they were able to do together. He was also bitter about the fact that she couldn't contribute to daily chores in any significant way. She heard over and over again his litany of complaints about what she couldn't do which fed into and reinforced her already established belief that she is "not enough." She called this "Jack's list."

Part of Jane's disabling agoraphobia included episodes during what she called her "freak out" period when her mind would begin to spin out of control with thinking about thinking. She always blamed herself for this but recalls that her mom and even one of her teachers reinforced that tendency in her:

> Ever since I was little—I think out of concern when I would have these weird scary things happen at night—my mom would always say, "Honey, you have to stop thinking so much. You're going to cause problems for yourself."
>
> When I was recovering and working to get out of this agoraphobia, this was the refrain that came a lot: "You've got to stop thinking so much. It's making you sick." Even the doctor who taught my phobia class made me feel guilty, like it was my mind that got me into this mess, like I had to learn to have control over it. And it was true—I did have to learn mental control. But somehow, either the way it was put, or the way I interpreted it, it made me feel like I was at fault for this problem and that the part of myself that is attracted to introspection is bad. So it was such a weird, hard thing to deal with because, on the one hand, I had this natural inclination, and on another hand, a certain channeling of that thinking was going to be my ticket out of here. And I wasn't able to separate out what was what and I just felt guilty a lot of the time.
>
> Another reason I couldn't really express where my mind went and what kinds of things I thought about was that I was afraid of criticism or feeling, "you're doing exactly the thing that's making you sick." And that's something I've carried. It's only been in the last couple of years that I've started making headway on constantly feeling the need to apologize for thinking deeply and being introspective.
>
> I know now that it is a capacity that was misguided early on. I didn't know how to use it and it was self-destructive in a lot of ways, but that capacity isn't the problem, and I've learned how to use it differently and continue to learn. It's not that I don't have any of those destructive tendencies, but it becomes clear that it is a gift, even if it's not a gift that I can appreciate all the time.

This is such an important point—and has been for me life changing: coming to understand that most, if not all, of our destructive tendencies are, at their base, positive impulses. If we can withhold our judgment and look more deeply, as Jane was finally able to do, we will often find gold buried beneath the rubble.

You Have Not Sinned

A friend said to me one morning, "Both my boyfriend and my former mate said the same thing to me, so I thought I should look at that. They both said that maybe I'm sick because I don't want to look at what I might do with my life if I were well." That hit me in a familiar place. In the early days of my illness several of my doctors suggested I go to a psychologist for help or that I was depressed and needed medication. I looked and looked at ways I might have made myself sick. And I *was* depressed. But I was depressed for a reason.

When my body broke down, my pain, weakness, and disability seemed at first to be centered mainly in my arms. I thought that I may have made myself sick so I wouldn't have to deal with the immense sadness and frustration I was feeling over the impasse between my husband and me in relation to having another child. I thought that perhaps in my deep subconscious some twisted logic reasoned: "If my body and particularly my arms don't work, there is no way I can hold or take care of a new baby. Therefore this tremendous block between my husband and me will not need to be dealt with and I will not have to feel this pain."

While these explorations into possible psychological explanations for illness may yield valuable insights into how we sabotage ourselves in many aspects of our lives, it also opens up a huge can of worms. The problem with this way of thinking is that at some point our bodies will fail. They *will* fail. We *will* die. And if we have subscribed to this line of reasoning, that failure will be seen as our fault. Even though we may know in our heads that everyone dies, we will feel in our bones that we must have done something wrong or our bodies would not be failing.

This is not, however, to say that we have no effect upon our state of health. That line of reasoning is equally fallacious. This kind of either/or thinking is usually not fruitful. Life is a mix of things and events, some of which we can affect with our actions, but over most of which we have little or no control.

In the larger sense, of course, we have no control at all, but in the relative world, in our everyday life, we must act "as if" we have some control. It is our job. The physical and the spiritual worlds are connected in some mysterious way, which we, as humans, cannot fully see or understand. We do not really need to understand or explain. We only need to live each moment from the heart. Sometimes it seems that it is not possible to do this. Something gets in the way. If we examine our belief systems, it may often be revealed that it is some negative false belief which stands in the way or blocks us from experiencing our true heart: "I am unworthy." "I am weak." "I don't deserve happiness." It is important to remember that pain and illness are not punishments, though this is a commonly held false belief. Mercy. Mercy on ourselves for whatever reason we are sick or in pain, whether we helped to create it or not. Mercy on the others in our lives on whom we may have placed blame, whether or not they helped to create our illness or loss.

Sometimes I still deal with heavy judgment around having a body that doesn't work, that seems so incredibly messed up in so many ways. Of course it's unreasonable, but some part of me still takes that on as a failure on my part.

Our entrenched belief systems do not go gently into that dark night. A little loving kindness and the withholding of double judgment (judging ourselves for judging ourselves) goes a long way toward helping ourselves with the eventual relinquishment of these insidious beliefs.

Relationships may reinforce our negative self-beliefs, but they can also be a vehicle to help us see and work with beliefs that we may have been adept enough at avoiding as a single person. Paul, another man in our support group, had dealt with diabetes and Parkinson's disease for many years but had avoided getting in touch with his feelings of "not enoughness" by avoiding relationships altogether. When a woman suddenly appeared in his life that he couldn't help falling in love with, he came face to face with his fears and deeply held feelings of inadequacy. His girlfriend had difficulty dealing with his health conditions, and Paul experienced anger at his illnesses for the first time. This was a very positive step for Paul. By getting in touch with his anger and fears, he began to free up the tremendous energies that had been bound up in their suppression. He also began to see the stories he was buying into that he is damaged goods, that he is unlovable, and that life is unfair.

False Beliefs and Fears

The following negative beliefs and fears seem to be the ones most connected to illness or loss and the ones that I and many of my ill or disabled friends have struggled with extensively. It could be anybody's list, but I think illness or loss accentuates them.

False beliefs and fears related to but not limited to illness and loss:

- I'm helpless.
- I'm incompetent.
- I'm small.
- I'm "less than."
- I'm damaged goods.
- I have no power.
- I need to be independent to be a worthwhile person.
- I need to do things to be a worthwhile person.
- I need to help people to be a worthwhile person.
- If I do the "right" things, i.e. choose the right healing path, meditate, be peaceful, love myself, etc. etc. I will get well.
- I deserve to be sick.
- I am sick because:
    1. I made myself sick.
    2. I have negative beliefs.
    3. I'm bad, stupid, defective.
    4. I'm not spiritual enough.
- If I have conflicts in my life, there is something wrong with me.
- I'm supposed to be able to keep up with things, i.e. keep my life in order, my house clean, bills paid, repairs done, pets vaccinated, laundry done, etc. even though I am sick or disabled.
- If I'm sick, there is something wrong with me in a much deeper way than simply physically.
- I'm letting people down because I'm sick and I can't get well.
- If I can't heal myself, I am a failure.
- People will think I'm irresponsible.
- People will think I'm a whiner.
- People will think I'm a fake.

- People will think I'm a hypochondriac.
- People won't want to be around me.
- People will think I just can't hack life.
- People will think I'm a quitter.
- People will think I'm lazy.
- People will forget about me.
- People will think I'm a slob.
- People will dismiss me as someone not viable.
- People will dismiss me as someone unorganized.
- People will get tired of me with my needs.
- People will leave me alone.
- I'm not enough.
- Life is unfair.
- Fear of being nothing.
- Fear of loss of control.
- Fear of chaos.
- Because of all of the above, I am unlovable.

I have the belief, "other people heal—I don't." "Other people get true love—not me."

But where *are* these "other" people? Most of the people I see around me are desperately seeking happiness or love or healing or the alleviation of the pain they are in, or some refuge from the chaos in their lives.

I was flabbergasted when I saw the power my unconscious negative beliefs and fears had held over me, and the depths to which I had to be pushed to realize this and take a stand against them. So how does one, in an ordinary life, have a chance to see and work with these insidious negative beliefs? Fortunately, you don't have to have a life-threatening illness to begin to work with false beliefs. You can begin small.

Labeling Thoughts

The first step is to begin to notice your thoughts. Joko Beck, who developed the Ordinary Mind Zen School and was, for many years, the head teacher at the San Diego Zen Center, taught a practice of labeling thoughts. This practice can be used during meditation or can be done anywhere, anytime you become aware of your thoughts.

Our minds are almost constantly churning out thoughts: mapping out a route to the store, making lists, arranging schedules and vacations, thinking about what we will say to our boss/child/husband, (or what we should have said!), telling us how stupid or incompetent we are, why we can't do what we want to do (we don't have the talent, courage, intelligence,) etc., etc. The mental activities of making lists and planning can be dealt with by making a mental note, "planning" and drawing the attention back to whatever meditation practice you are doing, or returning to a simple awareness of your body.

With other kinds of thoughts, it may be useful to be very specific with the labeling for the purpose of bringing to conscious awareness the negative beliefs that so severely limit our lives. Joko suggests prefacing the thought with the term, "having a believed thought that...." I haven't studied with Joko directly but have used this practice in my own work, so I will explain how I use it.

For example, I might say, "having a believed thought that I'm full of hubris for writing a book about spiritual practice and no one will want to read or publish it." I know right away that this is a particularly juicy and potent negative belief that is limiting my life, so instead of returning to my practice of wide open awareness[4] after labeling it, I take some time to explore the belief and to go more deeply into the feeling behind it. I try to experience how the body feels as I hold that belief, where the body is holding tension or anxiety, if there is nausea or increased heart rate. Then I look at the belief itself. On closer examination, I might realize that there's another belief hidden within the first. So I might say, "Having a believed thought that I'm not good enough," or "... smart enough," or "... deep enough," or "... people will never appreciate me."

By labeling the thoughts with the preface, "Having a believed thought that...," I begin to develop some distance from these beliefs, and may become able to entertain the notion that they are not necessarily God's truth. And I might ask myself after each stated belief, "Is this true?" And the answer, if I am honest, has to be, "No," or "I don't know." I go back and forth between labeling the deepening levels of beliefs I am uncovering and acutely experiencing the feelings in the body that seem to accompany the belief.

Special Circumstances in Relationship

The fact that some people may actually do the things in relation to us that we fear they will do, or have the negative beliefs about us that we fear they will have or that we have about ourselves, does not make our fears or beliefs true, nor does it change the way we practice with them. Marie's fear of not being enough and her belief that she would be abandoned because she wasn't enough were reinforced by her husband's beliefs that he needed her to do things she physically couldn't, and by the fact that he eventually left her.

This kind of situation made it doubly hard for her to see that her "not enoughness" was a false belief. Marie's work was to go in and experience the pain of the feeling beneath her belief and the grief of being left alone—both feelings that mirrored childhood experiences. By her willingness to experience the "raw" feelings in her body without clinging to judgmental thoughts about herself or her husband, she began, slowly, to clear the blocks being held in the body and the belief "I'm not enough" began to soften. It no longer had the solidity it had or the same power over her. Eventually it became a small vestige that surfaced only on occasion during low spots for brief periods.

When Paul began to work with his anger, the first thing he realized was that anger at his Parkinson's felt safer than anger at his girlfriend. By bringing a simple awareness to his feelings and beliefs and allowing himself to experience and see them without judgment, he was able to go deeper step by step, like opening a package layer by layer. Finally he reached the core of self-hatred. A loving kindness practice helped him to see that he was a being worthy of love and that all his life he had been depriving himself of it. When he began to befriend himself and offer to himself the love he so desperately wanted, things changed dramatically for Paul. His diffidence diminished; he smiled easily and there was a lightness and easiness about him—a shining quality.

Turning It Around

Any item in the false beliefs list, starting with, "People will…," could just as easily read, "I will…," and this is, in fact, the truer and more relevant statement. Truer, that is, in the sense that our beliefs about other people are usually more about ourselves. In fact, a very useful practice to try with any belief beginning with they, he, she, or someone's name, is to substitute "I" for the other person and ask yourself if this is not as true or truer.

Many of us personal-growth or spiritual-seeker types understand, at least theoretically, the idea of projection—that most, if not all, of the negative and sometimes even the positive qualities we see in others are actually projections, that is, these qualities are actually in us, but we can't or would rather not see them. Understanding something theoretically and really "getting it," however, are thousands of miles apart.

Byron Katie's simple system of turn-arounds has worked well for me in helping to ferret out many of my projections and limiting negative self-beliefs. And, in an interesting twist, some of these turn-arounds have also offered me a way to support myself against these negative holdings of mind. Here's how it works: The first thing is to write down everything that upsets, angers, confuses or disappoints you about someone close to you or anyone who has triggered anger, disappointment, confusion, fear, sadness, etc. in you (section 1 of the Getting-Really-Honest Exercise[5]). When I do this exercise, I let myself get really childish and petty. I even exaggerate sometimes in trying to get to the nitty gritty. I don't try to pretty it up or soften it in any way.

For example: when I was infatuated with a new love interest in 1999, I was struggling with feelings of rejection. Though I knew intellectually that these feelings were all projections, I could not experience it emotionally. I was feeling stuck so I decided to do Katie's turn-arounds. I wrote, "I'm angry with and saddened by John because he doesn't care about me like I care about him. I'm angry with John because he doesn't ask me questions or want to know about me. I'm angry with and saddened by John because he doesn't feel like he needs to be with me and doesn't think about me all the time." When I did the turn-arounds, I saw that it was all about me and my relationship to myself. I was angry and saddened with myself for not caring about myself enough to ask myself questions about how I'm really feeling, to want to know about myself and to give myself what I need, to want to spend time with myself and to be aware of my own body in the world at all times, that is, to be present to my own experience from moment to moment.

In another section (section 4), I wrote that John was emotionally unavailable, guarded and hidden. The turn-around was that *I* was emotionally unavailable and hidden. I had prided myself on being available and open, but when I really went deep and sat with the turn-around, I saw that there was definitely a truth there that I had not been wanting to see. Maybe I wasn't as emotionally available as I thought.

This is a simple exercise that seems to work for me. Somehow by just putting out the embarrassing primal truth of how I am feeling about someone in my life that I care deeply about or have strong negative feelings about, and do the turn-arounds, I am able to see things about myself that I can't access directly otherwise.

Section 3 of the worksheet asks us to list the things that the object of our strong feelings should or shouldn't do, be, think, feel in the situation that has upset us. This "shoulding"—normally anathema to relationship work or even inner spiritual practice—turns into a gentle or sometimes shockingly epiphanic finger pointing back toward the self. "John should be more emotionally available. John should care about me, want to be with me, want to know about me," becomes "I should be more emotionally available. I should care about myself, want to be with myself, want to know about myself."

The real gold came for me in section 5 when I was asked to list the things that John might give me or could do in order for me to be happy. I wrote, "I need John to want to know about me. I need John to respond to what I say, to ask me questions, to want to be with me, to love me." The turnaround was my prescription for what I needed to do *for myself*—"I need myself to want to know about me. I need myself to respond to what I say, to ask myself questions, to want to be with me, to love me."

I already knew I needed to love myself. I had been doing the loving kindness meditation daily for several years with very positive results, but I still forgot sometimes and needed to be reminded. This was my reminder. But the most poignant and life-changing statements for me at the time were the statements that directed me to ask myself questions and to respond to what I say. What a revelation: I need to act on my own behalf (!) and not expect others to do it for me.

Sometimes it may be impossible to see the quality in yourself that you are put off by in another. This doesn't necessarily mean that it doesn't relate to you. If you have strong feelings about someone or something, it always means *something* about you. If it's not that you *have* that quality and are hiding or suppressing it, it may mean that you are very weak in that quality and that it needs to be developed or strengthened in you, even though the quality you see in the other person may seem to be negative.

What may appear to be a negative or undesirable quality or action is often a distortion or an exaggeration of a positive or healthy characteristic. For example, if you are put off by successful people that seem to you to be braggarts or to be arrogant about their own abilities, but do not see these qualities in yourself, you may be reacting to the strong belief these people have in themselves and the stand they're willing to take to promote their own well-being. This could be a weak point for you.

Whether or not these other people actually believe in themselves is really beside the point in terms of the benefits you stand to gain by looking closely at your own beliefs and feelings in the situation. These "other people" may be covering over their own insecurities with bravado and not really believe in themselves at all, but the essence of the energetic and insight lesson for you are the same either way. Perhaps you see yourself as humble and unassuming, but that may be a cover for your own low self-esteem and your fear of exposure if you "put yourself out there."

I have had to do a lot of work with this issue in myself, and along the same vein I sometimes see myself react strongly to people I see as selfish or greedy, or may feel outraged when I see someone take advantage of those who are not in a position to defend themselves. While I'm sure this is partly due to the fact that I see the selfish and greedy aspects of my own self, I think it is also an inner response to or recognition of something that is weak or lacking in me. If these qualities, selfishness and greediness, are distilled down to their healthy essence, we find self-love, the willingness to take a stand to care for oneself, and the ability to maintain healthy boundaries. Having healthy boundaries and standing up for myself are things that I have had to work on continually.

Working with the "No" in Small Ways

Not everybody's NO will appear on the scene as dramatically and ferociously, nor as spontaneously as mine did. Sometimes we must choose to say no as we come to understand how our beliefs are running our lives. We can begin in simple ways in the more mundane happenings of everyday life. Once I was trying out saying no to a cultural belief that I had grown up with and subscribed to, that women are not supposed to call men, that men are supposed to make the first move in a relationship. I told myself that it didn't matter what the man's response was going to be, that it didn't make me "less than" if he didn't want to have a relationship with me.

So I called a man I had met at a conference and there seemed to be a positive response. But he was very busy, and I was very busy, so it seemed we weren't going to get to talk for a while. After a while it seemed to be getting awkward and I got the sense that maybe there wasn't going to be anything happening here. I still had no idea whether I would actually be attracted to this man if we were to get together, but some ancient feelings and beliefs arose insidiously and crept into my psychic and physical space. I experienced a familiar yucky feeling in the pit of my stomach—shame and wanting to run away, wanting to hide, wanting to somehow just get out of this pseudo relationship.

I started to call myself names: "stupid" for doing this; "flawed" for not realizing that this was not a good way to go about starting a relationship; "undesirable." And I watched my mind making up a story about how he wasn't interested; that he never had been interested and that it was because I am not an interesting person or I'm just too weird; because I was too "forward"; because I am sick.

All the old belief systems were arising. Even though I had forewarned myself, I forgot momentarily as I was gripped by the power of these old emotions and beliefs. I saw myself making what was really a positive step for me into something bad, something shameful. But in time I came to myself, and remembered that these were simply feelings *that needed to be experienced* and beliefs *to which I could say no*. So again I saw that the appearance of these seemingly "bad" feelings was actually a good thing—an opportunity for clearing old suppressed emotions and working with entrenched beliefs. I did learn that maybe yes, this wasn't the best way to go about initiating a new relationship, but I also understood that having done it that way didn't make me a bad or undesirable person.

It is important to remember that once you have had a strong experience of seeing your belief systems and working with them positively and saying no to them, it doesn't mean they are going to just go away. They are still there. They permeate our lives so completely and they have made tracks in our brains that are not going to just go away simply because we see them—though seeing them will definitely move the process along. It is guaranteed we will forget. We'll be caught again in our belief systems and in our old emotions. We must be diligent and offer ourselves loving kindness when we forget. This is a long process. We will not be a changed person with one realization.

The Myth of Consistency

Many of us spend much of our lives and energy shutting life out—living in a mode of self-protection because life seems just too dangerous to open to completely. When we open the door a crack, we inevitably meet pain or rejection because of our negative self-beliefs, which reinforces our perception that the world is dangerous and that relationships are destined to cause us pain, and we slam it shut again.

One day I realized that one of the things holding me back from being here now is the thought or belief that my emotions need to make sense—that I need to somehow be consistent or cohesive in my feelings. This is ridiculous of course, because I go back and forth between joy and sorrow like a chess piece on a chessboard. Still I have the idea that I "should" be consistent. Children do not have this limiting belief. Their emotions sometimes shift radically back and forth in a matter of minutes from laughter to tears and back to laughter again.

Perhaps those of us who share this quality may take heart in the biblical injunction, "You must become as little children." I see again, as I dig deeper, the close connection between beliefs and feelings. Beneath the belief that I need to make sense and be cohesive is fear—fear of chaos, loss of control, abandonment, and extinction. Who am I then if not a solid self? Who will love me if I'm not consistent in my feelings? How will I know what to do if I don't listen to my "shoulds?"

Getting to Yes and No—Taking a Stand Against False Beliefs

The inner guide or rudder which carries us across the ocean of life is hidden beneath the waters. It is a powerful force that cannot be denied, but we are reluctant to abandon our mental compass and give ourselves to that inner childlike knowing because we do not trust in the larger graciousness of being. We are often not willing to give over our illusory control until it is taken from us by some seemingly harsh hand of fate. This is the challenge—to let ourselves be taken—because life is continually, in big and little ways, showing us that we are not in control.

"The Man Watching"
by Rainer Maria Rilke (Barrows & Macy, 1996)

I can tell by the way the trees beat, after
so many dull days, on my worried windowpanes
that a storm is coming,
and I hear the far-off fields say things
I can't bear without a friend,
I can't love without a sister.

The storm, the shifter of shapes, drives on across the woods and across time,
and the world looks as if it had no age:
The landscape, like a line in the psalm book, is seriousness and weight and eternity.

What we choose to fight is so tiny!
What fights with us is so great!
If only we would let ourselves be dominated
as things do by some immense storm,
we would become strong too, and not need
names.

When we win it's with small things,
and the triumph itself makes us small. What is
extraordinary and eternal
does not want to be bent by us.
I mean the Angel who appeared

to the wrestlers of the Old Testament: when the
wrestlers' sinews
grew long like metal strings,
he felt them under his fingers
like chords of deep music.

Whoever was beaten by this Angel
(who often simply declined the fight)
went away proud and strengthened
and great from that harsh hand,
that kneaded him as if to change his shape.
Winning does not tempt that man.
This is how he grows: by being defeated, decisively,
By constantly greater beings.

CHAPTER 13

The Peace That Surpasseth Understanding

A Zen student once asked his teacher what enlightenment gave him. The teacher said, "Before enlightenment I was depressed. After enlightenment I was depressed."

IT IS NATURAL FOR HUMANS to strive to be happy, but I think we get confused. There is the "peace that surpasseth understanding," and there is comfort, the easy life—pleasure. We confuse the joy of Being with the small happiness that comes momentarily from getting what we want, the kind of happiness that dissolves the moment we lose our desired object or suddenly realize we want something else after all.

If we seek the peace that surpasseth understanding, it helps to know what it is not. Sometimes a concept is so vast or incomprehensible that it is impossible to define or understand in our usual, logical way of understanding. God, peace, and love, are some of those concepts. One of the ways philosophers use to know what or who God is, is to identify what he is not. There are experiences in our lives that can help us to learn this.

With my chronic illness, I experience great swings in my state of health, well-being and energy. One of the things I'm beginning to learn from this on-again off-again flirtation with wellness, with feeling good again in the body and then feeling bad again, is to learn what peace is not—what deep spiritual well-being is not—what God is not. It is not the surge of well-being that comes from the body—from bodily well-being. That good feeling is wonderful. When we feel it, all is right with the world. We feel alive and ready to take on new challenges, to be kind, to be generous to others, to clean the house, balance the checkbook, take a walk, fix that leaky faucet or do something creative. There's nothing wrong with this—and there's nothing wrong with enjoying it and fully entering into it when it is present. In fact, this is what our true spiritual aspiration calls us to do. The problem arises when we mistake this feeling for spirituality itself or when we think this is how we're "supposed" to feel and, if we don't, that we must strive to get that feeling again.

This kind of well-being is of the body and cannot last. It is easy to mistake it for spiritual well-being, to feel that we must be doing something right to feel this way. The downside of this viewpoint, of course, is that when it goes away, as it surely will, we will then feel that we must have done something wrong—that we have fallen from grace, when in fact it is just the natural rhythm of things. Every up has its down, every day its night, and each physical life of the body has sickness and death.

Life events or experiences that seem to elevate us into an extraordinary state of peace or euphoria bring the same teaching. Being "in love" is, of course, the magic elixir pursued throughout history as that which will finally bring true happiness and completion. The rock group The Eagles sing, "I've got to know if your sweet love is gonna save me," a song written by Jack Tempchin. And that's what we think—that love will save us—that someone or something will save us. And when we're in love, it does feel like heaven. The song from *The Sound of Music* expresses what we feel, "Somewhere in my life I must have done something right, because here you are loving me…" But when love goes—so goes happiness. I think the number of brokenhearted love songs outweighs the songs of love's fulfillment. But really they are two sides of a whole.

These losses that catapult us into crisis or despair often bring us face to face with what we need to learn or see. When I got the news that those two little lumps in my breast, which every doctor had taken pains to assure me were nothing to worry about, were, in reality, cancer, I was stunned and devastated. "How could this be?" I asked myself. In the previous fifteen years, every aspect of my life—physical, emotional, psychological and spiritual—had been carefully examined and turned toward a path of healing and spiritual opening. How could

I, all this time, have been growing a cancer? How could I be so off track? It seemed unfathomable. And how, I wondered, could I even be asking myself these questions? Hadn't I already learned that my happiness doesn't depend on bodily well being? I thought I had found my way to peace—to true happiness. But that peace was shattered in an instant. And for a short time I was thrown back again into confusion, self-blame, and a sense of failure.

The failure I felt from actually having the cancer paled in comparison to that which I experienced on an emotional and spiritual level when I saw the depth of my devastation from this new physical onslaught. I was supposed to be "spiritual." I was supposed to be beyond this kind of devastation. I remembered the time in the '70s when I took P.D. Ouspensky's teaching of the non-expression of negative emotions and misconstrued it into another form of suppression. It took me years to undo the fallout from that when I finally understood what I had been doing. And recalling the many other false starts and wrong turns in my spiritual path, I wondered if I had happened down another dead-end or veering side path.

Yet as I examined my life and my spiritual practice spanning the previous ten years, I couldn't see how I could have done anything different. I still felt that the work I had done was good. I had made bold steps and I had entered more and more deeply into my heart. I had uncovered deeply held false beliefs, old griefs, and ancient wounds that needed healing. It was painful but I knew it was cleansing and right. I finally came to the realization that this was not some big mistake I had blundered into, but part of a deeper opening on my path. "Perhaps," I thought, "I'm finally entering the basement—the place from which there's nowhere to go but up." It sure felt like it. But I knew that in truth, there is no "finally." The trap is always in thinking one has reached the final truth, the true understanding that will finally bring freedom and love from that time forward.

While the ups and downs of chronic illness had taught me many important things, it took cancer to bring me to the edge of the abyss and force me to look. I seem to always need to learn things the hard way. The cancer, now it seems to me, was a necessary condition for me to understand the basic fear at the bottom of existence—the fear beneath every other fear—the fear of death—the fear of nonexistence.

Perhaps not everyone needs to face cancer or death in order to understand this. I guess I did, perhaps because I'm a hard case.

Even though I thought I might die when I first became chronically ill, I lost that fear after a while, and saw that I would probably just be ill for the rest of my life. That was like facing death in a certain way, because it was the end of my life as I knew it. It certainly felt like death in many ways. I often felt that I was half dead and half alive. But after a long time I was able to grieve my lost life. My heart cracked open and I allowed myself to feel the pain of that—the pain of such a huge loss—and with it came the grief of a lifetime of losses, which I had not previously allowed myself to feel. I learned how to be with my life in the midst of my grief, how to be with life in its most basic forms—walking, lying, sitting, eating. It was a huge teaching. Enough for one lifetime, I thought. I came to a place of peace, of real happiness, perhaps for the first time in my life. And that peace and happiness seemed to sustain itself and to permeate my life even into all the dark corners and through all the hard balls life threw at me: divorce, loneliness, troubles with loved ones, financial crises—many of the things that commonly throw people into despair or depression—I was meeting them all, it seemed, with a certain equanimity. Though I had still struggled with all the old demons—fear, sadness, doubt, clinging, and even brief interludes of despair, they seemed to pass through fairly quickly and to be held in a larger context of loving kindness and acceptance.

Then came cancer. And at the same time love came knocking. I opened both doors and was thrown into an amazing place between heaven and hell—joy and devastation together. I kept opening my heart further and further as I had been taught. The love however, was short lived. I realized later that the love had helped me to bear the weight of facing the cancer. I also thought, on looking back, that perhaps the loving itself was fostered by the deep heart opening I experienced through facing cancer.

Opening to death and loss of love together, however, was too much, and the loss crushed me. I woke up one morning and realized I was unhappy. What a shock. I had been crying every day for weeks—after having been happy for a good number of years, perhaps eight or nine, for the first time in my life—after having experienced real happiness, real peace. "What happened?" I asked myself. I had thought, when I reached that place of happiness, that place of peace, it was forever. I thought I had crossed over that bridge. I thought that whatever was thrown at me, I could handle. I thought I knew how. I had opened my heart and allowed it to break and thought that nothing could ever shatter me again. But there was the face of death laughing at me. And there was loss of love mocking me. They seemed to be saying, "Ha, let's see if you really have equanimity. Let's see if your heart is really open."

I was devastated. I was broken all over again. I felt like someone had left the cake out in the rain, and I wondered how I would ever be able to open again, to trust again. The cancer had made me so open, so vulnerable. And before that the chronic illness had already made me so open and vulnerable. Chronic illness, and being alone had been my koan. I thought I had passed it. But now this was a whole new koan. I had thought I could handle anything—even facing death and loss of love. But one day in the midst of chemotherapy, I was overwhelmed by the incredible confusion and pain. It seemed too much to bear. I burst into tears and blurted out to one of my very compassionate doctors, "I don't want this life. I want a different life." To hear a statement like that coming out of my mouth, especially in front of a doctor, shocked me.

All of my life I had struggled with the deep pain of life and being who I was. Having grown up in a dysfunctional family with an alcoholic father and an emotionally wounded mother, I carried the wounds of the generations with me, as we all do. Yet somehow I managed to have a very rich inner life that kept me going. When I looked around me at all the people coming in and out of my life, I never could truly say I would exchange places with any of them.

Even when I was younger, very young—even before I started on this path, even before I had my big breakthrough and came to peace and equanimity, even when I was a miserable teenager—I never felt I wanted a different life. I always somehow felt that the life I had and what I was learning were more valuable than any of the people's lives I saw around me. Probably that was still true. If I really looked around me, I wouldn't find anyone I really wanted to exchange myself with. But that cry, that "I don't want this life, I want a different life," didn't come out of the thinking mind. It came out of the heart—it came out of brokenness and despair.

So though I thought I had reached the bottom with my chronic illness—that it had taught me what I needed to know about death and loss—there was more to learn. With the cancer, that feeling, that realization, was more imminent. With every new pain, with every symptom from the chemo, I saw the fear arise: fear around the body; fear of a life unlived; fear that I would go to my grave not having done the things that I really wanted to do. It seemed that something or someone—perhaps life itself—was intent on bringing me all the conditions that would help me to understand the ephemeral nature of this life, and the exquisite beauty of this life. That all will be lost—all things will be lost—our possessions, our life, our love, our joy. But it became clear to me that the answer to this dilemma is not to withdraw from life and from all things, but to release the desperate clutching, the clinging, and to enter each moment, each joy, each morning, each opportunity for love as completely as possible. Within this moment of entering, all things, all knowledge, all awareness is present.

One morning after I was diagnosed with breast cancer and realized the truth of my own dying, I was walking down the road that I had been walking most every day for ten years. I picked a sprig of fennel from the roadside and brought it to my nose. I wept with the sweetness of that smell. My heart simply burst open and I was overcome with love for this world down to the tiniest blade of grass. The awareness that this moment will pass, like in the Kate Wolf song, "Days like flowers bloom and fade, and do not come again," make them precious beyond all imagining. This understanding of the futility of clinging, and the experience of living each moment simply for itself is the exquisite teaching of life-threatening illness. I no longer harbored the illusion of being changed forever, but each moment of opening seemed a miracle to embrace.

Sickness puts us on the fast-track of opening our hearts and minds to love and wisdom. And life-threatening illness puts us on the ultra-fast-track. Dealing with cancer, I saw all the parallel lines in my life trying to bring me to understanding. It was intense, but I saw the wisdom of it all, the necessity of learning the lessons I was being given. There was facing the cancer, and having a taste of death, and at the same time experiencing a taste of love and then losing it. The black river of loss seemed to engulf me at times, and yet the preciousness of life was right there in the midst of it all. These lessons, these teachings, were bringing me deeper and deeper into myself, closer to true understanding and moments of pure joy and freedom.

Probably if I had been well when my love left, I would have gone out and tried to meet and get involved with someone new. I definitely see the wisdom in not being able to do that, but instead, circling the wagons—seeing what existed in my own little circle of life and understanding—taking stock, and entering myself completely once again in light of all the new learning that had flooded my being. I wrote in my journal:

> So this, once again, is my path—opening to this sadness, opening to this brokenness, accepting and loving this broken being, accepting and loving this scarred breast that housed the cancer, facing death—the ultimate loss—the loss of everything human. And then, as if to illustrate this, getting love, and losing it, or rather, glimpsing love, glimpsing the possibility of love, and then losing it. As if to say, "This is what it's like—experience it!"—the ultimate loss of life, loss of love.
>
> I guess I should feel complimented, that God thought I was ready for this. It feels like it, but when I really look again, I see it's still only a baby step. I see it's still only a test case. I'm not really dying. I have breast cancer. I have a good chance. I have a 75 percent chance—of the cancer not coming back. And I didn't really have love and loss. It was only a taste of it. Oh my God, how much bigger if I *really* had love and then lost it—which, if I had love, I surely would. At least this time I know what to do—open to this brokenness—let it crack me open another layer to see what's there. To open once again to this brokenness, to say yes to this apparent loss, to welcome this poor child into my heart... this scarred being—the outer and the inner converging. I want to make sense out of it for her and for me. I want to tie it up into a neat package.

But the teaching relentlessly destroys any packaging I devise. Having thought I knew some things at the beginning of this phase of my journey, I was thrown back into "don't know" over and over again. That place, where the love and who I had thought I was (all my identities, even the identity of the new "more open me") had been, was just a huge and empty space. And out of that space—out of that "don't know," when I truly surrendered to it—came the most incredible experience, an awareness, a kind of understanding that defied my ordinary mind, of those indefinable concepts: peace, love and God. And so I saw that peace and love were possible even in sickness, even when love had fled, even with the face of death staring at me like a crow from a leafless tree.

So life goes on. I see love from inside and outside. I see pain and illness from inside and outside. Getting and losing, getting and losing, in and out of the crucible. I am poured into the flask and heated. The flame is applied, and after a while I am poured out again, and it's like, "Hmmm, what have we here? This is a new compound." This is my teaching—to go back and forth, in and out of emptiness and fullness, until I finally see that there is no essential difference between them. I see how I desert myself over and over again when the pain comes. Then when I come out the other side I say, "What for? Why did I leave my true heart?" I begin to glimpse the truth of the essential oneness of all things and all experience. There is nowhere to go, nothing to do—we are always home.

Rumi says:

> Days full of wanting,
> Let them go by without worrying
> that they do. Stay where you are
> inside such a pure, hollow note.

The breath of the universe moving in, moving out. Which is better? The in breath or the out breath? One sees how ludicrous this is, and yet, we cannot see how ludicrous is our constant judging of our experiences—this is good—that is bad—I like this—I don't like that. And how futile our clinging or our pushing away of experience. Every good thing we get, we will eventually lose. Likewise every painful experience will eventually pass—like the clouds passing across the clear blue sky.

If we can just ride the breath in, out—enter the experiences of our lives wholeheartedly, whatever they may be at each moment—the bittersweet truth of existence can shine forth. It is not good—it is not bad. It is just what it is, and somehow that is wonderful when truly experienced. Stephen Mitchell, in his autobiographical novel, *Meetings with the Archangel*, describes the day he experienced this truth,

I discovered the secret of the Zen Masters. It happened in Sumi-sahn's interview room. There was no fancy explosion of my mind, only a small surprised Oh, as if I was noticing something that my eyes had passed over one million times before. It was all so very simple. There was nothing—no thing—that I understood, no content to the experience, though if I had been forced to put words to it, I would have said that for the first time I realized that everything in the world is just the way it is. This sounds inanely tautological. But it was a revelation. I felt lighter than air, suddenly freed from the gravity of must and should.... I looked at Sumi-sahn with tears of gratitude in my eyes (p77-78).

There is a well-being, a peace, that does not depend on the body feeling a certain way or on things being a certain way, or on any emotion or person being present or absent—that does not depend on any "thing." This is the power of Love, beyond life and beyond death. Look for that which does not vanish: what remains when all else is stripped away, the whisper beneath all of creation that always was and always will be. This does not mean the small "self" will go away or stop doing its thing—being happy, being sad, feeling hurt, angry, amazed or euphoric. The show will go on. The story will continue. But there comes a point where we can just watch it and smile.

My friend asked, when she read this chapter, "Why is love what is left? Why not despair?" My answer to him was that, in my experience, despair is still a layer—something added—and that when despair is truly and willingly entered, it too drops away.

Sometimes I still feel like my life is hurtling down a steep mountainside out of control, but something has changed. Someone somewhere in me remembers—no matter how faintly. Sometimes it is so faint it is like a distant smell, but it is there.

As spiritual aspirants, we may come at times to a place where we may feel that all our efforts have been in vain. We have striven, and driven ourselves incessantly. We have tried and tried and at times actually seen results, actually thought we were making progress. But then we hit the wall. We see our "self" as big or bigger than ever—doing the same thing it has always done, and a deep sense of shame pervades the body. I wrote to my friend one day, "Do you think we ever really do anything different?"

Well, the answer, I think, is yes and no. In learning what God is not, I also begin to understand what *I* am not. With this on-again off-again pain, with illness and loss, comes a growing awareness that I can't take credit for my energy or the good things that my body does. I see clearly that it's a gift. It's not mine, and therefore it's not *me* either. The same holds true for the "bad" things—the weakness of the body and the things that bring embarrassment or shame, like my messy house. When I come into a place of more wellness and my body is able to do more—especially if that lasts for a while (though this is extremely rare)—I begin to notice, after a week or two of having a little more energy, a little extra oomph to do something each day beyond the bare necessities, my house slowly getting cleaned up, neater. The piles begin to disappear one by one—big patches of floor appear—and again I realize that I somehow see myself as a "better" person simply because I was able to clean my house a little bit.

But that little bird on my shoulder, the watcher, is there to remind me how ludicrous that is. I see that when I have energy, cleaning up—making things neat—is a piece of cake. It's easy. You just do it, and the messes disappear. It just takes time. It's not hard. It's not something to write home about. It's fun. It's rewarding. The hard thing, when you can't do it, is living with that mess, living with other people's judgments about it and your own judgments about it, bringing to bear some loving kindness on the person who cannot clean up, finding some peace within the chaos and the loss. Or when you do have a tiny bit of energy, to have the discipline to walk past the mess and to nourish that little bit of energy and let it build toward more health, or even perhaps to use it for something other than cleaning, like a fun night out or doing something creative to nourish the spirit. What fantasy to think that I'm good or better simply because I have the energy to clean up!

Even more ludicrous is when the "small self," the one that calls itself "I," claims and takes credit for spiritual "achievements," creativity, or emotional "highs." These elusive wildflowers that sometimes bloom most exuberantly when the body is wilting are no more me or mine than the great ocean belongs to the baubles it throws on the beach. So now when I start feeling better and I start doing more and I think, "Oh, this is good, I'm really getting it together," or have an epiphany and think "Oh, I'm really spiritual," there's a little bell that goes on—a little alarm that goes off inside my head. It's like a joke.

It's like the trickster is there and I've been caught again. Because that's not what it's about—being able to do something or not do something, feeling good or feeling bad. That's not it at all. And so I smile, and I go on with what I was doing.

All this talk about what God or love or peace are *not* is somewhat misleading. The Heart Sutra, a Buddhist chant, proclaims "Form is emptiness and emptiness is form." So the great masters are saying, it seems, that even illusion, in a sense, is God—the dark side of God. One can say that there is no thing that is God, but really it might be more accurate to say that *everything* is God—the small happiness, the big peace, love and loss of love, bodily well-being and illness, openness and clinging. There is nothing we can experience that is *not* God. This is not something that can be understood with the logical mind. God is beyond logic, but we bumble along and try—thus the reference to what God is not to try to get across the idea—to get to the truth that God and love are inclusive of all, but cannot be defined by any of the parts.

All of our life, all of our lessons, all of our learning and our apparent changing and growing, it seems, in the end, are designed only to bring us home—to that place we have always been—to see that nothing has really changed, and to see that this is okay. It is not only okay, it is perfect just as it is—there was never any need to change anything.

> *We shall not cease from exploration*
> *And the end of all our exploring*
> *Will be to arrive where we started*
> *And know the place for the first time.*
> —T.S. Eliot, *Four Quartets*

Red Woman in My Womb
   After Viewing Mayumi Oda's "Nibitsu"

You, red woman in my womb, guide my bones
to the shore of your becoming.
A frog in the storm croaks softly at first,

then louder and louder until his love chant
fills the darkness. Rain gives
way to gray sky, sunlight dimly, shyly lifts

her skirt a moment at a time. Warrior woman,
so strong in the belly,
waits to be born. There can be no timidity here.

When the clouds are effaced to this degree,
She is ready. No more room
inside to grow—she must be in the world now.

Take up the bed clothes and bite if you must.
The pushing must begin.

—Diane LaRae Bodach

CHAPTER 14

The Warrior Path

We can't sit back and wait for miracles to happen. We are the miracle.

SO, OKAY, I wasn't going to have the life I wanted or expected to have, and at first that seemed like Death—it *was* like Death. Almost all that I knew life to be was no longer possible for me. Most of my identities were gone, deeply diminished, or threatened. What was left seemed very stark, very small; but the very starkness, the very smallness was a spiritual opening for me. And so I made peace with my chronic illness and even came to see it as a blessing. I felt strong and happy in my vulnerability. I felt at peace and very much alive. Love was a growing force in my life. I thought I could face anything.

But making peace with cancer was a whole new ballgame. To make peace with cancer is truly to make peace with death. I guess I hadn't done that yet, though I thought I had.

I had been struggling for months, but particularly strongly for about a week, with another one of those either/or questions. I knew unequivocally from my past spiritual experience that either/or questions are almost always a trap—especially the ones that seem particularly juicy and compelling. I knew the drill: don't fall for the polarization; just settle into the heart and this moment in time. Yet, I couldn't seem to get past the question: "Do I just surrender to this devastation that seems to be sweeping through my body, or do I use my Will to take a strong stand for life?"

I knew intellectually as well as on a deeper, emotional and spiritual level that the answer to these two questions was the same. Having read Stephen Levine's book, *Healing into Life and Death*, many years previously, when struggling with coming to terms with my chronic illness, I remembered again Steven's own question, "Where is healing to be found?" which he asked himself in a moment of deep introspection, having been confronted with a question similar to mine from a dying woman. That question and his answer were branded into my heart and soul and had started me down a path of deep inner healing that profoundly changed my life, my approach to spiritual practice, and my relationship to my chronic illness.

When I wrote out the question that had been hanging in my mind like a dead weight, I was astounded to see it was virtually the same one the woman had asked him that day. Her question was, "Should I stop trying to heal, and just let myself die?" (Levine 1987, 1). So there I was, full circle—seemingly back on square one. I asked myself, "Didn't I already know that there is only one true healing, and if I focus on healing, wherever it is needed, that is my path?"

Clearly, there were still emotional holdings obscuring the path to my heart, but when your child runs out into the street into the path of a speeding car, you don't consult the *I Ching* or stop to meditate before you run with all your might to whisk your loved one into your arms and out of harm's way. With my own life on the chopping block, and a thousand options being presented to me for cure both medically and spiritually, my own path was suddenly less clear than it had been for the past ten years, when my primary focus had turned to an inward healing, and that healing revolved around opening and surrender to whatever presented itself in the mind, heart or body. I had thought that "whatever" had included the possibility of facing death, especially since, at the beginning of my chronic illness, I hadn't known whether or not what I was facing was life threatening. Now, however, with that possibility much more prevalently present, I wasn't so sure.

I had also been focusing again on intention, and on praying for, asking for pure intention. I knew the importance of pure intention and felt that the cancer had obscured that—had tainted my pure intention. Did I now just want to live? Damn the consequences? Had I lost my pure intention, the intention of healing on a soul level? Of opening to the deepest Truth? Of simply being with my life as it is? Of serving? Still, there was that pesky notion that I somehow need a body to do this kind of spiritual healing. C.G. Jung said in a letter to a very sick man:

> We live in order to attain the greatest possible amount of spiritual development and self awareness. As long as life is possible, even if only in a minimal degree, you should hang onto it in order to scoop it up for the purpose of conscious development. To interrupt life before its time is to bring to a standstill an experiment that we have not set up. We have found ourselves in the midst of it and must carry it through to the end. That it is extraordinarily difficult for you is quite understandable, ... but I believe you will not regret it if you cling on even to such a life to the very last. (Vol.1 1906-1950, 434)

So it seemed he was saying we must hold onto life as long as possible to do the work. And then there was that image of the child running into the street. Wasn't it my job right now to focus on this body—to do whatever is necessary to preserve it, and therefore make it possible for me to continue my spiritual work?

I was so tired of being sick and miserable. I desperately wanted relief, wanted to go out and have some fun, to connect with people. But it just wasn't working. I would feel a bit better one day and then crash again the next. Perhaps, I said to myself finally, I need simply to turn inward for a time.

So with all these questions in my heart, I did an intense meditation session. Surrendering to my process, I saw clearly how I had been severed—divided against myself or against God—and I realized what I needed to do. The feminine, receptive part of myself knew how to surrender. This was the fruit of the spiritual work I had done over the previous ten years, the healing precipitated by my chronic illness and Stephen Levine's insights. And the masculine, warrior, willful, doing part of myself knew something about doing—accomplishing—yet mostly from the small, narrow point of view of the small self. This "power" part of myself, it seems, had been put on hold in recent years, sent into limbo, while the feminine/child side was nourished and strengthened.

This was a good thing. It was what was needed, but now something further was being asked of me. To let the warrior woman in me be strong, while still maintaining a path of surrender, acceptance of what is and harmony with the Divine, required a merging—a surrender, of my masculine, small, doing self with the larger Self. To bring these two, the masculine and the feminine archetypes in me, together into the Divine Will was to reconcile these two seemingly separate parts of myself, and to go beyond the seemingly either/or question that had been plaguing me.

My vision was that the rising power, the male, "doing" energy within me, when unfettered, mingles with the receptive female energy giving birth to the creative force. It has no agenda of its own. It is at the service of the Godhead—the greatest good. As long as I have an agenda for this power, it will be askew. If my agenda is that I—small self, Diane—live, I will be blocking the creative force that wants to manifest in service of the highest good. The agenda of the small self continuing to live is an impossible agenda and cannot, ultimately, be fulfilled. Therefore, it will bring only suffering. If I cling to life above all things, I will meet what seems to the small mind like defeat. However, if my intention or goal is Life itself with no motive as to its form, the energy will flow freely and with great power.

Of course, in the larger sense, ALL is given; nothing is mine. Yet sometimes my own ideas of what is true color or get in the way of what is actually there. The male doing, "power energy" is given, and is part of the Absolute Creative Energy. Yet my *idea* was that it was *mine* (small self, Diane)—so when I began to experience this budding power opening in me, I *thought* it was mine (small self i.e. ego-based)—something to put aside, to allow for God energy to come in.

So this mistaken notion kept me, and may, I believe, keep many people, small and powerless. Because we see how the energy can be misused in the world to wield power over others or for seemingly evil purposes, and because we believe this energy is our own and thus perhaps tainted or even "evil," we may be keeping our given creative power under wraps and waiting for the "True Power" to descend from above.

We are like the man in the story of the flood who is waiting on his rooftop for God to save him. As the waters rise higher and higher, various people come by to help him. First, when the water is up to his windows, a man comes by in a rowboat and offers a ride. But the man on the roof refuses and tells the other man he is waiting for God to save him. When the water is on the roof and lapping at his toes, the Coast Guard comes in a big cutter and calls to him to come aboard. He again says no and waits for God to come. Finally, when the water is up to his waist, a helicopter drops a ladder, and the pilot urges him through a loud speaker to climb to safety. He turns this down as well saying he has faith that God will come to save him. When the water is up to his chin he cries out, "God, I've waited and waited for you to save me. I had faith in You. Why have you not come?" And a voice from the sky answers, "I came to you three times. First in a rowboat, then in a Coast Guard cutter, and lastly in a helicopter. But you refused me each time."

So it is with the energies surging inside of us. It is *all* God energy. We cannot lay claim to it, but we can allow our bodies to be a vehicle for it. This delicate balancing act, I have found, must be pursued in the heart. The danger is that the ego (that is, the small "false ego" as distinguished from the healthy ego necessary for our personal beingness in the world), based in the mind, will be mistaken for the Will and take over the process for its own purposes.

So out of the swirling confusion of facing cancer and possible death, I began to have a feeling for the direction I was going and what my path was from there. The kundalini power in me was rising. I felt it every day—such inner strength in my utter weakness. I continued to give myself to it and to open. The physical and emotional suffering was like an auger helping me to go to deeper and deeper levels of inner knowing. I think this power that can arise when we are pushed against the wall and feel we are about to be crushed can be very strong. It is like lion energy:

> "The lion," says Nietzsche in *Thus Spoke Zarathustra*, "says no to any dutiful carrying-on, or comfortable inertias. The spirit lion leads out of marginal, dependent existence into the danger and blankness of the desert.... In most instances the lion is the point of necessity that comes at a certain moment, the fierce intensity that destroys ego-imprisonment, and opens one out into light and another field of being. Lion energy is the bridge.... He roars. He speaks strong language and wants, above all else, for the truth to come out and be seen. When the lion enters, the revolution begins. Lion energy and warrior energy are close." (Barks, 1991)

My friend, who is so debilitated by chronic illness that she rarely leaves her house, talked about a kind of energy that arises for her: "Sometimes I sit in my chair and wonder how I will make it across the room. Then an energy arises from somewhere—it is almost not physical. It's like I slip under the radar."

Yet, even when there is no physical energy at all forthcoming, there is still an inward energy, an inward power, available to do the great work. This inward power in me was growing stronger and stronger. The warrior path continued to deepen. I later saw it as a kind of warrior woman in my womb gestating, getting ready to be born. I also saw clearly, and remembered as well very vividly from the birth of my daughters, that giving birth is anything but passive. So it seemed I had again come to a new stage in my inward journey—not square one as I had thought, but a new place on the spiral, circling very close but a significant step up from the former "yes" of acceptance. This path now pointed to a more active role for this center of beingness called "I." Something new was being asked of me: to open to this new mysterious power energy of creativity and birthing, to journey with God energy in a new way—perhaps almost a partnership—a merging.

The youngest of five children, with siblings considerably older than me (my oldest brother was thirteen years older), I grew up believing I was little and incompetent and that all the people around me knew more than I did. I went through life trying to change myself to be like them—to be an adult as I saw them to be. I was rebellious, true. I even ran off to California and became a hippie in the late sixties, then developed a lifestyle quite different from my family of origin. I had had inclinations all my life to be creative. I wanted to be an artist, a musician, a poet and dabbled in all these expressions, but it was half-hearted. I was holding myself back somehow.

It wasn't until I got cancer and had such huge upheaval in my inner world—tectonic plates going berserk—that I realized I was still doing it; I was still in many ways trying to live a life that resembled my siblings, or would perhaps be somehow approved of or even admired by them. I was still believing I was little and incompetent. What a shock. But I saw then that the child Diane had a rich inner life—a rich fantasy life—a rich musical and artistic life—a rich communion with nature. And that has never changed. I realized that I've had it all along.

This childlikeness—this deep opening into heart—is a gift. Others on the spiritual path I'm following would do much to have these things that I have. I tried to change myself to fit the mold I saw around me as I grew up, but I finally saw that I have within me a being of great value and that my job is not to change myself, but to be myself fully, and even to give this gift to others if I can.

Illness and loss are great teachers. They are different from other teachers in that they are closer to us than a physical human teacher in one way and farther away in another. More like a force of nature, a hurricane or a flood, they are harder to blame and impossible to reason with. In this way they are more "other," even than a personal teacher, but also part of us physically (as illness or disability) and thus intrinsically "me" and impossible to avoid. Being "me," then, the intrinsic illness or loss is a door through which we can open to our own inner truth and guidance. And yet even this teacher/teaching can become something we cling to and rely on and consequently, something that can keep us from our true heart.

Whether I live or die is not the point. This body will, of course, die. It is not in my realm of responsibility or business to know when. But my job, as I see it, and the fruit of the deep questioning with which I had begun, is to enter my life completely in each moment, to take up the sword that was thrown down, and to be a warrior woman, to dare to be really alive, to feel my feelings fully and deeply, and to dare to *do*, in both the physical world and the inner psychic world, to truly *be* the creative and vibrant person that I already am. This opening in me has created a sense of myself which is completely opposite from the passive victim or "poor me" mentality that had sometimes appeared in relationship to my chronic illness and the cancer as well as earlier in my life. We must, at some point, accept the responsibility of co-creation with God. We can't sit back and wait for miracles to happen. We *are* the miracle.

CHAPTER 15

On Not Being Able to Do

Oh great Sun, what would your joy be without those for whom you shine?

—Nietzsche

THE COMPLETION OF A THOUGHT is usually an action, be it to carry out a plan to clean the garage, write a symphony, go to the store to buy milk and bread, write in a journal, or simply to share the thought with another human being. The natural progression of events for humans is usually a thought followed by an action. A normal person can decide to do a project, and the major things that stand between him and the completion of his project are his will power or planning and time constraints. To become ill or disabled often blocks one-half of the equation.

This is a huge loss, much larger than most well people realize. We humans love our plans and, though we often don't actually carry them out, we have the idea that we *could* carry them out and that perhaps in some future time we *will*. When we are very ill or debilitated for a long time, or become disabled, that illusion may be shattered. Descartes said, "I think therefore I am," but to be alive is also to do, and not to be able to do can feel like death. There comes a time when plans are useless. There is a hymn in the Orthodox Church, "When his breath departs, he returns to his earth. On that day all his plans perish." When our body is incapacitated, we can make all the plans in the world, but they won't do us any good because we can't carry them out—they only make us sad.

Life in the Slow Lane

Being ill or disabled makes one see time and accomplishment in an entirely new light. At first there is a tendency to think that because we can't do things as quickly or efficiently as others, that we can't do them at all, or that it is not worth doing them. A job that takes a well person ten minutes to complete may take a chronically ill person an hour. Something that "should" take a day or two might stretch out to be week or a month. We are snails living in a world of antelopes or tigers. The world is set up for antelopes. We snails must learn to use a series of tricks, jerryrigs and come-alongs to get anything accomplished in this environment.

In the world of getting things done, it seems that things work best when they have a certain continuity. While others can accomplish things using momentum, we cannot rely on this force. If I try to do something at a pace that I can sustain, I find that by the time I get halfway through the project I have forgotten a vital part of what I learned in order to complete the task, or another task comes up that takes precedence and I have to abandon the first before completion, or maybe I forget why I started the stupid project in the first place.

For example, trying to put a room or a desk in order, I start by making stacks of things to put away. Within half-an-hour I usually have to stop because my arms are hurting. Maybe I can continue in an hour or maybe not until the next day. The next day I might be too sick to do anything and the day after that I have to go to the doctor, which uses up all my energy for that day. Two days later I am having company so I have my aid move everything I've started sorting into a back room. Finally, a day comes a week later that I can continue working on my sorting, but the dog has walked through the room and the piles that remain standing look unfamiliar. By the time I figure out what order I had in mind for the piles, clean up the mess made by the dog and add two or three more bits to the various piles, I am exhausted again and need to stop for the day. The next day the pump goes out on the well and I need to call a repair man to get water for drinking. You get the idea.

A well person reading this may think, "Sounds like my life." And it's true—we all have interruptions, and many of the things described here happen to everyone. We're talking about an order of magnitude and that order of magnitude can make a life seem from a different planet. A person with what may be called "normal" energy can usually spend an uninterrupted two- or three-hour period working on a project. For people with limited energy, ten minutes at a time or maybe ten minutes a day might be all they can manage.

And what is *not* apparent in the above description is the desperation that often forces the halt of activity for those of us with extremely limited capacity, and how that leads to doing things that may seem totally inappropriate, lazy or downright weird. In this desperation state I have put half-eaten food and empty containers in the refrigerator because I couldn't deal with putting them away properly or washing the dish. I have left my clothes or spilled food or even broken glass on the floor overnight, and stuffed trash in a nearby drawer rather than walk across the room to a trashcan. I have abandoned shopping carts full of food or goods, that I had spent a considerable amount of time collecting, in the middle of a store aisle to head for the nearest exit because I simply didn't have any energy left to wait in line and pay.

When my body is collapsing, it can happen very fast. Sometimes I don't get a lot of warning; I just run out of energy or whatever combination of hormones and muscles that make my body work. Say in the sorting situation, I may be close to finishing when I notice that I'm wearing down. Within five minutes I'm so desperate to lie down, to just *stop*, that I'll do anything. My mind becomes jumbled as the body seizes whatever remaining blood sugar or hormones that are necessary for functioning and/or sends some kind of red alert to the brain which says in blinking neon, "You have thirty seconds before melt down … bzt … bzt … bzt…"

If it is imperative the papers be put away, I may simply have to stack them up again in any order and start over the next time. Similarly, in cleaning out a cabinet or the fridge, I might get everything out and realize I am too tired to do anything except put it all back. I think Sisyphus[6] probably ranks in the top ten patron gods for those of us with chronic illness. Sorting papers or cleaning cabinets and putting things away are relatively small tasks. What if we need to do something bigger? When I was going through my divorce, the rest of my life virtually came to a halt while I dealt with the issues at hand.

My sister, who also has a chronic illness, mops her own floor, but it takes her a week or more to do it. She mops for five minutes, then rests for an hour. She may get three cycles in before her body says to stop for the day. Is it worth it? When you consider the alternative—doing nothing—the answer has to be yes. So you move on, realizing that you can still do things; you just can't do them as fast or as much as other people. On the plus side, you get to really work on priorities. When there is no possibility of actually keeping up with what may seem to be the necessary chores of life, one gets to choose where to invest one's tiny quota of available energy.

After a number of years experiencing the frustration of trying and trying my hardest to "keep up" with the most basic "obligatory" tasks of life, i.e. keeping me and my family fed and clean and our house and affairs in order, and never even coming close, I began to understand why destitute people sometimes spend what tiny amount of money they can lay their hands on, on candy, liquor, or some extravagance.

I know that people sometimes judge me when I go out to social events, yet can't seem to keep my house in order or take care of what seem to be more "pressing life concerns." What they don't know is how hard I have worked day in and day out at this Sisyphusian[7] task. The problem is, I can use up a whole day's worth of energy in fifteen minutes on sorting and cleaning, and what I have accomplished is laughable. In the meantime, the end of my life is rushing toward me. I never have enough energy to actually get the elementary work that "should" get done "done," so that I can move on to something fun—something that brings joy—in the way that well people give this to themselves as a reward after a hard day's or week's work, or to do something "meaningful" in the sense of what I see my larger life purpose to be.

The category of people for whom "not being able to" has poignancy is very large and manifests in many different ways. There are many reasons besides physical illnesses or disability that render people unable to accomplish plans or even do simple physical tasks.

Speaking of dealing with agoraphobia, my friend Jane said,

> As far as my outlook on what my purpose was or what was in store for me,. I really didn't know. I did't know if that was because I'd forgotten

or because I almost couldn't let myself wonder. The scope of my life had become so narrow that I never knew how big it was going to get, so it was hard to imagine things because I didn't know what was really going to be within my reach. I could be wrong, but I think I often didn't try.

Something that I really, really missed, probably more than anything when I was housebound was that the sense of possibility was just gone. I think that was the hardest thing, to be right in the beginning of adulthood, just breaking in and suddenly, I couldn't even allow myself to imagine future possibilities. I couldn't imagine what they could be because I didn't know if I'd ever get out of the house. So to say, I'd love to do this or I want this, certainly wasn't in my realm of possibility then, and I never really knew if it would be.

Depression is another illness that can be much more debilitating than many people realize and is very widespread in today's world. I was terribly worried about my daughter during a severe depression she experienced in her twenties. Her social life disappeared. She sat at home for months doing virtually nothing whenever she wasn't at work. I recall painful phone conversations when she would have nothing to say. It was question from me: one word answer from her,

"How are you?"

"Fine."

"What did you do today?"

"Go to the store."

And then there would be silence. It was impossible to get a conversation going. I worried about her all the time. It was painful to call and painful not to. I didn't know how to help her.

New Look at Priorities

Yet somehow, within the sorrow and difficulty that arises in the depths of our illness or loss, if we look deeper, we find a recompense or more. We may find a new way of looking at our lives. There is poignancy to life in the slow lane. We learn about priorities from a new perspective. We learn to savor the sweetness of the smallest piece of candy. I believe we were not made for drudgery. We were made for joy. I know the cleaning will be waiting for me again the next day and the next and the next. Sometimes I simply opt out and go fishing (metaphorically speaking)—do something I really want to do instead of what the inner critic is telling me I "should" do.

When I got sick, my husband took over the garden in which we both delighted and had previously worked together. When we separated, I couldn't bear the thought of not having a garden at all, so I schemed against all odds to have one, albeit a very small one. After planning how much time I could spend each day without having a relapse, arranging for reasonably priced yet competent help for the digging and other things I couldn't do, getting plants and painstakingly putting them out one at a time perhaps at the rate of two a day, it began to seem a bit ludicrous—especially when I considered that in order to do the garden, the whole rest of my life had been put on hold.

The mail sat unopened, the kitchen was a mess, clothes were piled high on my bed, and friends were neglected. But the joy of working in the soil—getting my hands into it and smelling the sweet humus, putting seeds and tiny plants in the ground, watching them grow, tending to them in the ways that I could, being somehow a partner in God's creation—fed my soul more than my body and met needs that were deeper than the need for order in my physical house.

Another time I took the kids camping. It took us two weeks working every day to get ready to go. My daughters, six and nine, did almost everything under my direction. When we were within a hair's breadth of leaving, my older daughter got sick and we had to put all the perishables back away, unpack all the food and utensils we used every day, and live for a week stepping over boxes while she got better. Then we spent another four or five days getting it together again before we could leave.

I began to wonder if I might be crazy putting us through all this just to go camping, but when we actually got there and felt the sun on our faces, heard the wind singing in the trees and dipped our toes in the river, I knew it was worth it. I took a deep breath and laid down by the river, exhausted but happy, recuperating while I watched and listened to my girls giggling and splashing in the clear mountain water. It took us two more days to get the campsite in order and the tent up, but at that point it didn't matter. Sleeping under the trees and stars was an adventure, and arranging the campsite slowly at our leisure, to the chatter of chipmunks and jays, was like play.

I pretty much gave my life to my kids after I got sick. There was so little of me available that I wanted whatever tiny amount there was—or at least the lion's share of it—to go to them so they could have some semblance of a "normal" life. I tried hard to keep my husband happy too, but it was an impossible situation given that some days my quota of energy for the day allowed me to walk to and from the kitchen from my daytime bed in the dining room and *perhaps*, to read a paragraph or two from a story to the girls at bedtime.

At one point I was spread so thin and the amount of the available "me" as in "mom" and "wife," which basically included everything that I had to give, was incredibly tiny. It certainly wasn't enough to provide two growing children with anywhere near what might be considered a rich or fulfilling life, let alone an adequate one, or to keep a husband happy or even minimally satisfied. I also realized that none of this "spreading" of the me involved anything enjoyable or enriching that was strictly *for* me.

I decided that maybe it would be a wise idea to try to give Diane at least one small piece of the tiny pie of Diane energy I was dividing up among the family. When an opportunity arose for me to join a small group of singers forming around a talented music teacher from my children's school, I decided to try it. I had no idea whether or not this was something I could actually do, but I loved to sing. In fact, singing is one thing I can truly say brings me deep joy as well as good old-fashioned fun.

My husband felt hurt and slighted. "Why do you have the energy to go out and sing when you say you have absolutely no energy for me for lovemaking?" he asked, angrily. I in turn was hurt, wondering why he couldn't support me going out and having a little fun when he knew how hard my life was, and how little I did for myself in the way of enjoyment.

Lovemaking since the illness hit had been problematic at best. I was exhausted and hurting every night, in fact, almost all the time. It's pretty hard to enjoy lovemaking under those circumstances and it's pretty hard to make love if you are not enjoying it. If you are tired and hurting, you can make yourself do a lot of things. You can take out the trash, do the dishes, drive the carpool or fold the laundry, maybe even go to the movies or a party. The quality of it may not be top notch, but *something* might get accomplished, or in the case of a movie or party, you might get distracted or fulfill an obligation. With lovemaking, however, I don't want to be distracted and I certainly don't want to feel that I'm simply fulfilling an obligation, though I actually came close to doing that plenty of times because I knew my husband needed it. I tried to frame it for myself that I was doing it for love, but I wasn't enjoying it. I wanted to be present to give and receive love and pleasure, but physically I just didn't have it in me.

I wanted him to understand that my level of energy was so low that no one—not me, not my friends, not him, not even the kids—could get what they needed or wanted from me. It just wasn't there. What *I* didn't understand, I think, is that what I thought I needed from him, an inordinate amount of compassion and understanding, wasn't there either because of the severe stresses he was under. We were all getting much less than what we thought we needed.

Of course we didn't *really* need these things but we thought we did. It was the epitome of the age-old story of lack and loss and blame. On an intellectual level, one could look at the situation and see that certainly there was not enough to go around—we were all stretched to our max—and that a quality of compassion and loving-kindness was called for—first for ourselves, and then extended to those around us. What neither my husband or I understood at the time was that this sense of lack, the sense of loss, of deprivation is not intellectual. It is from deep emotional wounds stemming from childhood that have never healed. So instead we took it out on each other in unintended unconscious ways that were hurtful and alienated us from each other. I withdrew from him even more, emotionally and physically. He acted out with anger or sarcasm. And we both did a lot of blaming, externally and internally.

For the children, the situation was very different. They were children—they had no thoughts of need or lack. They didn't complain I wasn't giving them enough attention. They got cranky, and acted out in their own ways to the maelstrom of destruction in which families dealing with severe loss or illness often find themselves enmeshed. Mostly, though, they went on with their lives as children do—exploring their world, finding mud and sticks and rocks in the ditch to play with, holding tea parties for the dolls, making houses for the kittens, creating their lives without Mom and Dad for the most part since we were both so overwrought—me with sickness, my husband with all the extra chores he needed to do to make up for what I couldn't do—that there was not much time or energy left over for them. However, even though they, with the resilience of children, went on with their own work—the work of childhood, which is play—underneath it all their own wounds of lack and loss were forming.

Writing the Book

When I first began to have an urge to write this book, there were times when it seemed ridiculous and flat out impossible. After all, I couldn't even take care of myself and my family, let alone add in a huge book-writing project. But again—there was my life staring me in the face asking, "What are you going to do with me?" Also, there was still that deep desire to somehow be of service to others. I knew on a very deep level that I *was*, in fact, serving by bearing children and creating a family as well as an environment to nurture them. But something was still pushing me to contribute on a deeper or wider or perhaps more universal scale—to reach outside the circle of my little family to the wider community.

After I decided to go ahead, I spent two years trying to get my affairs in order so I could devote myself to the task. Well, "big surprise," I finally saw that I could have spent another five years at it and never have gotten there. About halfway up that "Sisyphusian" hill, on say, the five hundredth round, I let go of my boulder and started the book, one day, one paragraph at a time. I figured even if I only wrote a half a paragraph a day, it would eventually get done—if I lived long enough!

It has been interesting to note that in regard to writing this book I have faced a real conundrum: the more physically able I am to write, the less accessible is the real knowing, the real understanding of what it really means to be ill or disabled. So I encountered another paradox, another lesson. Because my energy level fluctuates considerably from week to week, month to month and sometimes from year to year, there are times when doing is much more possible than at other times.

Sometimes when I am having a relapse, I have to totally withdraw from life, from activities, from any contact with my friends or anyone. My life virtually goes on hold and this can go on for weeks or months. It's a black hole out of which nothing can come. In writing my book, this is an impossible situation, because I want to describe what this is like, but I can't do it when I'm in that space; I'm simply too weak. Sometimes I furtively put something on the tape recorder or on a little scrap of paper, so I can remember. It's kind of like notes from the underground, because when I get better, I don't remember what it really felt like. Was it really that bad, I wonder? Then I read my note. Yes, it was.

One day I was sitting, feeling depressed and frustrated because I had all these plans for the book, and my body just wasn't working. Mentally, I had decided (when in a more up phase) that I was going to do certain things to make sure I kept moving on the project: do one interview a week; meet with my advisor once every two weeks; begin to type up what I had already written; work for at least one hour total per day on things related to the book. These were not overly ambitious goals, but actually reasonably geared to my state of health the previous week. But at that time I couldn't do any of them. I was in a low spot physically and from the looks of things it was going to last for quite a while, probably months. I felt stymied, defeated.

Suddenly I realized that my body was teaching me exactly what I needed to learn: how to live with chronic illness. It was making me an expert on the subject about which I intended to write a book. Thank you! So going out into the world for answers was not what I needed right then. The world doesn't have the answers for me; it doesn't know the rules under which I operate. My illness constantly throws me back into my own deep knowing.

But on a deeper level it is teaching me something even more important. I was very identified with this project. Writing this book had become *me* in a sense. And in my self-importance I believed I could be in control. Both of these assumptions are wrong, and life was teaching me again: "Stop! See who you really are—more than just writing this book. Stop! See that the flow of life is not in your control (Thank God!). It has its own agenda. Give up your agenda. Give up that false sense of control. Relax. Enjoy your life in this moment—each moment, just as it is."

And so it is with all of life. If we look deeply, our present condition is teaching us exactly what we need to know in each moment. And as for the "doing," which can often feel so futile given the seemingly pitiful amount we can accomplish with our small quota of energy—this doing itself can be approached with a new attitude and purpose and a new appreciation for the teaching of illness or disability: the joy of doing simply for the sake of doing but with no concern for results.

Animals do this—a friend once told me he used to watch birds flying and think they flew with a sense of purpose. "They fly so straight and strong," he said, "as if they know exactly where they are going." But one day he was watching a duck fly across an expanse of sky with that kind of strength and intensity as if it were intent on getting to some known destination and getting there fast. A few minutes later, however, this bird turned in the sky and flew in the opposite direction with equal intensity.

What would it be like if we lived our lives like that? What if we could put our hearts and souls into every act regardless of whether or not we were sure of reaching a certain goal or attaining the object of our desire? When I was so sick and doing my garden alone, I learned to savor each moment with the plants and the soil, not knowing for sure if I would be able to continue to care for them long enough to taste the fruits of my labor. When we do things simply for the sake of doing, there can be joy in the act of doing that has nothing to do with whether or not we achieve a certain result. Our chronic and terminal illnesses give us constant opportunities to learn this lesson.

Lightening the Load

My adult daughter always says, "Mom, you don't have to do that," when I make a nice meal for her or put myself out in some other way to do something nice for her. She has some idea of how much it takes out of me to do these things. I know I don't have to. She would not fault me if I didn't cook for her. And I don't have to keep the house clean; I don't have to call people or go out to visit them. In truth, when it comes right down to it, there is not that much that I really *have* to do. But on one level, every physical thing I don't do in the world seems to make me that much more of a non-person. This is not necessarily *bad.* On the spiritual path, the wise ones say, the less of us there is, the better. And we learn that—we really do—if we're alert and willing to surrender to the teaching.

My friend Mort shared a poignant story of being laid up with a back injury for several years. When he finally began to have a little mobility, he walked down the street to the local health food store to get some much-needed supplies. On the way back he realized his pack was too heavy and as he continued to walk under that heavy load, he realized that he couldn't continue and he would need to lighten his load. So he took a cabbage out and put it in a nearby trashcan. Slowly, as he continued toward his apartment, he had to forsake, one by one, almost all the items he had bought in order to make it home. As he told me the story, we cried and laughed together with the common understanding of this experience: the sadness, the loss, the poignancy—and the grace infiltrating—the lightening of the load.

My parallel experiences flooded into memory: I remembered walking down a deserted beach, filling my pack with beautiful rocks and, on my way back, needing to slowly return them all to the beach; feeling the loss and the freedom mingled—the exact perfection of giving the rocks back to the sea; I remembered finding myself during uncountable numbers of walks within sight of home or my destination but lacking the strength to walk the last fifty or a hundred yards, being forced to lie down by the side of the road to rest, and noticing how much more beautiful it was there than in my house where my destination lay; and I remembered being stranded over and over again in some far corner of Penny's, Costco or Yardbirds and having to find some out-of-the-way place to wait out my exhaustion so I could walk to my car and drive home, and in the process being forced to see how my rushing and always needing to be somewhere else keeps me from experiencing the preciousness of each moment.

Hard Truths

Still there seems to be some deep pull, perhaps beyond ego, to inhabit and use this body for *something.* And there are certain feelings, love in particular, that long to be expressed in a physical way. I long to do things for my daughters and other loved ones and it is extremely painful when I can't. I understand that doesn't mean I am not still part of the huge cosmic process or that God doesn't love me, or that I am not a being in the spiritual sense, but the hard truth is that, in the physical world, I am a person to the extent that I have a physical body and I use it.

If I stop calling people, people eventually stop calling me. If I don't invite people over, they stop inviting me over. We make our friends through involvement in some activity, through "doing" something, even if that something is simply talking. When someone dies, the world goes on. But that person is no longer part of the active exchange that goes on in this physical plane. There may still be connection on the spiritual plane, but on the physical plane the person no longer exists. As a person's body fails, he becomes less and less connected in the sense of worldly activities. This is a hard truth to be faced, but it is simply a truth of this world—our physical bodies will eventually fade and die.

Jean Dominique Bauby described his yearning to be part of the camaraderie in the physical therapy room of the hospital where he lived. Strapped to a board and suspended for half-an-hour a day in a vertical position, he sought contact through the one part of his body that still worked—his left eye. But the more fortunate "tourists," as he called those who would actually be rehabilitated and eventually leave the hospital where he lived, would turn away, as he said, "feeling the sudden need to study the ceiling smoke detector" (*The Diving Bell and the Butterfly,* p. 33).

Sometimes I feel like the walking dead. There, I've said it. It sounds so morbid, but I know many of us have felt it—all those times when we felt more dead than alive, or at least half dead. My niece said to me, if she got sick and couldn't do the things that she loved to do, she would rather be dead. I said to myself, "Just wait 'til you're there." Still, I remember feeling that way in the beginning of my illness. It took me years to begin to appreciate my new life with its severe limitations. The quadriplegic man on whose life the movie, *The Sea Inside* was based, spent twenty years fighting for the right to die. For him, life was not worth living with the limitations of his broken body—and he never changed his mind.

What Is the Essence of Being Human?

There have been times, especially in the beginning of my illness, when I was so weak I had to spend weeks mostly lying down. Much of this time, I was so gravely weak or exhausted that I could not lift my little finger and, more importantly, I could not talk.

These were lonely times. To be trapped in a body with nothing but thoughts tumbling around and around inside my head with nowhere to go can be extremely depressing. Sometimes as I lay there with only my thoughts for company, I asked myself, "What is the essence of being human? What is the essence of being alive? What is the essential thing that makes life worth living?" I decided that communication or *connection* was the thing that makes us human—or maybe the thing that makes life worth living. We seem to be wired with the desire for connectivity with others of our species. The film *The Amazing Newborn*, reveals footage of a newborn baby moving arms and legs in rhythm with the mother's voice. Phyllis Klaus writes,

> One of the newborn's first responses is to move into a quiet but alert state of consciousness. In this state, the baby is still; her body molds to yours; her hands touch your skin; her eyes open wide and are bright and shiny. She looks directly at you.
>
> This special alert state, this innate ability to communicate, may prepare the way for the future attachment between the newborn and those who care for her. The intensity and appealing power of this little bud of humanity meeting the world for the first time are all but irresistible. (1998, 22)

I still remember the exhilaration of meeting the eyes of my firstborn shortly after birth. It felt like falling in love, and it was a love affair completely out of the realm of anything I had ever experienced.

Robinson Crusoe (or the real traveler he represents) lived on an island for years without so much as a glimpse of another person. But the urge to communicate was strong. He kept a detailed diary with pictures to tell and show the world his adventures and troubles. Whether this tale is actually truth or fiction doesn't much matter. Few would dispute the human inclination played out in the story. This mythic traveler had much to communicate and the ability to do so, but no one to listen. Yet, in the irony of life, during my worst times, there I was with people all around me and an abundance of thoughts and feelings to share, but no way to communicate them.

The Longing for Purpose

One could argue that the most essential thing to being human is to take care of the body, i.e. survival. Without a body there can be no life, no human and no thought—nothing to communicate. This is true, but for what? A car uses gas to go, but one needs a destination. The human being, it seems, longs for purpose, or something beyond simple existence. What does it mean to be a worthwhile person? To have a worthwhile life? We tend to think of it in terms of what people do. "He's so nice. He went out of his way to drive me home." "She's such a good person. She donates time every Saturday to cook for the homeless," or "She's such an angel. She takes care of her invalid mother and rarely takes time for herself."

For some, a worthwhile day might be a day in which a lot has been accomplished, such as cleaning the house or doing the shopping and the laundry. If one is an artist or a writer, a good day might be painting a beautiful picture or writing a chapter in a book. But what happens when we get sick? What if we *are* the invalid mother or child or spouse that some "angel" must care for? Does our life cease to have worth? Sometimes it feels like it. One of the most difficult hurdles an ill or disabled person faces is the feeling of being worthless, of being nonproductive, of not being able to help or do for others—or, worst of all: being a burden.

We live in a world in which, for most people, time is the most valuable commodity. There are some, however, bound in bodies that don't work, for whom time is an interminable wasteland to somehow be gotten through. Though I don't now feel that way, I have been there and I understand. The man in "The Sea Inside" felt this way. He lay in his bed and refused to be put into a wheelchair or even be carried outside.

I noticed when I watched the movie that I had judgments about his choices—that he was pushing life away, that he was turning his back on love and a chance for happiness. This was good for me to see. It was good to see the arrogance of my judgment—the idea that I can judge another's experience and decide what is right for him. No one can judge another's experience. No one can decide what is right for someone else. And no one can ever truly know what is being perceived or experienced—what is actually going on—inside the skin of another being.

And yet we think we do, or we want to. Perhaps it is in this wanting that the seeds of empathy are planted, and in this thinking that judgment enters. This is the bud of loving kindness. This is the precursor of war. This is the mystery—the beauty and the pain of humanness—the conundrum of opposites that seems to arise out the same basic impulse. It is that impulse to reach out, to love, to want to help and understand another fellow being, it seems, that can also lead to the desire for control or judgment.

And again, it comes back to "know thyself." If we don't know ourselves, if we don't know what we're up to, if we don't know *who* we are in our deepest self, that impulse to serve can be distorted and lead to harming instead of helping. And here again, illness and loss can be our helpers and friends. In taking everything away, even sometimes the ability to be of service, they can help to purify our intention and our desire; they can help us to know who we really are (which is love), so that when we *are* able to help, it will come from a place clear of ulterior motives or distorted desires.

The inability to do for others, to be of service, is for many, one of the most painful aspects of chronic illness. This is a deeply ingrained human yearning. Not being able to fulfill this yearning is a huge loss. The feeling of being useless can be overwhelming and devastating. Shondeya, a woman in my Attitudinal Healing Center chronic illness support group who suffers from debilitating migraine headaches, shared that she didn't picture her life turning out in this way. She said, "I keep thinking I could offer so much more if I was well—if I didn't have this pain all the time."

Not being able to do for others has been one of the greatest griefs of my illness. I remember being overcome with grief and sorrow one morning as I took a short walk. I felt I had so much to offer, so much heart and wisdom, so much feeling for others, ironically much of it learned from my chronic illness. Yet, I was locked in a body that couldn't do. It seemed such a waste of abundance. So un-ecological. There is such a deep belief ingrained in us that being of service to others means "doing" in some way. It just seems true that in order to show love for someone, one needs to do for them. This was especially devastating for me when my children were very young, and I was so sick that I could barely read a paragraph to them before I needed to lie down and rest.

One morning in particular, grief came in waves, along with the deepening awareness of the need to be with the truth of the moment and of my life. I had learned enough to know that one can't argue with "what is" and that "what is" is somehow "right" in the larger picture of things. "This is what I have," my inner voice said. "It must be what God wants me to have. The situation must have some basic and intrinsic goodness to it, because it is what is happening. It is the truth."

I groped for understanding. I asked the deep heart question, "What is my role here?" And my heart, in deep wisdom, answered. Something opened up in me and, as I looked around, I was filled with appreciation and wonder at the beauty of the world. It welled up in me as a deep gratitude for my life, for the natural world, for friends and lovers, for the man passing me on the road who offered a friendly hello, for the teachers of the children—the teachers who actually love them, and who reach deep within to go the distance each day to try to find ways to make a difference in their lives, who teach them to add two plus two, and inspire them with stories of Gandhi or other great persons—for the gift of music, and all who make it, for the writers of all the wonderful novels and poems that have touched my heart and changed me in some basic and mysterious way, for all the volunteer workers who give of themselves selflessly with no expectation of return, except the inner satisfaction of knowing they have made a difference in someone's life.

I thought of the woman at the local swimming pool to which I took my girls on hot summer days to cool off and stretch and grow into their young bodies and emotions. She stood at the counter of the steamy locker room greeting long lines of youngsters day in and day out with a cheerful "hello," seeming never to tire of seeing their eager faces, dispensing keys and band-aids and down-home wisdom, comforting or finding lost little sisters and brothers, settling disputes, consoling the forlorn, and offering a suggestion about where one might find a lost towel, or how one might deal with an angry father.

She knew the names of many and treated all with obvious affection. She was the substitute mom for two hundred kids for the afternoon. I remembered being overwhelmed with gratitude for this simple woman, uneducated, probably making minimum wage, who put her heart and soul, and the love of a saint into her lowly job. And she did it all completely without fanfare. I saw her job as one of deep importance to the well-being of the world. I thought she must be one of the richest people I had ever seen.

As I pictured in my mind's eye all these people for whom I felt such gratitude, I wanted desperately to be one of them: a creator, a celebrator, or a helper. But that, it seemed, was not to be—at least not at this point in time, perhaps not in this lifetime.

Learning to Receive—Being Love

I realized that my illness had deepened my appreciation of the world and all the wonderful, good, beautiful and crazy things in it a hundredfold. Like the apostle Paul, who, on his way to Damascus, fell from his horse surrounded by white light, and felt that he had become "nothing but eye," I felt that I had become one huge receptor, and could receive all the things that needed receiving.

For every doer, there must be a receiver. The woman in the locker room needed those kids as much as they needed her. It was a totally natural and mutual exchange of energies. The conductor of a great symphony, though perhaps not actually *needing* an audience, still wants to share his experience of the music with others. People in grief need someone to listen. Nietzsche said, "Oh great Sun, what would your joy be without those for whom you shine?" Even God is powerless in manifesting that which He desires the most—our love. Shondea, the woman who has suffered for many years with migraines, said she realized after many years of struggling with the pain of not being able to do, that "it is by our being that we influence people in the world, not by what we do." So, though this wasn't the role I chose, it was the role given to me. I wanted to be the doer, but instead, it was given to me to be the receiver, the appreciator, the lover.

When illness comes, often we have nothing but time on our hands. And that time seems to stretch out into an eternity. You are there and you feel the world is passing you by. You feel you might as well be dead. You feel you have nothing to offer, or that your life is so difficult that it just isn't worth living. Your life seems so small, perhaps almost non-existent. You may ask yourself, "What good is it for me to even exist? All I can be is a burden to others."

A woman in my wellness group came in one day in despair. Her life wasn't working: her assisted housing had fallen through, her friends had fled, her doctor couldn't help her, and she needed to haul an oxygen tank around with her in order to breathe. She asked God and the universe why she was here because she, herself, saw no reason. She was close to suicide. The next week when she came to group she related how some man in the grocery store, some stranger, had opened himself up to her. His overflowing joy of life wanted to be shared with someone and she somehow was there to receive it. In that simple act of receiving, something changed in her. The deep searching her illness had evolved in her, the question she had posed to the universe in her deepest anguish was answered: We are here for each other.

During the year of 1982, when I was separated from my husband the first time, I was very ill, and every day felt like an insurmountable obstacle. I felt that what I was doing was impossible—i.e. trying to raise my two daughters alone with my chronic illness. Physically I was just not making it. Each day I felt so sick, so exhausted and in pain that I whispered a silent or audible prayer nearly every minute of every day. This prayer was a million miles away from asking for the perfect life, for finding true love, for happiness, for a great vacation, or even for being able to go out to the movies with a friend. It was simply "Please, Lord, help me make it through this day. Let me be able to do what I need to do for these kids and this dog, without collapsing or having a major relapse, so I will be able to get up and care for them again tomorrow." Often it was simply, "Please, just let me make it through the next five minutes." I do think that during that period it was only grace that got me through.

I remember one occasion very clearly. I was lying on the couch in the living room. My two girls, ages five and eight, were playing on the couch, on and around me. I was feeling so miserable, and so exhausted, that I could barely interact with them. Despair was sweeping over me like a giant wave. There were my beautiful children, wanting to be with their mother, and I had nothing to give.

And it wasn't like this was an occasional occurrence. Day in and day out, I struggled to put healthy food on the table for them, to keep them in clean clothes, to get them to the places they needed to be, and to try, somehow, to get some enrichment into their lives, because God knows I couldn't offer it. I read them a paltry story once a day at bedtime, before I collapsed, exhausted and hurting into my own bed. I wanted desperately to play with my children, to sing with them, walk with them, paint with them, laugh with them. But I was too sick and weak to do any of these things. When we went somewhere in the car, I needed my older daughter to help with the steering—that's how weak I was. I felt utterly useless, and worse, I felt deep grief and shame that my children were not getting what I thought they needed. Yet there they were, gathered around me, playing happily, wanting to be where I was.

Suddenly it dawned on me. No one in this wide world loved these beings in the way or to the depth that I did. No one cared about them enough to devote every stitch of available energy to their welfare—except me. No one would be there day after day, year after year, to watch over their unfolding, to listen to their hopes and their dreams, to cheer every achievement, to kiss away their tears of rejection or defeat, except me. I realized then, that though they would have to get much of their learning, experience, and the physical help they needed from other sources in the world, they would never lack for someone to love them.

I take another look at the word "essential." The root word is essence. What is essential? What is the essence of being? The essence of our being is love—the ultimate communication—the highest level of connectedness. Mary Oliver, the poet, asks, "What is it you plan to do with your one wild and precious life?" There are worse things to do with a life than love.

Doing Versus Being—The Practice of Being a Tree

As I lie on the grass and breathe in the tree energy,
I become more tree-like: strong, still, serene, rooted,
and the wind blows through me on the breath gently rustling my inner landscape.
Nothing to do, no one to be, just this moment, life as it is. Beautiful, perfect.
I cannot hold onto this perfect moment.
It will pass, as everything does. But this tree's grace sustains me for a while.
A tree never moves—things, animals, weather, come to it;
Birds fly into its branches, nest there; people sit beneath it for a time—
rest in its shade, seek protection from the wind.
When I become overwhelmed, when life seems too much,
when I think I need to act, but the body prevents me,
when it seems my life has crumbled to nothing,
I remember tree energy. I say to myself, "Now I will become a tree,"
and I lie still in some degree of peace and dignity.
It is only my overactive mind that thinks I must do in order to have worth.

—Diane LaRae Bodach

CHAPTER 16

The Practice of Being Without

We live in a finite world with finite bodies and we live under their laws.

WHEN A ZEN STUDENT GOES TO SESSHIN, or a Christian enters the period of Lent, there is a feeling of giving something up, putting oneself under some restriction, or depriving oneself somehow. Yet when the period of restriction is over and the person comes out the other end, there is often a lightness of being and a joy that defies explanation. Chronically ill or disabled people do not make the choice to put themselves under restriction—they *are* under restriction. This is both an advantage and a disadvantage. It's an advantage because they don't have to make the choice, a choice that could be put off indefinitely and more than likely would never have been made—it's already been made for them. It's a disadvantage because they may not have the same attitude of openness and willingness necessary to benefit from the situation that they have when they have made a choice to participate in something.

Of course the truth is, we are all under restrictions all the time. We live in a finite world with finite bodies and we live under their laws. We are always running into situations we wish were different. People and things are always disappointing us and we are always disappointing ourselves. There is always something we want that we can't have. Maybe the love of our life has just left us or the neighborhood deli has stopped making our favorite sandwich. In big or little ways, life is always disappointing us.

Sometimes just a slight twist or change in perspective can shift something that seems negative into something positive. One can do this with big things or little things. For example, it is my habit to drink milk with cafix (my coffee substitute) and mineral water with fruit juice. On my way home from an outing, I realize I am out of both, but too tired to stop at the store. Or, let's say, after looking forward for months to a trip with my family to the east coast, I go to one event too many or walk a block too far and trigger the chronic illness that lurks in the shadows like a feral cat at the edge of my civilized life. Suddenly I am light years back to the incapacity I had climbed slowly out of over a period of months or years—the trip now an impossible dream.

I could see these situations as deprivations—or I could see them as opportunities for practice. This is not a trick to talk ourselves into being satisfied with something that's sub-par. It's not putting a happy face on something bad. It is rather an exploration and inquiry into the deep truth of our situation. Is it true that we need what we think we need? Is it true that not having what we want is bad? To begin to question the rigid belief systems that seem so obvious is to begin to open to a new way of looking—a new way of being with our lives that can be refreshing if not life changing.

For this exploration, one could start with the premise that all states of being are equal. That is, every state of being, everything we experience, is equally valid and valuable. Not only that, but each state, if we really allow ourselves to enter it completely, has within it the same qualities of joy and peace that we have experienced in our most "high" states. This is a truth I have experienced deeply, though I don't always "know" this truth in the body. Sometimes I may only remember intellectually, but I have begun to have a deep belief in its veracity through many encounters with the actual experience. The practice of being without helps me to "remember" or experience it anew. Even if you don't believe this premise is true, you may decide to try the "what if" practice—that is, to set aside for a moment your tightly held beliefs about what is true or not true, to ask yourself "what if" this premise were true, and to imagine it might possibly *be* true.

I used to get upset or maybe just a little peeved when I didn't have something I thought I needed: scotch tape for wrapping a present, some ingredient for a recipe, candles for a special evening, my milk or mineral water, etc., etc. Even if I didn't get peeved, I still *believed* on some kind of emotional level that I needed these things and, if I had enough energy, would make a special trip to the store to get them. This was fairly easy to do when I had good health—considerably harder with chronic illness. So, again, illness or scarcity are revealed as props or tools to help us delve more deeply into truth.

I am a person who loves to eat good food, and even though I am not a fussy eater in the sense of the range of foods I will eat (I like almost everything), I do want my food to taste good. So when I'm cooking a dish, I like to have all the ingredients and have been known to use my last ounce of energy to drive to the store to get the missing lemon and tomato or whatever ingredient that will add just the right taste to make a dish (in my opinion) delicious.

I wouldn't attempt to count the number of times since I've been ill that this tactic has left me too exhausted to enjoy the hard-earned meal. I still do this, by the way, but more often these days I will find myself rummaging through the frige to see what I have on hand instead. Since I've hit upon the idea of the practice of doing without, I have discovered hundreds of new taste sensations and ways of cooking dishes that I never would have dreamed of before. I have sometimes chastised myself with the notion that I'm not *really* practicing doing without—I'm just filling up the hole left by one wonderful thing with an equally wonderful thing.

Going more deeply with this inquiry I realized that there are two great ways to practice being without. The first way, the way of using what you have on hand to create whatever it is you have the impulse to create, is called the "Practice of Being Satisfied With What You Have." The second, "The Practice of Being Without," is a practice of *simply being without*—no substitution, no tactics to get what you want through another avenue, no way to fill that craving—just experiencing what it feels like to not have what you want and existing in a naked intimate relationship with your desire.

The former is lighter and allows for creativity and a sense of play in using materials one has on hand. It has also turned me on to ways of dealing with common situations that occur in my life that are more sane (or less neurotic) and has made my life a lot easier and more fun.

I let my inner wisdom guide me to whatever aspect of practicing with scarcity will be most beneficial for me being in my present circumstances. If there is a "charge" that seems disproportionate to the situation, or I sense that my need or desire is based on grasping or the avoidance of feeling some feared emotion, the practice most likely to be aligned with my highest good will usually be the "Practice of Being Without."

I find this usually the best place to start regardless, as we are usually not "on to" the great lengths our false egos will go to keep us from encountering these feared emotions. For example, if I have the necessary ingredients to make a very acceptable substitute dish, or, given my state of exhaustion, the need to rest would, upon rational examination, pre-empt the need to go to the store but I am about to go anyway, the "Practice of Being Without" often reveals deeper levels of holding—the need for control or perhaps deep fear of rejection or unworthiness (if I don't make a dish that tastes really delicious).

So, instead of running to the store, when I come up short of something, I imagine that this is just the way things are: maybe I am sick or dying and can't get out to get what I need; maybe I am in a wilderness and there are no stores; maybe I am poor and cannot afford to buy supplies. We in the West are so used to simply getting in our cars and going out to buy whatever we want or think we need. And indeed, I think this tendency extends into many other aspects of our lives as well. We are always running out into the world to fill some need we think we have, whether it be physical, emotional, intellectual or spiritual, and this modern world is only too ready with events and activities to fill them. So instead of running out to attend the first singles event that presents itself when my boyfriend says he needs space, I try allowing myself time to sit quietly with whatever is presenting itself in mind and body.

I think these are very good practices for us. You may think, "Oh, it's about cooking! It can't be about anything very deep or important." Or "I can't sit quietly with myself. My mind is screaming at my boyfriend. And that's all that's there." Or "I'm just too sad to do anything."

You'll be surprised to find that in every action, no matter how minor or overwhelming, our whole being is present, though it may be hidden. Our whole system of false beliefs and repressed emotions are active. That may seem like bad news. Well okay—that's the bad news, but that's also the good news—because it means that no matter where we go or what we do, we always have an opportunity to do the work and to heal into our true and joyful heart.

If you decide to experiment with this, try not to distract yourself with diversions. Don't turn on the TV so you can forget about your desire. Let yourself experience your sensations and your inner dialogue. No doubt, "this is a stupid exercise!" will be one of them, but when you go deeper, you may discover a rich arena for inner exploration—a goldmine of repressed emotions and restricting negative false beliefs awaiting your exploration and the healing light of awareness. Notice your body—what do you feel and where? Notice your inner talk without judgment. Do the steps for practicing with negative emotions from Chapter Ten.

If you don't have a big charge or you are feeling playful or you are simply not wanting to go deep at the moment, you might decide to use "The Practice of Being Satisfied With What You Have." Look around at what you have on hand and use it to fill whatever need or desire is animating your action. Be creative. Be playful. Be willing to go in a different direction from your original impulse.

My practice with dying has led me to question the necessity of a lot of things, and has opened me up to a new way of playing and being creative in my life. Instead of stretching myself to the breaking point by running to the store every time I come up short of some supposedly necessary item, I more often rummage through the fridge and take out what I have to put together into a meal, or look around the house for some string or discarded piece of raffia to hold the wrapping onto a present. This has been fun, satisfying, and easier on the environment, as well as saving me a lot of time and energy. If it is an emotional desire that is being thwarted and I've decided to do "The Practice of Being Satisfied With What You Have," I might ask myself if I can offer to myself what I am desiring from someone else. Sometimes it is simply my stubbornness that is keeping me from being satisfied with what I have.

Once I was feeling sad because I was alone, i.e. without a mate. I was thinking about how simply having a lover/partner in the house with me—sharing the space and my life, even if we are not interacting—has changed the experience of whatever I happen to be doing into something almost magical. Then I started thinking about all the things that are done separately even when one is in relationship—which is really a lot. I realize that what I was doing at that moment I felt so alone (taking a bath) was something I would have been doing alone anyway and that I wasn't really being with myself in a loving/caring way. I wasn't offering myself the loving kindness and attention I had learned to offer to myself or to attend to the magic already impregnating that very moment. And suddenly, like a switch had been flipped, my reality opened to some kind of magical matrix in which *I* was imbedded. So again here was a time I was expecting someone else to do *my* job—to take care of me. Though it is wonderful and magical to love and be loved—to share a life—we must be aware of our unconscious tendency to fall into dependency on others to meet needs we could be providing for ourselves. But most of all it behooves us, at all times, to be present to each moment, in which case, we will have no unmet needs and our experience will be filled with the magic that is always permeating reality, *if* we are paying attention.

Let's talk about another example—I love to go out and have a good time with friends or go on trips with my family. There have been many times when, because of my illness, I have had to miss events or trips on which I've really had my heart set. This kind of situation presents us with a great opportunity to use both practices. First use "The Practice of Being Without" because there is sure to be some serious emotional reaction to being left out or behind; again do the steps for "Practicing with Negative Emotions." When you've completely mined the gold from your deep holdings, move on to "The Practice of Being Satisfied With What You Have."

Some of the best times I've ever had have been situations like these where I've had something planned that has fallen through and there has initially been a huge disappointment. When I have gotten past the disappointment, I suddenly have a huge open space I didn't expect to have. It is like I have a huge blank canvas I can fill up in any way I choose. It's an unexpected date with myself. Since I have no obligations, and I hadn't intended to accomplish anything in that particular space of time, I can play without feeling guilty.

I have many examples of this, but one that really stands out in my mind is from a time early in life when I was a teenager, before I started practicing, at least in any conscious way. It was New Year's Eve and I didn't have a date. I had already gone through a huge funk, but when the big night actually descended on me, I had the time of my life with myself. I put on some rock and roll music, peroxided my hair, put my goldfish in the bathtub with his seaweed and all his pretty rocks and accessories while I cleaned his bowl, wrote in my diary, danced around the whole house (since my parents were out and I had it to myself), and generally had a great time that I remember very explicitly with pleasure to this day.

CHAPTER 17

The Way to Be Happy

May all beings be unaccountably happy.
—Rosemary Rau Levine

MY MEDITATION TEACHER once asked us all to tell what meditation was for us, what we wanted from our practice. One woman answered, "I want to be happy all the time—forever." We all long to be happy—and that is right and good and natural. We were born for joy. The problem is that we have a picture of what that happiness should look like, and we'll rot in hell before we allow ourselves to experience joy without that picture. We block our happiness by comparing all our experiences with our picture and rejecting anything that doesn't match. All of our unhappiness stems from our requirement that life be something other than what it is. But life can never be anything other than what it is, moment by moment by moment. This life fits us perfectly right now.

Having had a chronic illness for twenty-two years, which is sometimes better and sometimes worse, I have learned to deal with the ups and downs of being ill, weak or in pain much of the time, but it is never easy.

The only way to be truly happy is to be happy with things just the way they are, and that is the one thing we refuse to do—the one thing, above all things, that we don't want to do. And if we get really honest, if we dig deep, we must acknowledge that this is the one thing we do not want to be true—that is, the idea that we *can* be happy with things just the way they are. However, we are often in deep denial about the fact that we do not want this to be true and that we are generally unwilling to consider the possibility that it might be. We claim we want to know the Truth, to open to God, to trust our process—but only if it fits our picture of what we think it should be. Anthony De Mello, S.J., says, "If people were not actively engaged in making themselves miserable, they would be happy."

But to be happy with things as they are means to learn to be happy with our broken bodies, our broken hearts, our broken dreams. How can this be? This pain in our bodies, this longing for the love that would fill us up and make us whole, this wanting our bodies to do what they just won't do, this longing for what has been, but is no longer possible, this deep shame that washes over us when we do the thing—again—that we have vowed never again to do, these unwanted feelings and thoughts that live in the shadows of our psyches and pop-up when we least expect or want them. To be happy while these feelings are present is just too much to ask, isn't it?

One evening I had a sing-a-long at my house. I was watching my friend, who is my age, play guitar and sing all evening long after having worked all day, and it was like watching a miracle. For me, living as I do with chronic illness, it would be a true miracle to be able to do that. But I still sometimes long for it, even after twenty years of not being able to do it—especially when it comes so close to home, like it did that night.

When we are in pain, either physically or emotionally, all we want is relief. To even entertain the notion that we can be happy in the midst of one of these miserable moments seems impossible, not to mention unreasonable. We would much rather think that at some future time we will be out of pain, that we will heal, that we will be in love, that we will become that loving, giving, funny, uplifting, or peaceful person we have dreamed of becoming, than to imagine we can be happy in the midst of our pain, our illness, our loneliness, our messy lives.

Many have probably heard the Buddhist teaching story about creating our own room. The scenario starts out innocuously enough. We have a room and we begin to fix it up to suit ourselves. We pick out furniture we like, put pictures on the wall that please us, play the kind of music that suits whatever mood we happen to be in, stock the refrigerator with all the food we love to eat, paint the walls with our favorite colors. What could be wrong with this? We all need a place of our own, don't we? A place to call home? A place that brings us comfort? Well, yes of course. So far so good.

We invite our friends over—only the ones we're really close to—the ones with whom we feel very comfortable. And we have a very good time together. But when we go out, we see and hear things that disturb us. We meet people that rub us the wrong way. Some of them just plain don't like us, or we don't like them. The streets are messy and dirty. The air is smoggy. It's noisy out there. Bad things are happening. It's good to get back home to our room where we can be comfortable and not see the bad things. We go out less and less. And pretty soon, we don't go out at all. We have become a prisoner in our own room.

We can't have it both ways; we either create a world for ourselves and live in that narrow little world we have created, or we throw open the doors of our heart and soul to what God and the Universe have cooked up for us, accepting and experiencing the immense totality of it, the good and the bad, moment by moment. Once we begin to pick and choose—there is no end to it.

Even if we have a strong spiritual practice, and believe the mantra we have heard a thousand different ways: "Be here now," "Open to this moment," "Give up attachment to past or future," etc., we still have a belief somewhere in the back of our minds that, if we do this practice "right," we will get relief, we will be out of pain—maybe even that we will be in bliss. And, for those of us with chronic or acute illnesses, behind that belief is another hidden belief or agenda that says, when the body and spirit are properly aligned, the natural and proper consequence will be that we will be healed in the body, and thus be able to again do all those things we long to do.

Once we have gotten an intense jolt, had a deep opening, or "hit bottom," and learn something very valuable, we think things should change. Our reasoning goes something like this, "Okay, I have learned this lesson. Now I don't need these conditions any more." And we expect them to change. We expect things to get "better." Our determination and the imaginative contortions we will go through to get what we want are really quite amazing. But the truth is, if we had really learned our lesson, we would not *need* things to change. Though we may prefer certain things over others, we would not require them for our happiness. We would understand that the truth underlying all existence is constantly manifesting itself in myriad forms, each as valid and deep and true as any other.

Instead, we continue to cling to the idea that there is some future time, some future "me" that will be better than the one I have now, and my job is to strive toward that—to change somehow to make this better me, this better moment, materialize. If only I could find someone to love, then I would be happy. If only I could walk, then I would be happy. If only I could find a better, easier, or more rewarding job, then I would be happy. If only my child would get off drugs...if only my husband/wife/boss/friend/lover weren't so critical...if only...if only...if only. If we are spiritual practitioners, the "if only" might be: " if only I were enlightened," or "if only I could drop my attachments..." etc. etc. Of course, if we actually got that thing that we think would make us happy, there would just be one more thing to replace it.

Before I became chronically ill, I could get on a roll and spend three or four hours cleaning and organizing my room. At the end I would pretty much have it done. I would survey my handiwork with an eye of satisfaction. Now I look sadly around at the stacks of papers and clothes and feel the hopelessness of the situation. I work for ten minutes and become so tired I have to rest for two hours. I get through one stack—thank God—but then have three bad days. The mail, the dishes, the clothes build up. Then there are three stacks to replace the one I have conquered—like the seven-headed dragon who grows two heads to replace each one that is cut off.

But if I suppose for a minute that I could have that healthy body again—that impossible dream—that I could get my house cleaned up, get all my work done, organize everything and have order in my life, or perhaps relative order—even if I could play my guitar and sing all night, would I be one centimeter closer to true happiness than I am now? No, I don't believe I would be. Was I happy before I got sick, when I could do all those things I so long to do? No, I wasn't. There was always something lacking, something I thought I needed before I could be happy. The truth is, I am happier now, with a body that hurts and doesn't work much of the time.

I love Adyashanti's insight into this phenomenon of desires. We think, he said, that certain objects, people or circumstances that we don't have will make us happy if we could only get them. And actually, if we get the object of our desire, we *are* happy—for a short time. And we think that we are happy because we have the object of our desires. In reality, he says, this is a false conclusion. We know it is false because if it were really the object that made us happy, we would continue to be happy as long as we have the object. But of course we all know that this is rarely, if ever, the case. Usually within some period of time, very short for a piece of clothing or a car and somewhat longer for a new friend or lover, we begin to have desires again. We begin to wish things were other than what they are. There is something else we need, or our friend or lover doesn't quite fulfill our desire any more.

So if it isn't actually the object, person or circumstance that make us so happy for a while, what is it? Adyashanti says it is the absence of desire. For a time after we get what we have desired, we are *desireless*. We bask in the happiness of what we have and thus we are happy.

I once knew a man who dreamed of being a success. As a child he dreamed he would be successful and have nice things, and that dream was epitomized for him in owning a metallic blue Mercedes convertible. The man grew up to become a successful businessman, raised a family, and built a beautiful house in the country. He went on great vacations and bought his family many nice things, but he still wasn't happy. Then one day he decided it was time to fulfill his dream and he bought a blue Mercedes. Within a month, his family found him dead—he had taken his own life.

We have an idea that if we could get this or that thing we would be happy. It may not be a blue Mercedes; it might be a new job, new husband, or in the case of the chronically ill, our health. It's easy to say, "Oh, of course, a car can't bring happiness." It's not so easy to see that all the objects of our desires are the same as that blue Mercedes—essentially empty, and incapable of bringing us the happiness and peace we so desire. And not only is it the *objects* of our desire—the external circumstances of our lives—that cannot give us lasting happiness, but the internal world as well—our high emotions, our lofty thoughts, our epiphanies, all of our experiences. These too are transient and in time will pass.

All that striving—all that yearning—is keeping us from experiencing the only thing we can ever have: this present moment and the love that is inherent in it. And it also means simply putting off the inevitable—when we finally have to come to terms with the fact that our bodies will eventually fail and die and that the bodies of our loved ones will fail and die. We will lose it all one way or the other. So, we begin to learn to live with the disorder and pain in our lives and even with the highs and lows of our emotions. We begin to reside and to rest on that "hard and icy couch" which is our life in just this moment, and which fits us so perfectly. And we begin to experience for brief moments a peace that defies understanding.

To be happy with things as they are means to give up the notion that things need to be different in order for us to be happy. And to give up this notion means there's nothing that has to be done or changed. To simply BE with life as it is really is all that is required of us, and the only thing that is actually possible. To truly understand this and the strength of our resistance to it, is to begin to get a grip on the immensity of the task before us, and, at the same time, of its utter simplicity.

One day when my doctor was giving me an osteopathic adjustment for the pain in my back and neck, I asked her how she was doing. She said she was unaccountably happy. She added that she looked for reasons but couldn't find any, so she hypothesized that it might be the lovely fall colors, or some hormonal change or other strange unknown factor. I said, "I think it's wonderful that there's no reason. If there were, then when that reason went away, your happiness would too."

She said, "The Buddhists would probably say, 'May all beings be unaccountably happy.' I'm not a Buddhist, so I always look for reasons." I loved her statement so much that I decided to make it a personal mantra—*may all beings be unaccountably happy, may all beings everywhere be unaccountably happy.* As long as we need something from life, we will never be free. As long as our happiness depends on some condition to be met, we will never be truly happy, for we will always live in fear that that condition will never be met, or if we have it, that it will be taken away.

No matter how much money we save, no matter how much knowledge we manage to accumulate, no matter how much weight we lose or how many facelifts we have, whether we are beautiful or handsome, well or sick, we are all naked against this very moment in which we exist. It is all we have—our awareness, our love, and this instant in time. We think life is supposed to be for something, but it's not for anything. It is just for itself—this precious moment. If we come to this understanding, it doesn't mean we stop doing or striving, but we can enter our lives in a new way, a lighter way, a more playful way. Life can be a dance. To live the possible life that is right in front of our noses, instead of yearning for the impossible one from the past, or in some distant future, is the path of peace.

> *What will you do, God, when I die?*
> *I am your pitcher (when I shatter?)*
> *I am your drink (when I go bitter?)*
> *I, your garment; I, your craft.*
> *Without me what reason have you?*
> *Without me what house*
> *where intimate words await you?*
> *I, velvet sandal that falls from your foot.*
> *I, cloak dropping from your shoulder.*
> *Your gaze, which I welcome now*
> *as it warms my cheek,*
> *will search for me hour after hour*
> *and lie at sunset, spent,*
> *on an empty beach*
> *among unfamiliar stones.*
> *What will you do, God? I am afraid.*
>
> —Rainer Maria Rilke

CHAPTER 18

The Inner Healer

Our higher inner self knows what to do in any circumstance; it's just a matter of getting out of our own way so the higher self can manifest.

OUR DEEP INNER SELF is very wise. One could, depending on one's belief, make the leap and say that our deepest, truest, highest self is God speaking to us, trying to order our life in a sane, even divine way.

Usually people have cut themselves off from their true selves. Most often, the disconnect happened when we were tiny babies and we needed to protect ourselves from some external or perceived threat. Prominent family therapist, teacher and author, John Bradshaw says most people in the West come from dysfunctional families. But even if our families weren't exactly "dysfunctional" and our parents loved us very much, they still weren't perfect (no parents are) and probably did things at times that were unloving—things that reflected their own disconnection with their hearts, their own true selves.

Perhaps these unloving actions were even done "for our own good," as parents all over the world have done horrendous things to teach their children lessons. Governments have even tortured their own people to "help them see the light." In addition, as we all too sadly know, wars are often fought "in the name of God" or righteousness. When we are disconnected from our true selves, there is no limit to the damage we can do in the name of "trying to do the right thing," and this dysfunction, this disconnection, gets passed down through the generations.

If those of us who have had some kind of physical or mental breakdown look back to the time when we were well, especially if we have begun to do inner work and to make connection with the wise knowing part of ourselves, we can often see that a deep inner voice had been trying to speak—had been trying desperately to tell us something about our life that we, equally desperately, tried to block out. We just didn't want or couldn't bear to hear it.

I almost want to cry when I think of how hard I pushed myself during those years before my body broke down, how unloving I was to my physical body, and how ruthless I was with myself on an emotional level. The inner child must have been crying out, but I wasn't listening. I thought I needed to be strong, to be pure, to be "spiritual." My intentions were good, but I was going about it like a ruthless despot, so it came out in the shadow form against my own self as with Jung's warning that, if we do not deal with our shadows, they will become our fate. But we can break the chains of dysfunction and disconnection. We can reconnect with our own true self and begin our own healing, and thus the healing of the world.

The Divine Child

There are two archetypes that are closely aligned with the inner healer: The Divine Child and The Wise One. Jesus said, "Unless you become as little children, you cannot enter the Kingdom of Heaven." Surely he is not implying here that we should go back to being completely helpless and dependent on others to take care of us, or forego qualities which may have developed in the wise adult, such as discernment and compassion. What then is that essence of child that Jesus admonishes us to embrace?

If we look at a baby, we see a being who is naturally trusting, and who seems to live almost completely in the present moment. She is totally open except for the short period of time when face recognition begins (i.e., a baby begins to differentiate her mother's face from others and may cry when strangers try to pick her up).

Babies and toddlers are remarkably free from the kinds of social inhibitions that keep adults who don't "know" one another from connecting. At several parties I've been to lately, babies who have never seen me before have come to climb on my lap or have grabbed the edge of a stranger's cup to peer in and see what was inside. These activities would be unthinkable for the normal adult. Often we are suspect if a stranger approaches us or treats us in a familiar manner. But once in a while if we are feeling particularly open, a person may come up to us and start talking to us as if he knew us—and it feels good. It feels really good. It feels like we're home—like we've known this person all our lives. We laugh and chatter and feel like a kid or a teenager again. We go home and think about what a good time we had.

    A baby is not concerned with being consistent. He can go from tears to laughter in a matter of seconds. He does not notice distinctions of good or bad, man-made or natural. His senses are filled with wonder at the colors and movements, smells and textures before him, whether they are flowers waving in the wind or silverware from the kitchen drawer being clinked together. One of my oldest daughter's delights as a baby was to sit in my biggest canning pot and bang the smaller pots on the kitchen floor. You could see the joy emanating from her, the sense of power she inhabited from her tiny throne.

    A baby is innately playful. Any kind of experience can be made into a game. Give a baby a spoon and then put out your hand. Soon the game of handing the spoon back and forth has been created. A baby is completely enthralled with the sound of her own voice. She delights in singing and making up nonsense songs and words. She doesn't worry about singing in tune. She is a natural born actor/artist. She takes pleasure in hamming it up or in putting color to paper, unconcerned about what other people think of her or whether what she has painted resembles anything in the outside world. If you go to any concert where there is dancing and mixed generations, you will undoubtedly see several toddlers out in front of the band bouncing and wiggling and opening their hearts with absolutely no consideration for how they look and whether they are doing it right or wrong.

    As we grow up, we lose much of that capacity to be delighted by the world and our willingness to give ourselves to our joy or to reach out to others for fear of appearing foolish. What kind of a world would it be if we all talked to everyone as if we already knew them—when in fact we do. We've all known each other from before our mothers were born—because we are all connected. We are all one, but we have forgotten.

    We begin to make distinctions: good/bad, me/them, natural/man-made, win/lose. We begin to be concerned about results and how we will appear to others. We begin to question and doubt ourselves constantly. Do I have talent? Am I competent? Will people think I'm a fool? We begin to think we need to make everything count for something. We begin to be so concerned about what's going to happen in the future or what's already happened that we miss the precious moments of our lives. We forget how to play.

I can't even count the number of people I have met who have told me a story about how someone, usually a parent, sibling or teacher, told them in one way or another that they couldn't sing or draw or dance or play sports—and that this one-time occurrence changed the course of their lives. Basically they swallowed the story, hook, line, and sinker, and from that time forward avoided the activity they believed they were incapable of doing.

These experiences can be very direct and real, like when a woman friend of mine, at the age of nine, brought a picture she had painted to her father and asked him to frame it. He told her the picture wasn't good enough to frame and from that time forward she never set color to paper. Or the experience can be much more subtle or indirect or even completely constructed in our own heads out of the insecurity we already feel. For example, a man I know used to love to write as a young adult and had even had an offer from a publisher friend to publish several of his short stories. Before this came to fruition, however, his publisher friend went to a workshop with a famous writer who told him that a person will never amount to anything as a writer unless he puts his whole heart and soul into his writing—unless he *has* to write. When my friend heard this story, it scared him. He thought, this friend was telling him *he* didn't have what it takes to be a writer. Even when his friend called to inquire again about the possibility of publishing his short stories, he never responded. Thirty-five years later he tells me he now understands that what his friend told him was about him (his friend), and that the story he heard was his own made-up story about himself. At least he finally *got* it. Many go through their whole lives believing the made-up stories from their childhood.

Recovering my relationship with my inner child and with my inner wisdom has been a very important part of my healing. Losing my ability to be in the world as I had learned to be as a well person, and even losing much of my personality through the loss of physical abilities, have been useful in helping me get back in touch with the true essence of me, the wild, creative, playful part of myself that loves and enjoys life and knows what it wants and needs. And having cancer put me in very intimate touch with my mortality: the hard truth that I will lose everything in this physical world at some point (maybe very soon), thus revealing the utter preciousness of this life and the value of my time here. I have learned to play again and to take great delight in simple things.

Still, even now, sometimes I forget and revert to my old ways of fearfulness and doubt, or I get so caught up with the utility of things that I again lose contact with my true self. For example, I go for a walk every morning. Sometimes that can start out as a very joyful, wonderful thing, a connection with nature, being truly present and grounded in my senses. Then, before I know it, it turns into a chore—something I am doing with a goal in mind: suddenly it feels like an obligation, building my muscles, toning my heart. When this happens, I notice some of the joy has gone out of my walking. I may push myself to maintain a certain speed (for cardiovascular fitness) and forego stopping to talk to the donkeys or study the colors of a bird.

If I deeply want to maintain contact with my Divine Child, I have to keep checking in, I have to keep asking, "What is it that you really want?" I need to converse with myself in every way, through talking, through the body, through music or art, through dancing, free writing, nature, or simply sitting silently with myself wherever I might be.

This touching into the playful and creative part of you is not utilitarian. It is not useful in the normal sense of the word. You can't *get* something out of it. You don't get "ahead," nor do you obtain money or prestige or muscles. These things might ultimately come out of our playfulness or our creativity, but if we're going for them in the first place, we will not find that wild, free, creative place within. Play doesn't try to *get* anything. Play is just play for the sake of the delight that arises when we do it, though it may ultimately also lead us to a deeper satisfaction, peace or sense of aliveness.

If you have a person inside of you saying, "But I don't have a playful and creative person in me—I'm more of a utilitarian type of person—I'm not creative," *this is not true.* Everyone has this part of themselves. Remember, unless we're completely integrated (unlikely) or "enlightened" (more unlikely) we have lots of different "I's" in us—various selves who do not really even know about each other. Maybe you're barking up the wrong tree (looking to the wrong "I")—a case of "mistaken identity." The "dull, uncreative" part of ourselves was never meant to be wild and crazy, but has other very important functions to perform, like thinking, planning, analyzing data, etc. I used to think I was one of those dull, uncreative people. But I've discovered that while I certainly *do* have one of those in me, she's not all of me.

I am not talking about taking up a hobby, collecting things, painting preformed ceramics, or even singing with a choir, though these kinds of activities can be very beneficial in the sense of being calming, heart opening, or very satisfying. I am talking about the edge that says, "I don't know where this is going to go. I don't know what I am going to do next." Whether or not your singing would enthrall an audience, or your artistic self comes up with a finished product that you would want to show someone or sell or publish is an entirely different story. That's not the point. The point is to develop a connection with yourself—the inner creative, playful, alive part of yourself.

This doesn't have to be dramatic. It can be something very small and simple or quirky. Some of these things I have discovered almost by accident and seem almost like tricks because they appear to "work" in a magical way. I will try something or imagine something almost on a whim and suddenly my whole experience of reality and/or myself opens up. I seem to be transformed from a dull, ordinary person in the midst of the doldrums into a very alive, playful, magical person, at least momentarily, simply through some subtle shift of awareness or willingness to do something different. More often than not I find that these opportunities open up when my normal routine is somehow disrupted. (Remember—the one in charge of setting routine is *not* the playful creative aspect of ourselves.)

One day I wanted to save my morning walk for later because I felt a desire to go to the park and yet I still wanted to wake up my body before breakfast, so I decided to dance. This is something I often do, but it's almost always a surprise when I do it, *if* I do it in the way of the playful child—that is, as a kind of free-form dance that just tunes into my body, that just lets my body move in the way that it wants to. In this way of dancing I let go of any kind of thought of form and just allow what wants to come out in any particular moment to come out.

Another time I was having a "leg relapse." I didn't want to completely lose the small amount of cardiovascular conditioning I had managed to build up so I tried to use the rest of my body to move aerobically. I found myself going into another wild moving/stretching/dancing on the floor that ended up having some free form chanting and singing with it which ultimately evolved into an original song. So what started out as a utilitarian exercise ended up as playful creative expression.

Somebody in you, however, has to be *willing to follow* that wild, playful, creative energy as it arises. Someone in you has to be willing to suspend the work, to leave the "to do" list behind for a short time and enter the magical realm where time and getting things done have no importance. It may seem frightening and out of control to "the planner." After all, she has business to attend to, work to do. But as you see in this example, the "planning I," though very distinct from the "creative I," can, in spite of its fears or reservations, be inadvertently involved in opening up the "creative I" or at least move aside so the creative I can come forward. Since it is the inner adult who decides things and implements actions, it will be some aspect of the inner adult that relinquishes control to the wild, creative self, an aspect of The Divine Child.

When we've discovered and reconnected with our playful, creative divine child, the aspect of ourselves that we may have labeled dull, stilted, and uncreative—which is really a distorted or wounded aspect of our adult—may begin to be transformed or healed into the wise adult. Or it may be the wise adult already and, as noted earlier, we have simply mislabeled it.

I am motivated to share a few of the simple things I have discovered because they have brought me such joy and aliveness. I believe these are things that anybody can do. However, though the activities I am going to suggest will often bring a feeling of joy, it's important to remember that the Divine Child isn't always "happy" in the sense of what we normally think it means to be happy. So it is also possible that difficult feelings may arise, such as anger or grief, because opening to the Divine Child cracks open the armoring we have built up around our heart and may expose us to feelings we have suppressed.

Nonetheless, doing these practices is a very loving and kind thing to do for yourself and often leads directly to *"experiencing,"* which lies at the heart of being completely present to life as it is, the greatest healing. Of course, none of these practices take the place of the major practices of *loving kindness,* *experiencing,* and *working with false beliefs* described in earlier chapters, but they do contribute to them.

Practices for Connecting with the Inner Child or Creative Self

1. Free Dancing

Put on some music. It could be any kind of music—hip-hop, rock-and-roll, reggae, classical, folk, or some deeply spiritual kind of music. You could choose by your mood or even better, just let your finger point to something and let your body move to whatever you have chosen. I often like to use the music of Deva Primal because it seems to go to a very deep part of me and elicit the natural-healer-movement person in me.

But this is always changing, open, flowing—this relationship with myself, with my body. So what may be true one day is not true the next. It is easy to get into a rut and think, "Well, this worked so well yesterday, I'll do the same thing today." This is the ego legislative aspect of ourselves, which is what we are trying to sidestep for a few moments. It is the ego trying to "get something," to make us a "better," more alive, more playful person. This is the antipathy of playfulness. Be willing to just try something different, to play with it—to imagine you're performing or to be sensual, to try new music or to interact with the music in a new way.

If your body is too weak to dance, you can stand in one place and make slight movements. If your legs don't work, you can get on the floor and wiggle around. I know a woman who was so sick she couldn't stand. She got on the floor and imagined herself a snake. She was snake from the inside out. This gradually opened up her body and she became crocodile and eventually many different animals. She is now an amazingly energetic performance dancer/actress.

See what your body can do. Get on the floor; use all the space around you. Feel the rhythm. Have fun! Or not. Maybe what wells up in you will be a great sadness or anger. Don't try to direct. Your inner director will lead you, show you what to do, where to place your feet and your body parts in each moment as it arises, and will evoke whatever feelings are yearning to be evoked. Let it be. Let it all come. Open the floodgates.

2. Morning Pages

Morning pages are another way of accessing the inner child—or the wise one. Julia Cameron coined this phrase (morning pages) in her book *The Artist's Way*. It's not exactly journaling; it is more like playing on the page. It is leaving the judging mind on the doorstep and dancing onto a page where there are no rules. Well, okay, there are a couple of rules:

1. After you put your pen to the page, you don't stop writing until you have reached the end of three pages or fifteen minutes, or however many minutes or pages you have decided on ahead of time.
2. When you first start, don't read your morning pages for at least one week. Then make it a point to not read them at least until the day after you've written them.
3. When you are writing, don't censor yourself in any way. No one *ever* needs to see these pages, not even you! Write whatever comes into your mind or, better yet, bypass the mind completely. Actually, this is one of the major reasons for keeping the pen or pencil moving—it doesn't give the mind time to form thoughts. In this way, the wisdom underlying the conscious mind has a chance to come forth. Let yourself say things "you" would never say and in ways that you would never say them. Make things up. Make up words. Put them together in ways that don't "go" together. Try on different voices, different personas. You may be surprised at what comes out.

3. Free Singing

Begin with "las" or "ahs" or some other sound that is comfortable to you. As with the dancing, simply let your voice float and allow the music to come out. You may need to push yourself a little at first, especially if you are one of those people who thinks they can't sing. I believe music is a natural human inclination. My first-born used to sing constantly as a young child. Granted, she went to a Waldorf school where singing was always a big part of every day's curriculum—"the pump was primed," so to speak, but there was water (music) in the well, and original music poured out of her pretty much all day every day.

I was in a singing group once where we experimented with vibrations by simply singing a single tone—all of us the same. With careful listening we could sometimes hear the harmonics, that is, the tones that vibrate in harmony with the note we were singing. Where did these tones come from? It's a phenomenon that I'm sure some scientist could explain, but I prefer to think of it as a wonderful mystery: music floating in the universe waiting to be found. Music exists in the universe. Certain tones cause vibrations that elicit sympathetic vibrations from nearby objects that have vibrating capacity. We can *find* the music.

Begin without thinking that you need to be singing any kind of song or melody. Play with the sounds, with the tones: high, low, loud, soft, slow, fast, or any kinds of variations you want to play with. Listen to what pleases you. Or experience the vibratory qualities and go with what feels good. Where does your voice want to go with the next note or tone? We know a lot more about music than we think because we are innately musical beings—and have listened to it all our lives—but don't get caught in the trap of trying to make something "right." Whatever you create is just right for you right now.

You can add words if you feel like it. Music can help you access or process your sorrow, your disappointment or your rage. It doesn't have to make sense or be melodic and it doesn't have to rhyme, though rhymes may come. Or you might want to play with rhyming or making different melodies just for fun.

4. Free Painting

You do not need to be an artist to do free painting. Even if you think you have no aptitude for art whatsoever, you can benefit from free painting. Get three tubes of watercolor paint in the primary colors and mix them up in three jars of water to the strength that pleases you. When you begin, try to do a short meditation, prayer or centering exercise, or simply ask the colors to speak to you. You are going to interact with the colors, letting them move and mix in the way they want to flow.

Begin with a color that wants to start and put it on the paper in a way that seems true to that color and your interaction with it. Rinse your brush thoroughly before dipping into a new color or use a fresh brush for each color. Fairly big, soft brushes are best for this purpose. With the new color start on a new part of the paper and let it move toward or away from the other color as it wants to. Feel into the colors. Eventually, the three colors will meet and then you will discover what they do together. By experimentation you will find the amount of paint and wetness required to keep the colors from turning into mud brown (unless of course they *want* to turn into mud brown).

5. A Date with Yourself

We make dates with other people and think it is important to keep them. We develop relationships with others and go out of our way to nurture them. Sometimes parents make dates with each of their children so they can have special time with them. But when it comes to our relationship with ourselves, we don't give it much thought or intention. Our own self is the one person we have spent our whole lives with, but we don't often remember to make special times with ourselves. We may just take whatever is left over after we have taken care of everyone else.

Making a date with yourself once a week is a good way to spend quality time with yourself. You can ask yourself what you would like to do and make a plan to give this to yourself. It could be a movie or dinner or a walk in the woods. It might be a leisurely bath with scented bath oil, candles and music. I like to think of different things that my inner child might want to do. Once I took a bus ride on a city bus, rather than using my car. I take a walk every day, but for my date I might decide to bring a lunch and make a picnic under a favorite tree.

I think it is good to schedule a certain time each week, but you can vary the time to fit your plans. It is surprisingly hard to do this— or rather, not so hard to do, but hard to keep up. Something always seems to come up to get in the way of keeping my date with myself, or I may think I want to do it with someone else. If I keep my date with myself, however, and follow through with my intention, it is incredibly rich and rewarding.

6. Taking a Vacation (Being on vacation 365 days a year)

We all look forward to our vacations. Whether we get a month in Tahiti or a weekend up the coast in the redwoods, it's something to look forward to, a respite from the ordinary, a time to leave all our worries and cares and troubles at home. When we're on vacation, we seem to enjoy our time moment by moment, whether we're surfing the waves, climbing a mountain, training our binoculars on a rare bird, gazing at a beautiful sunset, cooking a meal over the campfire or just relaxing in our hotel room or tent.

Once we put that last box in the van and turn the key in the ignition, a sigh of relief escapes our lungs; a smile creeps over our soul and we drive off feeling like a bird who has just flown through the open door of his cage into paradise.

As we drive along we are happy, relaxed. We chat with our travel mates, look at the map, dig around in the cooler for a sandwich. Or if we're lucky enough to be on our way to some exotic paradise, we sit in the crowded airplane amid noise and confusion, happy as a clam.

What makes these experiences pleasant, while a drive to work in the morning or a business trip across country are experienced as dull or tedious? What makes cooking a meal over an open fire, with primitive tools in semi-darkness as flies buzz around, exciting and fun, while cooking a meal in our well-lit and equipped kitchens often seems like drudgery?

I used to feel really jealous when I would hear my friends planning trips or describing their adventures after they returned home. I wanted so badly to go on these kinds of adventures, but I was stuck in a body that just didn't have the energy to do most of those things. Once when I was lying on my deck feeling sorry for myself, I looked up through the backyard mulberry tree leaves at the blue sky and it dawned on me that this was the same sky that vacationers in Maui or Alaska were looking at. I remembered from the one time I had gone to Kauai with my family (many years before) how much the vegetation and the geography there had reminded me of Sonoma County where

I live. I had been sitting on the deck of my cottage in Hawaii enjoying the afternoon shade.

So there in my own backyard, I allowed myself to imagine I was on vacation and my mood miraculously shifted into a more relaxed, spacious state. Instead of feeling jealous or sorry for myself, I tripped out on the beautiful trees and sky and reveled in the summer breeze wafting across my face.

Of course, I still couldn't go hiking or surfing, but I surely could enjoy many of the other experiences of camping or vacationing there in my own back yard. Even in my house, there are times when I can bring a certain adventurous frame of mind to my activities and suddenly I am on vacation. I am present in this moment and I have no other obligations but to enjoy it, which I think is the distillation of what makes a vacation a vacation.

We've all experienced "magical moments" when we're on vacation or with a special person—when the moon is shining on the water just right, or the wind blowing through the trees seems to be blowing right through our souls with the warmest and tenderest of breaths. But vacations are not always relaxing, fun, or romantic.

When I was heading down to the UCSF Breast Cancer Center to have surgery for cancer, the sky looked like something out of *Gone with the Wind*. There was an amazing array of pinks, blues and grays. The car was packed up with clothes and supplies for my stay at the hospital. A dear friend was driving and I thought how different this experience would feel if we were heading off for some sunny vacation instead of into the eye of the storm, as it seemed that night.

At some point, however, I dropped into my experience, releasing future and past, and though we were still heading into the eye of the storm, it was an almost unbearably beautiful storm. The poignancy of the situation helped me to ride the edge of my experience, like a wave down to the hospital, and even later, being pushed through the halls on a gurney, there was a beauty to the experience that defied logic.

Our life is really always like this, but we don't know it. There is really never a past and a future, but we make them up and they interfere with our present "vacation"—our enjoyment or appreciation of this moment. Sometimes we need to trick ourselves into experiencing what is already present, so we can imagine we are on vacation. But of course, even vacations get old—then we are back to the "trick" of being able to experience life as it is.

I believe that bringing magic into our lives is no trick. It is already here. We only need to become aware of it. We are always with someone special—ourselves. We can be on vacation 365 days a year.

7. Being Silly

Being diagnosed or having a loved one diagnosed with a serious chronic illness or potentially fatal disease such as cancer, or losing a loved one to death or separation, can be devastating. The impact of such losses are deep and usually life-changing. Facing seemingly endless medical appointments and procedures, important, sometimes life-and-death decisions, and a quality-of-life that may be considerably compromised due to illness or treatments, all leave little room or energy for the activities that used to bring us joy. These challenges, along with the concern and fear we see reflected in the eyes, words and actions of our friends and family, contribute to a milieu of emotional constriction and/or heaviness which add to the sense of world weariness, fear and loss that we already feel.

In the case of dealing with losses endured by a friend or loved one, the emotional experience may be somewhat different but devastating nonetheless. The all-consuming task of caregiving or the devastation of dealing with funeral arrangements, etc., are overwhelming, and common emotions such as guilt or anger are usually pushed aside or viewed as unimportant in relation to what the loved one is experiencing. Living with these truths over the long haul can lead to a life that is weighty, serious and dreary.

Allowing ourselves to experience all feelings that arise is, of course, the cornerstone of loving self-care, and must remain the priority in long-term deep healing. Maintaining and feeding a healthy sense of humor can also be very helpful in winding our way through these difficult times. After all, who says one can't feel genuinely playful and silly when dealing with cancer? This is another place we might want to take a close look at the belief systems that get in the way of joy. Laughing, watching funny movies, listening to or telling jokes, and goofing around with friends might seem inappropriate or irreverent considering the circumstances, but a little lightheartedness or even some "gallows" humor may help to lift the pall of tension and anxiety that can weigh us down and drain the joy out of whatever life we still have. At least this has been true for me.

Jokes and funny movies are good medicine, but going beyond this to a bit of plain silliness or even make-believe can do wonders. What could it hurt to break out of our fixed repertoire of behavior to do a few things here and there that may seem a bit... well—silly? In fact, what better time to begin breaking old behavior patterns? Or maybe even perhaps crossing some boundaries of what society deems "appropriate"?

Just before I was diagnosed with breast cancer, I had begun a new relationship with a man from another state. We had developed quite a deep and intimate relationship through lengthy correspondence and phone conversations. When we finally got together, it was the weekend after I got the diagnosis and we spent several days together due to the distance we would have to travel to see one another again. When he left, I teased him about having perhaps missed out on the opportunity to feel my left breast, since I didn't know at that point whether I would be having a mastectomy. I knew it was a bold statement, but I was feeling pretty uninhibited due to the little bird of mortality sitting on my shoulder, as well as the incredible feeling of intimacy that had developed between us. He later shared with me how much he appreciated my humor and the lightness with which I was able to touch the prospect of a life-threatening condition.

When I lost my hair after chemotherapy, it all came out in one weekend. I was so debilitated and lost from the onslaught of chemicals, which seemed to be killing me faster than they were killing the cancer, that I swallowed my pride, called my (by then) ex-lover and asked him to take me camping. I just wanted to get away from my life as it was with the seemingly endless doctor's appointments and procedures as well as the constant realization that my new love had ended almost before it had begun. I wanted to go to some beautiful place where I could forget all that—where I could pretend life is beautiful, that I was a normal person, that I didn't have cancer, that I still had love. I didn't care that it was pretend.

Of course there was no way I could actually pull off the forgetting or the make-believe. My hair pretty much all fell out while we were there. I would find big nests of it in my hat or on my pillow in the morning. I said I looked like a drowned rat, with wisps of long hair hanging here and there on a mostly bald head. When we came back from the weekend, the make-believe was over. My ex-lover was still my ex-lover. He finished off the job on my hair with scissors and a razor. I looked into the mirror and saw someone I didn't know—a completely bald woman, someone who always, every time I looked, reminded me that cancer had invaded my body, that this was no weekend holiday sickness, that I was fighting for my life.

It was a beautiful weekend nonetheless—one I still treasure. The beautiful earth nurtured me. My new friendship with my ex-lover nurtured me. And I saw that beauty and love still existed in spite of the devastation I was experiencing. What started out as make-believe led me to a deeply profound experience of peace and beauty. In fact, what started out as make-believe *turned out to be true* in the most deep and profound way.

The next weekend I went to visit my friend. He had bought me a present: a neon blue wig and blue star sunglasses. I put them on and we went out to a concert in the park. I felt like Lucy in the Sky with Diamonds. It was a warm July evening and, as we walked toward the park, I noticed that people were smiling at me: big beaming smiles. Some were laughing—not *at* me it seemed, but simply in delight. Some were saying things like, "great hair," or "I love your hair," or giving me thumbs up signs. I found myself beaming back, returning the thumbs up.

One woman came up to me with her daughter (maybe eight or ten years old) and said, "My daughter loves your hair. She wants to have hair just like yours." I whipped off my wig and said, "Well here. She can try this on if she wants." The daughter was too shy, but it was a wonderful interaction. All of them were—from the simple exchange of smiles to heartfelt sharings about cancer and loss. It was an amazingly fun and beautiful evening with many delightful connections with people, strangers I would never have interacted with had it not been for the cancer—and my new blue hair.

That was only the beginning. After that, I wore my blue wig and star sunglasses everywhere I went. And everywhere I went, people laughed and forgot their problems for a few moments. Many were touched and/or inspired by my story and the blue wig. The nurses, doctors and patients at chemotherapy looked forward to my coming. The nurse took a picture of me and put it in my chart. Sometimes, when I didn't wear my wig, people would be disappointed. "Where's your blue wig?" They would ask.

When the cancer recurred five years later, I promised myself I wouldn't do chemo again. But I should have learned by then: "Never say never." I did end up doing chemo again, albeit a milder version, and I did lose my hair again—very slowly. I mostly wore hats, because my hair was hanging in there, only much thinner. Finally I got to the point where I was saying, "these little wisps of hair look worse than no hair at all," so my daughter shaved my head. I resurrected the blue wig and went off to poetry group. Turned out that a friend of mine, who had told me a few months earlier about a red wig she wanted to loan me if I should need one, wore the red wig to poetry group that night. What a time we had passing wigs around the group. And of course I went home with the red wig.

It was a huge, curly, bright red, Janis Joplinesque wig about twice as big as me (well, at least my head). But somehow it looked like it belonged on my head. Many people actually thought it was my real hair. The color was perfect for my skin and eye color. Now, I had promised myself five years earlier that I would never use a wig for hair loss that tried to look like real hair. Tsk, tsk, there's that "never say never" thing again. I guess I'll qualify that with, "unless it turns out to be really fun and outrageous, and people have to ask whether it's your real hair or not (if they have the nerve.)"

It's a tough call to say which was more fun, the blue wig or the red wig. But I have to say they have both been *a lot of fun*. And part of the fun of the red wig was that, in addition to making people laugh, I think it was really attractive on me and made me look quite a bit younger. In both cases, it was actually quite nice being the center of attention for reasons other than, "Oh, how sorry I am that you have cancer and might die." Mostly though, it was amazing how wearing both of the wigs made me feel completely different. As soon as I put them on, I felt my mood change, either subtly, or not so subtly. I felt lighter, more free and open. I felt like I was *playing*. I felt like *I* was more fun.

Sometimes I find there's great resistance to doing the practices described above. Sometimes the old curmudgeon in me says, "Grr ... I don't *want* to play." There seems to be some force trying to keep me from entering into this relationship, from entering into this joy. I think this is what Gurdjieff called "denying force." Jungians may call it ego or shadow. It may also be the true meaning of what Christians call the devil. This force comes up whenever we take a step toward truth, light, or joy, or toward our own power or authenticity. Don't give this force too much acknowledgment, too much energy. Just simply do the thing anyway. I'm amazed that when I slip through that little door, my entire being so easily responds, "Oh, here's *this* again. Here's freedom. Here's playfulness." It's always surprising.

Of course you can spend lots of money and go to all kinds of workshops that are already planned for you to do many of the things I am suggesting here. There are Sweat Your Prayers workshops, Trance Dance, play workshops, authentic movement workshops, writing workshops—you name it, someone is giving a workshop on it (especially in Sonoma County, California, where I live). I'm not at all putting these workshops down—quite the contrary. I have been to many of them myself and have found them extremely useful. They have the added advantage of putting you in touch with a community of people who may be trying to do what you are doing.

What I am encouraging people to do, however, is to be your own creative director! No one has the time and money to take official training in everything that inspires them, but that shouldn't keep you from exploring your desires and going where your joy leads you. Feel into it. Go to workshops if you can afford it and are moved to go, but also try your hand at tuning into yourself. Begin to develop your own intuitive sense. Don't just do the practices suggested here—make up your own.

Jane describes how, in her long struggle with agoraphobia, she used the piano to access her spontaneity and heal herself.

> I hated the piano as a kid. I hated practicing, I hated lessons. But I came back [to my mom's house] and there was a piano there. So I started

just closing my eyes and putting my hands on the keys and seeing what came out. That was something I would do every day after that. There was just this soothing... I could allow some spontaneity, which was so hard for me, especially in the worst phase of my agoraphobia. There were so few opportunities for it, too, because my life was so limited. But I think somehow closing my eyes and letting my fingers do something, when I didn't know what they were going to do, was an exercise in [spontaneity}, and an exercise in not judging the outcome of whatever came.

Bring your inner child into your everyday activities. If you have had children or been close to friends with toddlers, think back to the time they were beginning to walk and talk. Remember the joy and sense of power with which they took their first steps, the lack of inhibition with which they jabbered, not caring if their words made any sense but only delighting in the sound of their own voice. When you move, try experimenting with walking in the way of a child without direction, without knowing where or how the next step is going. When you talk, try talking without having any idea what you are going to say. I experimented with this at my attitudinal healing group check-ins and I was actually amazed at the wisdom and deeply felt experiences that came forth in this spontaneous expression. And, contrary to my fear that speaking in that way, completely without forethought, would reveal a bumbling idiot, my words often came forth quite coherently and with an aliveness that touched the group much more deeply than my normal, more thoughtful mode of expression ever had.

It requires courage to do this, but if we are present to ourselves, the words we need will be there—and if they are not, perhaps we don't need them. Or make that another experiment to try with communication: Simply keep silent until you have something to say. At his retreats, Ekhart Tolle is often quiet for some time before he begins to talk. He once said that the reason he was quiet was because he didn't know what to say. He pointed out that if he thought he "should" have something to say, or if he thought he was stupid for not having anything to say, that situation would be uncomfortable. But he didn't have those thoughts, so he just waited until he knew what to say.

I have also drummed up the courage to act more often on my impulses, like voicing some remark that comes into my head in social situations before my inner critic has a chance to convince me that it's stupid. This has lead to more playfulness in my interactions, which is something I've been seeking.

There's a healer in you. There's a healer in the earth. There's a healer in the universe. And there's a healer in each person you meet. But they're all the same healer. So whether we get our instruction from inside or outside, it is the same. Someone deep inside knows what we need.

Challenges of Tuning into the Inner Healer

This can be a little tricky when we first begin because we may think we are opening to the inner child or wise one and "feeling into" what's right for us, but may in fact be simply following old dysfunctional patterns that have become comfortable. We have been doing things in a certain way for so long that it may feel as if it's the "natural" way for us. This is one very good reason to begin with a teacher or perhaps a spiritually oriented therapist so he/she can call us on our self-deception, and perhaps give us a little push into new territory.

Remember what it was like when we learned to drive a car or ride a bike or a horse? It was very hard at first. We had to use our minds to tell us what to do; it was awkward, and we had to practice it over and over again. But as we practiced, it got easier and easier. Pretty soon our bodies started doing it automatically and we didn't even need to think about it. When we are learning to play a musical instrument, we need to practice and have our fingers learn certain patterns. Whenever we are learning something new, we need to practice at first. Our mind lays down tracks in the brain of what we're doing, and if we do it over and over again, the tracks get stronger and deeper, like ruts in a road. The body and mind get used to the activity and naturally go along those same tracks.

I saw my children doing this when they were developing their personalities. At a very young age I noticed them "trying on" different personalities. I didn't know what was going on at first because their initial attempts at some new way of putting out their personas to the world were understandably a little—shall we say—awkward. But after I realized what was happening, I found it quite hilarious and extremely interesting.

We also learn other things this way. We learn habits of mind. We learn ways of thinking and being. Our first disconnection with ourselves was based on a decision we made—a decision that perhaps life was too dangerous, or people were too dangerous, or we were too weak, or something along this line, and we began to act in a different way based upon this belief. After a while we forgot that it was based on a belief that arose in us following some traumatic event, and it became our "natural" way of being. It became easy.

To unlearn something or to do something in a different way than we're used to doing it may seem very hard or very "unnatural" or even frightening at first because our minds and bodies naturally want to go along the same tracks that they've made over all those years.

To really tune in to our inner healer, we *must listen very carefully*. As with toning when you find the music that already exists, you are listening for the wisdom that exists in the universe and in your body. So this is a very subtle listening that we need to do to the inner body—to the very, very inner body. This is a wisdom that is not really "ours" in a sense, at least not if we are still identified with our ego or the physical body as "I." I think that's part of the reason the denying force comes up so strongly when we're trying to do something different, when we're trying to tune in our natural body, because what we're listening to does not have to do with ego and so the ego may feel threatened and try to stop us.

The Dangers of a "Teaching"

Working with a teacher is very important, especially in the beginning of one's spiritual journey, but as with all things there can be dangers as well, so I think we need to be careful. And we need to be just as careful learning through reading and especially in learning about a teaching second-hand through a friend or from a student of a teacher. It is vital to remember that language is not the thing itself. Language is a pointer. It is a clue to help get us to the place in ourselves about which the teacher or teaching is referring. There can be misunderstandings because language doesn't always mean the same thing to everyone.

When we are using concrete words that refer to something we can touch or see, we can be more certain that we have a common understanding of what is being said. If someone says cat, the picture we have of a cat is likely to resemble the one in the mind of the speaker. However, when it comes to feelings, concepts, and experiences such as love, compassion, peace, joy, hatred, and energy, or attributes such as, mean, nasty, kind or good, we can never be sure that what we are seeing in our mind's eye or experiencing is the same as what someone is describing. Descriptions of spiritual practices are particularly subject to misinterpretation.

We can look at the teaching as an analogy of a map. On a real map, routes have numbers and names, and in the real world, names and numbers are posted on street signs and roadways. We can be fairly certain that we are taking the right turn when we take the numbered turn indicated on the map because it corresponds to the number on the street and the city name or the highway and so forth.

In the soul world, however, maps are a little different. They are more like vague directions: "You come to a green church and you turn left. Then you come to a big rock on the right, and you go on past that to the next rock. You turn right at that next big rock and go around it, and follow a path up the mountain." I think we can misinterpret what the map maker above and the spiritual world is saying a lot more easily than we can with a real physical map of streets and highways.

When I moved to San Francisco in 1969, I moved in with a man who was using LSD as a spiritual tool to access higher states of consciousness. This was life changing for me because it showed me places and experiences I never could have dreamed existed, and stimulated a desire in me to want to live that experience all the time. We even went down to Esalen to a workshop with Stanislaus Grof, a famous scientist who was working with using LSD to help neurotic and psychotic patients access higher states of consciousness. The problem was I always came down. The other problem was that it also had shown me some terrifying aspects of my inner world in which I felt hopelessly lost. I needed a teacher.

After I read *The Master Game,* I called the author, Robert DeRopp, and asked him to be my teacher. He sent me to a group that was forming in San Francisco, led by his student Ed Van Tassel. I immediately saw that this was an entirely new way of approaching my life. I also saw in it hope for a way out of the quagmire of my mind and a way to access the high states I had experienced on LSD. After a few meetings, I joined the group, gave up drugs and began the work in earnest.

Choosing a teacher is one of those places where our inner wisdom must come into play. Even if we have not yet developed our wisdom, the bud is there. There is something in us that can lead us to the teacher or teaching we need. P.D. Ouspensky called this our "magnetic center." Yet even when we find the right teacher, there are pitfalls to watch out for. Our own inner wise one can never be put on automatic pilot. There will undoubtedly be places where the teacher is still stuck. Even assuming that the teacher is wise, fairly aware of his stuck places, and has great depth of being, and that we are pure in our intentions and fairly open to the teaching, we can *still* do ourselves a great deal of harm simply through misunderstanding or *mistranslation*.

My first guru taught that in order to do inner work we need energy and that our bodies are the vessels which hold the energy. But, he said, we have all kinds of leaks and the energy is constantly draining out through the leaks, thus inhibiting our ability to do spiritual work. According to this teaching, one way to plug up leaks is the non-expression of negative emotions. The premise is that through expressing our negative emotions we are just throwing away energy. Since I was a sincere aspirant to the spiritual path, I took these things very seriously and tried very hard to do them.

The instruction in this case was not to express negative emotions either externally *or* internally. What the teacher *didn't* say was what we *were supposed to do* with these emotions. Maybe it was supposed to be understood that one was to *experience* them, but it wasn't understood by me, and I didn't have a clue how to do it. I realized many years later, through my practice with experiencing, that even though I knew the danger of suppression, I actually *had* been *suppressing* my negative emotions instead of simply not expressing them.

I learned the hard way that an important part of the non-expression of negative emotions is allowing yourself to *experience* them even though you are not expressing them either externally or internally. If you are not expressing them and not experiencing them, you are suppressing them and this is very dangerous.

But this was how my mind interpreted the instruction. It was an honest mistake but an unfortunate one. However, with diligence and perseverance in my practice over many years, and continuing to have the intention of waking up and being open and honest and sincere in my practice, I finally realized what was happening. I began the process of clearing these suppressed emotions and others from a lifetime of suppression through the process of experiencing.

Another danger, along these same lines of mistranslation, is when the teaching seems to contradict something we have already learned. I may stumble upon a very useful and true practice or simply a deep truth, a way of opening. Then perhaps I will hear a great teacher saying something, teaching something, similar. My mind, however, interprets her way of saying it as something else and I think, "Oh, I am doing something wrong. I should be doing something different." When I met Gangaji, she said we just need to stop, just stop. She talked about dropping our story line, our ceaseless inner conversation about who we think we are, what we should be doing or should have been doing, and our judgments about everything and everyone we encounter.

After the public meeting that day, in the smaller private meeting I had been allowed to attend, a woman asked, "Can our story ever be of service?" Gangaji said no. But I disagreed—I thought yes, I believe it *can* be of service. I believe *everything* can be of service. Yet in spite of my own inner understanding, I immediately began to doubt myself. At first I thought this teaching was negating all the work I had done with experiencing, because at times it seemed I was *using* my story to get to experiencing. In this case, however, my doubting didn't go on very long because my "knowing" was deeper than my doubting. I knew the work I had done was true and good.

For me the story has been part of the compost out of which my opening spirit has been fed. And my story, like my negative emotions, leads me to the places I am stuck, blinking like a neon sign every time I drive past—until I finally decide it's time to go into that seedy dive and look around. The story seems to be a cover for the long-held resistance against feeling the pain of my life. Illusion? Yes. But I cannot know this until I finally enter that place and see that it is empty.

It seems to me that perhaps the story itself is not so bad. It is my *belief* in the story that keeps me trapped. If I make a map of myself—if I understand my story, then when it comes up again, which it surely will, I will not be shocked. I can say, "Oh, that's my story." I can say, like Stephen Levine, "Big surprise."

I still trusted Gangaji's teaching explicitly but it didn't negate my own understanding on a gut level, which felt very strong. I felt quite certain that it was a matter of mistranslation or misunderstanding, while still remaining open to the possibility that my understanding could change with deeper exploration.

Even when the teaching comes from our deepest self, we can be fooled in this way. We may be following a path that seems to be flourishing and deepening when we suddenly discover something that seems to prove we are on the wrong track—like when I got cancer and fell into the trap of thinking I must have been fooling myself with all that "good work" I had done, because there I was with cancer. In the shock of having a life-threatening condition and dealing with it, I simply forgot what I knew: *that being sick did not make me a failure, or mean that I was doing something wrong.*

Trust Yourself—Developing Your Intuitive Self

I believe the major thing is: *trust yourself.* If your deep knowing is telling you to do or not do something, listen. It may not be the final truth. It may be wrong ultimately, but like the labyrinth which sometimes curves back on itself seeming to take us farther from the center before it turns back again to take us home, if we follow our deepest wisdom, are sincere in asking for guidance and open to its manifestations, something we need will undoubtedly be uncovered to bring us closer to our true heart. This of course is predicated on the premise that you are giving to your practice the time, energy, and serious attention that will allow you to access your own wisdom.

And, yes, this gets sticky. Don't we have blind spots? Haven't we also been talking about how we have lied to ourselves our whole life? Don't we need someone to set us on a true path? Yes, yes, and yes. But ultimately the buck stops at our front door. There's no one but you who actually knows the whole truth about you. And no one but you who can decide finally, in the end, the true path for you.

It's easy to become a self-improvement or spiritual work junkie—reading book after book for years, going to meetings, talking the talk, following the path laid out by a particular teacher, and imagining that we are growing in self-awareness, knowledge, and spiritual depth. But in reality, we may have done all this without ever actually penetrating one centimeter beneath the surface of the protective coating we have constructed around our tender heart. Or we may have had a significant breakthrough at one time and then run back under the protection.

Every practice at some point becomes a hollow form. When we find ourselves struggling with a practice that seems empty or shallow, and we just can't seem to find our center, often the real practice or action or non-action that would lead us back is right before our eyes. If we sincerely ask ourselves (or the Divine Presence inside of us) questions such as: "What is needed (or what is truth) in this situation?" "What is my practice right now?" "What does my pure heart want me to do?" or "God help me to know what to do?" and if the asking is not an intellectual question but a deep soul yearning to know, the wisdom inside of us will often provide the answer. Sometimes, I simply put the yearning or my deep heart question into my heart *without* any words and tenderly hold it there, with love and awareness throughout my days and nights until an answer appears.

It may be an answer we don't want to hear. It may be that it is much more comfortable to continue the practice prescribed by our teacher or spiritual guide or to read another spiritual book or write in our journal—to do practices which have become comfortable or at least practices with which we have developed some familiarity or experience—but our process, like reality, is changing every instant, and our teacher may not necessarily know what we are experiencing in this moment. So if these practices are not alive for us in this moment, they are empty and useless.

On the other hand, perhaps we have been resistant all of our lives to receiving any kind of teaching from anyone, and what we really need to do is to open to a teacher—to give over our tightly held sense of power to someone outside of ourselves. If we are sincere in our intention, our inner teacher/healer will help us to see this truth and lead us to our teacher. And again this doesn't mean we abdicate responsibility. We may have to work very hard to find a teacher and to follow the teachings.

The real use of a book, a speaker, a teacher, or any external stimuli or input of any kind is to stimulate our own inner creative response so that we may discover or uncover the truth of our own nature. Sometimes we need this kind of stimulus or a group of like-minded seekers to provide a map or encouragement along the way, but if we are using these external things to avoid doing the necessary inner work, we might as well go to the movies or a party for all the good they will do us. I don't think we ever actually "learn" spiritual wisdom from anyone. We know it all already, but often lack the tools to access it. But it takes a great deal of work to uncover the truth within ourselves—work that we would often rather not do.

Actualizing a Teaching

When we read or hear something—something that seems wise or true, that rings some deep bell or resonates with us in a deep way—we may think we know it. This is actually true in one sense because we do have the truth and deep wisdom within us, and the teaching is resonating with the place in us that knows. We recognize it. And we think then that we have been changed, that we have learned something or that we already know it. But, though we have the truth deep inside of us, it has been covered over by the layers and layers of protection we have laid down around our hearts over many years.

The teaching we have read or heard has opened us momentarily to our own deep knowing, but unless we act on the knowledge presented to us, the armoring around our heart will quickly close again and we will forget what we have seen. We won't really know it or be able to maintain the opening that has appeared until we interact with the information and use it. We may remember and understand on an intellectual level, but perhaps it has not yet become part of our being. We do not yet truly embody the knowledge. It's kind of like setting dye in fabric. When fabric is in the dye bath, it looks beautiful. It takes on the color of the water. But if the color is not fixed by taking certain steps and adding the fixative, or the fabric has not been cleaned or prepared properly beforehand, the color will disappear after a few washings.

To make any teaching a reality in our lives requires action and discipline because the walls we have built and the ruts we have created with repetitive behavior and thinking block the truth from manifesting. So again, sometimes what we need to do is to *unlearn* things that are keeping us from experiencing our own deep truth. Byron Katie calls this the "great undoing."

When I was reading Stephen Levine's book, *Healing into Life and Death,* the first time, I read it a few paragraphs at a time because I found so much there that I wanted to work with. I didn't move on to the next section until I felt I had really digested that teaching and had applied it in my life.

It is possible a certain teaching will not "take" because we are not ready for it. Perhaps we do not yet have the "being" to be able to embody it. If we continue to practice in the ways that we know and to open in whatever way we can to the opportunities presented to us, our being will gradually be deepened, and perhaps we will be ready for the lesson next time around.

The Wise One

All this talk about practice, work, and discipline may begin to sound antithetical to the idea of just moving and *being* in a playful way. But these aspects of the inner healer have more to do with the wise one, the one who sees, the one who knows—the discerning one who makes wise decisions to guide us on our path. Sufi teacher and transpersonal psychologist Atum O'Kane says that we need both the playful innocence of the Divine Child and the discerning eyes of the Wise One on our journey. His teacher, Hazrit Inayat Khan, told him the child is born innocent, not wise—that wise eyes come in older people.

Atum maintains that, to become wise, one must have touched life very deeply, to have experienced suffering and loss, confusion and clear seeing, grace, abundance and abandonment, been lost and found, to have lived by the heart, to have let life in and let it touch you and impact you on the deepest levels.

The archetype of the Wise One, according to Atum, holds the following attributes:
1. Discernment—knowing what goes where and when, knowing the right time and the right season, knowing the appropriate way of holding or meeting something, and having clear boundaries.
2. Acceptance of life and humanity.
3. Compassion as the natural response to life.
4. Detachment—life is not reduced to one's own drama.
5. Witness—the capacity to witness life and respond compassionately.
6. Meaning—the capacity to reflect and harvest our experience in order to share it with others.
7. Ego (in the positive sense of ego)—standing in the right place for service—i.e. service that doesn't arise out of the need for the ego to serve itself (except in the larger sense of service to the soul) and is not bounded in identity to results.

It is through allowing ourselves to experience our lives on the deepest levels that we begin to access the archetype of the Wise One. This archetype is closely aligned with our healthy inner adult—the one who acts in the world on behalf of the inner child and for the highest welfare of the self.

The Devil and God Are in the Details

The spiritual life is made up of the substance of everyday life. There's nothing that occurs that is not a spiritual occurrence. There's nothing we can feel or experience that is not fodder for our spiritual path—grist for the mill, as Ram Dass calls it.

We tend to think of the spiritual path as something lofty. The words of spiritual masters often include things like emptiness, peace, and love. We think that if we're experiencing anger, jealousy, depression or despair, we're off-track, we're not "holy," we're not in a spiritual place—like the words of the Leonard Cohen song, "If you're not feeling holy, your loneliness says that you've sinned." But for some, it might be: "When you're not feeling sinful or worthless, your negative self-beliefs keep nagging at you that you must have missed something." Yet often this point—when we are at the lowest of the low, when we're feeling small and mean, rejected, unworthy, unlovable, or just plain selfish—is the time when we are closest to our true heart.

We may sit in Zazen and achieve very high and/or peaceful states—or we may come to deep insights in our meditations or be filled with rapture when we are in a beautiful place. But when the baby is sick and the cat does his business behind the couch for the third time in a week, or our husband has left hair in the sink again and then comes home from work cranky and tired, expecting supper on the table at six sharp, our peace is nowhere to be found. There is a saying, "The devil is in the details," but God is also in the details. This is our life. This is our work. This is our path to God—in the details of life.

We don't want to think that the simple act of stopping eating when we have had enough is a spiritual act, but our spiritual world is made up of such details. How much easier is it to go on a prescribed diet, something laid out by some health guru, than to simply tune into our bodies in the middle of a meal and ask, "Am I really still hungry right now, or am I simply indulging my addiction to eating? Or trying to dull my sense of inner emptiness?" How much easier is it to just follow a prescribed practice—to sit in meditation at 6:30 AM and 9:00 PM, go to regular sesshins, go to regular meetings with a teacher and/or therapist—than to take responsibility for our life in each moment, asking ourselves what we're doing to keep us asleep right now? Where are we taking the easy way out? What old dysfunctional pattern are we falling into? How are we ignoring some inner voice at this very moment? What is alive for us in this moment and how can we serve that?

Of course there are great risks in directing our own practice. We all have blind spots, which by definition means we can't see them. The force of sleep in the spiritual sense is so strong that it is very easy to slip back into old patterns or to continue doing some external form of practice that was vital at one time but has gone onto automatic pilot and to which we are no longer present. So we still need wise teachers or true friends on the path to show us where we are stuck and to give us a prod when we have fallen asleep, even after we have moved to directing our own practice. If we are alert, however, the conditions of our lives often give us the jolts and the information we need to self correct.

I think we often have a sense of something amiss when we are doing or about to do something contrary to our true spiritual path, but we have not been empowered in our own intuitive knowing and we generally don't trust it. Tuning into our bodies during meditation and other formal spiritual practices can be a great help in this regard, but we can also gradually learn to take back our intuitive power, starting in small ways using the activities of everyday life. When we notice that inner voice saying something, or that discomfort that signals something amiss, we can listen and we can act.

When my own children were very young, I resisted having a TV in the house because I believed it to be detrimental to their developing minds and souls. As they grew older, I finally gave in to having one. I saw myself slowly being drawn into watching certain programs even though I don't generally like to watch TV and believe it to be fairly addictive. It was especially hard to resist when I was very tired.

I was torn because watching TV became a way to be with my husband when we sorely needed more togetherness, and I *did* in a way enjoy certain programs. I was uncomfortable with the situation, however, because I knew deep down that it wasn't what I wanted to be doing with my life—at least not to the extent I was finding myself doing it. But I continued to sit there and watch TV just because we had started to and it was easier than getting up to do something more satisfying.

At a certain point, I started tuning into that little discomfort when it pricked me. I resisted watching and went for a walk instead. Sometimes in the middle of a movie I would suddenly realize that I wasn't *really* that interested in what was playing and that I was on autopilot. Resisting or stopping an action that was already started (inertia) was harder—especially if I was very tired, and I have to acknowledge that there was a certain amount of subtle social pressure involved as well. This was more complicated and went deeper than the simple fear of embarrassment over changing directions or resisting my husband's emotional and physical pull to stay sitting next to him on the couch. I didn't want to look at the implications it had for our marriage. But I began to listen and sometimes I was able to overcome the law of inertia and just get up and go to bed or do something else that I would, in my deepest heart, rather be doing. Big deal, right? Well, it actually *was* a big deal, because it was honing that spiritual muscle—the one that acts on behalf of soul.

I want to emphasize that this practice is different from "making a resolution" to do or not do something. Making a resolution is just more of the same—using our ego to brow-beat ourselves into some sort of specific behavior under the mistaken belief we can make ourselves into better people by changing our behavior. The decisions and actions I'm talking about cannot be preplanned. They come from our intuitive self which can only be accessed in the present moment—"now." These little actions make more of a difference than we might think. If we start tuning in to ourselves in little ways, the bigger ways begin to open up.

One day I was in the car with my ex and he said something I was about to react to. In that split second, I noticed the reaction about to arise and decided to take a different route. I had been reading Erica Chopich and Margaret Paul's book, *Healing Your Aloneness,* and had been struck by their assertion that there are only two intentions: the intent to protect and the intent to learn. So I decided to resist the urge to protect and instead go with the intention to learn and I began asking questions. I asked what he meant by his statement and I asked for other examples of his criticism of me. I kept asking questions with genuine curiosity and it was amazing how the charge went out of the situation for both of us as the conversation turned into a very heartfelt interchange. The moment of decision, however, was a very difficult one. The pull toward reactivity was so strong that it took a huge act of will to turn and go a different direction. I think the practice of listening to my inner voice in less charged situations helped me to make that turn.

Sometimes we are not called to do anything except to allow ourselves to experience whatever emotion is surging in us. It may be helpful at these times to ask ourselves more basic questions like, "What is going on for me right now?" or "What is happening here?" or "What is this?," and simply allow ourselves to feel. At other times, just to notice what we are doing is enough.

Small Efforts

Sometimes life presses down on us so hard that we almost have no choice. We have to surrender. I think of the times I came to my big Yes and No. These are the times when we are like coal under the earth and the weight presses down on us so hard that it seems we are turned into diamonds with almost no effort of our own. There are other times, however, when we are in the soup. Helplessness and confusion swirl around us. Things are bad or difficult, but they are not so bad that we simply give over and let ourselves be turned into diamonds. The weight on us is not that strong.

Our life is swirling around us and we feel that we are not the diamond, but we don't know where to turn, don't know what to do—there are too many factors. Gangaji says, "give up the search." My first guru said, "Man can do nothing, but if you try, something may happen." One seems to be saying, "stop trying," while the other says, "try." One aspect of our inner healer says play; another says practice. There are so many different things being said, and many of them seem contradictory. So what is the way?

Sometimes when I don't seem to be capable of doing something big, or I am in such confusion that I don't know what to do, it seems skillful for me to do two things: one is to remember my first teacher's admonition, "Confusion is a state and out of the state of confusion, nothing but confusion can come." So, I try to be patient with myself rather than make any important decisions from that state. The second thing I have found useful is to make one small step—perhaps, setting myself the task of doing a regular meditation.

Since my meditations are usually done lying down because of my weak body, I make a pact with myself to sit up in meditation two times a day for five minutes and to make this a ritual by lighting a candle first. Or, I may decide to leave one bite of food on my plate at every meal as an offering to the gods, to the universe, to my practice. These small things sometimes create a subtle shift that opens me to something bigger and often brings an intensified awareness to my everyday life.

The Relationship Between Play and Practice

Of course the ego mind that wants to control everything, and have things for itself, gets greedy. It thinks that more is better and decides that, if this little effort can produce something good, then let's heap on more and more efforts. It says, "Let's try *really hard* and maybe we can *get* something." But the whole point is to do the small efforts, or any kind of effort, without any intention of getting something—do them perhaps as an offering, or (what a concept!) as play. As I mentioned in the chapter "The Practice of Being Without," sometimes just a slight twist or change in perspective can change something that seems to be negative into something positive.

This is the meeting point of two diametrically opposed ways of looking at the spiritual path—"play/practice" and "try/give up the search." To give up the search, to stop trying, does not mean to simply let it all hang out. It means to follow your joy, to do your practice, to live your life, as if your life depended on it, to give yourself completely to each action, to each moment, without any attachment to results, without any expectation of return. My work is my play is my practice is my reward.

Sometimes when I think I'm really getting it together—doing the things I want to be doing, fulfilling my intentions, meditating regularly, going to spiritual events, working on my book and my poetry, doing morning pages etc. etc.—I may suddenly notice (if I'm paying attention) that there's tension in my body. I'm leaning forward ,metaphysically speaking (*and* physically speaking). I'm not at rest in my body or soul. I'm not truly enjoying the moments of my life but instead looking ahead to what I'm going to be doing in some future moment. I'm formulating some "really good realization" that I should put in my book. I'm not really being present to my life right here, right now—to delight in the taste of a bite of food, the feel of warm water on my skin in the shower or bath, the smooth soapy water in the dishpan, the myriad sights and sounds of the day, the faces, bodies and voices of people I encounter, the feeling of the air in and out of my lungs, and the sense of aliveness in my body. I have forgotten to play.

Our practice is a moment-to-moment act. We do not simply set something in motion and then sit back to watch as it unfolds. We are faced with choices in each millisecond. We are called to make each moment both a prayer and an act of play. Are these things contradictory? I don't think so. When we truly play, we are allowing ourselves to enter the sacred space where there is no mover—only movement.

Healing Exercises

The following exercises and meditations are ones that I have found helpful for accessing my own inner healer or the healing power in the universe.

1. Healing Touch

According to the ancient art of Chinese medicine there is a very powerful energy center in the middle of the palms of our hands. Some people who are naturally tuned into this energy or those who have discovered it and learned to use it have become healers. Yet we all have this power to some extent and can use it for our own healing.

Put your hands together, palm to palm. Bring your awareness directly to the point of contact. Feel the sensations in the touching. Slowly and gently rub them together, continuing to maintain your awareness of the sensations. Move them slowly apart an inch or two and back together several times. Notice the connection between your hands even as they separate—the space between, a vibrant field, a magnetic aliveness that ebbs and flows with the movement. Notice how this vibratory aliveness moves down your arms and into your body. Play a little with the space. See how far you can move your hands apart and still feel the connection, still feel that energy field.

Place your hands on various parts of your body, your face, your arms, your legs. Caress yourself as if you were your lover, or your mother—your divine healer. Run your hands up and down your body, paying special attention to the parts of yourself that are hurting or weak. Leave your hands on those parts for as long as you are drawn to do so. Using the tips of your fingers, gently touch your face. Run your fingers over all the contours—around your eyes, nose and mouth. Touch your lips and your ears. Feel the sensations, the healing qualities, the loving touch. Take it in. Every so often bring your palms back together and do the movements described at the beginning of this section. Notice if this enhances the energy emanating from your hands.

2. Healing Visualization

For years after I got sick, I went to doctor after doctor, trying to get help, trying to get a diagnosis. The Western doctors were either stymied and told me flatly they didn't know what was wrong with me, or they told me I was depressed and needed psychological help. Alternative doctors gave me remedies or herbs that may have helped infinitesimally, but at that point the effects of the illness loomed so hugely in my life that it was like giving me a fly swatter in the jungle. I also poured over medical books and kept mentally recycling my symptoms and the onset of my illness, which were unusual but very definite, to try to make some sense out of it all.

The year I gave up going to doctors and directed attention toward my own healing powers was the year I improved the most. Please do not take this to mean you should stop going to doctors if you have not exhausted every avenue of possible help. There are many illnesses that can definitely be helped by doctors. I certainly continued to take my thyroid medicine and herbs when I began to do these visualizations. It's just that sometimes I think we get caught on the track of searching everywhere outside of ourselves for help and forget the obvious: that we have a healer inside of us.

Every day I did two half-hour healing visualizations. I didn't know exactly what in my body was making or keeping me sick, so I just used my imagination to come up with several healing scenarios to encourage my body to heal itself.

One scenario was based on the fact that my entire immediate family had toxic pesticides in our blood. So assuming I had poison in my system, I visualized a watery environment that was murky and had decay or other nasty things in it. Into this environment came white watersnail-like creatures that took the murky water into their bodies and expelled clean, clear water behind them. Gradually, the water became more and more clear. They would also descend en masse upon the decayed areas and slowly eat the nasty creatures, thereby transforming them into healthy white cells. I had another scenario with white Pac-man-like creatures that went around eating nasty toxic things and generally cleaning up the place.

When I came out of my visualizations, I felt very high and extremely focused. It felt as though I had gone to a very deep part of myself. If one of my visualizations began to get stale, I would make up a new one. I had four or five altogether.

When doing a visualization, you must get very particular about the details. Picture everything as if it were happening: the rotted wood in the walls of a broken-down house being torn down and replaced with fresh strong wood; the heating system being replaced with all new pipes, so the air flows freely around the building and the exhaust or bad air is carefully vented out of the house etc., etc. Picture the repairmen making all these repairs, and the house being transformed into a beautiful, strong, solid house.

I had an autoimmune disease, which meant that my body was attacking its own cells, so I devised another visualization with a circle of Dianes who let in only healthy Dianes but not the foreign-looking ones. Some were disguised, either with hoods or make-up or sickness, but the Dianes in the circle developed the ability to distinguish which ones were really Dianes and which ones weren't.

3. Healing Meditation in Nature

You don't have to be in a pristine wilderness to do this meditation. You can do it in your backyard, a park, while camping or even in the grass at your workplace. Lie on the ground, preferably in the open with as little between you and the earth as possible: just your body, naked or clothed, is preferable; a light blanket is okay, but try not to use a pad—the more in physical touch you are with the earth the better. Orient your body comfortably in North/South direction with legs slightly apart and arms/hands on the ground (palms down), touching the earth if possible.

Allow yourself some time just to lie there doing nothing—aware of the energy fields and your breathing, but not focused on anything— all senses open, alert, enjoying the show. Birds may circle overhead or sing nearby. A faint breeze may brush your face; clouds may fill the sky with one of nature's grandest art forms. Stay grounded—in the present and the physical body, but softly—and enjoy. You can close your eyes if you want to, but the basic posture of your being is one of gentle openness. I like to keep my eyes open. Take a few deep breaths; allow yourself to just be. Allow the universal healing energy to fill you up. Open yourself to all things. Look up at the sky, if your eyes are open, and stay in the present moment as much as possible. You are a child of the Universal Life Force—and this force is here to support, nourish and heal you. You have issued from this miracle universe. *You are part of it—not separate from it.* Let the energy that is there heal and form you.

Feel the energy pulsing in the earth. It comes from a place deep in the core radiating up through the outer layers. Visualize and feel it entering your body through the palms and head, flowing down through your body and exiting at your feet, creating a continuous current with the earth. Or you can reverse the direction and visualize the energy entering your feet and exiting from the head and palms. Feel it enter your body, run through and go back into the earth, constantly replenishing itself—a current connecting you to the universal energy field.

As a variation, try running the colors of the rainbow up through your body, from feet to head, spilling down at the neck, into arms and hands, still like a current coming from deep within the earth—colors flowing, one after the other: red, orange, yellow, green, blue, purple. Take as long as you want with each color and notice how it feels as it flows up through the chakras.[8] Notice if any particular color lights up or wants to linger in any particular part of the body. If it does, just let it stay there. Your body knows what it needs to heal.

Now turn your attention to the vastness of the cosmos, Universal Life Force, God, or Tao—whatever works for you. Breathe the energy coming from the cosmos into your lungs. Let it fill you to the tips of your fingers and toes. Visualize, or simply feel this life force of the cosmos entering your body, penetrating you, filling you with life, and moving through you into the earth. Fill again and again with the life-giving breath of the universe, allowing it to fill your being and flush from the body any negative energies, images or blockages held there. Imagine yourself as a grand receptor whose only function is to receive the loving, healing, creative energies of the universe.

Do this exercise as often as you are moved to do it—especially if you are tired, sick or weary of life. You will grow to love it if it is given as a gift rather than seen as an obligation or a something you "should" do. Try to do it in a soft, loving, voluntary way—never by force.

4. Retreat

Try, if you can, to attend a retreat or make your own at least several times a year. When I can't seem to catch my breath, when my life is swirling around me and pulling for my attention from every direction, it is important for me to *take* time out to be separate, to see myself again as a simple being on the earth—living, breathing, being. This can be a formal retreat, arranged by a teacher or center where you sit in meditation without worldly distractions; it is the simple experience of being here.

Or, it can be getting away from your day-to-day distractions by going somewhere and making your own solo retreat, perhaps in formal meditation or in a wild place where you can experience yourself again as an animal living on this planet—smelling the smells, touching the earth with bare feet and hands, feeling the wind, the breath of the earth mingled with the breath of The Divine.

We may seem smaller, in one way, without all the connections that seem to make us significant and *somebody* in the world. And yet we experience ourselves as so much larger in a much more important way, as a part of a world, a life, that is so much bigger—huge—in comparison to that tiny world of affairs in which we have been enmeshed.

5. The Practice of Being a Tree

Using the same preparations and instructions described in Healing Exercise number 3, read the poem, "The Practice of Being a Tree" at the end of Chapter 15. Read it to yourself, or listen to it on a tape recording you have made, while you lie on the ground beneath a tree or sit in some place where your gaze can rest on a tree. If neither of these options is available, simply envision a tree from your memory that has made an impression on you.

CHAPTER 19

New Order

To go in the dark with a light is to know the light.
To know the dark, go dark. Go without sight,
and find that the dark, too, blooms and sings,
and is traveled by dark feet and dark wings.

—Wendell Berry

A New Way of Looking

MANY SPIRITUAL AND RELIGIOUS TEACHERS talk about our lives as a dream from which we must awaken. Waking up in the spiritual sense requires, or actually *is*, a whole new way of looking at the world and at our lives. This new perspective is so revolutionary that it seems to have nothing to do with life as we usually know and live it.

The way of the world, of the ego, of traditional learning, is to build on an ever-expanding base of knowledge. The way of the spirit seems to be a radical departure from that model. We must constantly let go of the old—of any understanding we think we have—and continually open ourselves, continually be beginners. As Shunryu Suzuki Roshi said, "In the beginner's mind there are many possibilities but in the expert's there are few." (21) He exhorts us to always have beginner's mind, which means we are empty.

You've heard the expression, "Think outside the box." But, how can we when we live our lives within that little box, or like a chess piece on a chessboard? To step outside the box, to think outside of our enclosed little world, to step off of the chessboard onto the grass, requires something more—something different, something to jar us out of our traditional way of thinking and seeing. When you get a chronic illness or experience tragic loss, life is turned topsy-turvey.

Old rules don't seem to apply anymore. Your world as you knew it is gone and replaced by a strange new world.

When a well person becomes ill, he doesn't think about whether or not he will get well because he has unshakable trust in his body. This trust is stronger than belief; stronger than assumption; stronger even than what we usually think of as faith, because until that faith is challenged we have no idea it even exists. These words—faith, belief, assumption—imply a feeling or a recognition of something that could possibly not be true. They all seem to apply to a concept or possibility we've pondered and made a decision about; something that has entered our field of awareness, however peripherally or briefly.

The invincibility of the body is not something we have given thought to and decided we would believe. When we come down with the flu, we don't do a deep soul search and then reaffirm our faith that we'll recover. We don't think about it. We go to bed and "know" that in a few days or a week we'll be better, just like we don't think about whether the sun will rise in the morning. In our mind it is simply true. So, when we get sick and don't get better, when that "truth" turns out to be a lie, it rocks our world in a way that few things can. We have taken a bite of the apple and can never go back to that same innocent trusting. Yet there is something expedient in the leaving of paradise.

Create Your Own Myth

Joseph Campbell, the New-Age prophet who brought a cornucopia of myths and ancient teachings to the awareness of modern man, implies that these stories are a kind of road map for the psyche, and even perhaps for the collective evolution of universal consciousness. Many of the myths contain descriptions of a descent into some kind of underworld or dark place in which something very valuable is learned or obtained. This common theme comes to us from such diverse geographic locations and times that it seems there is something much bigger going on than simply a random assortment of imaginative stories from isolated times and places. For example, the biblical story of Adam and Eve's expulsion from the Garden of Eden has been interpreted by many in a mythic rather than literal way as a necessary means for spiritual evolution instead of the punishment of a vengeful God for the disobedience of His creatures.

In a taped conversation with Campbell, Michael Toms makes the point that we humans generally see dark places as huge problems in our lives and we relate to them as problems rather than as opportunities. Campbell replies, "Mythology tells us that where you stumble, that's where your treasure is." He gives the example of the tale of the Arabian nights where someone is plowing a field. When his plow gets caught, he digs down to find what it is caught on and discovers a large cave with many jewels in it. Campbell tells us the cave is equivalent to our own psyche: our psyches have the jewels but we are not letting their energies move us and consequently we get stuck. He says, "The world is a match for us and we are a match for the world. And where it seems to be most challenging is where the greatest invitation lies to find deeper and greater powers in ourselves."

It seems that Campbell is telling us that when our lives head into a downward spiral, when everything seems to be going wrong, we may be entering a time of great opportunity.

Ann Ulinov, professor of psychiatry and religion at The Union Theological Seminary in New York City, says that the spirit wants to be embodied. God, the Bible tells us, sent his only son to incarnate a human body and suffer the ultimate humiliation of human death to save us from our sins. The Orthodox Church teaches that Christ then descended into Hell and opened the tombs to release all the souls who were being held there. Inana, a goddess from ancient Sumer, the Queen of Heaven and Earth, was stripped of everything during her descent to the Underworld, including the "me," the divine attributes given to her by her father, Enki, the god of wisdom. There she was hung on a meat hook to rot—a dead piece of meat. These stories end in resurrection or ascent from that place of no return. But the resurrected ones have been changed by their descent.

Those who were closest to Jesus didn't even know him as they walked and talked with him on the morning following his resurrection. They thought he was the gardener. And when he visited the apostles in a closed room, though he still had a physical body bearing the holes from his crucifixion, he walked through the doors without opening them. Inana, too, emerged from the dark region changed, more complete. Having undergone the mysteries of death and rebirth, she expanded her realm to include the underworld as well as heaven and earth and claimed for her own the gifts of the "me," which before her descent had simply been adornments. That even the celestial and divine beings have forsaken the heavenly realms to humble themselves to a fleshy body, even unto death, and have descended to the dark regions by choice, must point to some greater good.

So when you hit the roadblock or crushing loss that marks the beginning of your own descent, perhaps you are following in the footsteps of Innana, Persephone and, yes, even Jesus. Perhaps you are participating in a story of cosmic proportions. If we are following the maps that seem to be sent to us from some deeper wisdom, we can hope that resurrection will indeed be in store for us as well; that we will come through the darkness intact but transformed. Yet when you come to that dark place, it can feel hopeless. Even Jesus, we are told, felt forsaken on the cross.

A Different Set of Laws

When you are facing a life that may be permanently changed by illness or disability, your world is turned upside down. All the ideals, the maxims, the rules and ideas you used to live by no longer make sense: work hard, play hard; keep your life organized; work first then reward yourself with play; exercise regularly; push yourself beyond your limits—it will make you stronger; laughter is the best medicine; spend quality time with your loved ones; giving is better than receiving; take a vacation and you will come back refreshed; reward yourself after a hard day's work with something really fun.

These maxims are all wonderful and true, but when you are sick, or your body doesn't work, suddenly, all these ideas, though certainly sensible and worthy, become ludicrous and utterly useless because you can't do them. Even the rules and maxims you have learned through the school of hard knocks, in therapy or through deep openings in your spiritual practice, no longer apply: don't keep things locked up inside; talk about your feelings; follow your joy; do the things you love—sing, paint, hike, etc.—it will feed the soul; take care of yourself—stay clean and well groomed, eat healthy, take vitamins, find and go to the right doctors. All the things that could theoretically help you to heal are often beyond reach physically or emotionally.

One evening when I was exhausted from trying to get ready for a trip, my housemate playfully quoted Nietzsche saying, "If it doesn't kill you, it will make you stronger." Then, having become somewhat familiar with the laws under which I operate, he paused and added, "Of course, in your case that may not apply." Which, of course, was absolutely true. The laws under which many of us with chronic or life-threatening illnesses operate are not the same as the laws that govern healthier physical bodies.

My mother-in-law has a recipe for some delicate, delicious pastries. "Take them out of the oven just before they brown," she says. "How can you know when the time is 'just before they brown'?" I probe. "You just know," she says. "After you make them enough times—you will know."

The way to "knowing" our limitations as ill people is sometimes a long and difficult one. Usually when a healthy person exercises, he must make an effort, push himself a little beyond his limits, in order to grow stronger or increase his stamina or fitness or whatever his personal agenda might be. It may not necessarily be "pain equals gain," but there is an element of pushing oneself beyond one's comfort level and getting some benefit from that.

For the chronically ill person, the situation is often very different. We must take ourselves out of the oven before we brown, or we will get burned. Going just five minutes too long at something physical, even if we are not necessarily feeling tired at the time, can put some of us in bed for a week or, sometimes, even months. The same is true for almost any endeavor that requires physical, mental, or emotional effort, including most social events. We cannot simply *do* something—anything—with abandon, no matter how benign or enjoyable it may seem to a well person, without considering the possible consequences.

My friend John, who experiences chronic pain in his shoulder and back, found himself in the frustrating position of discovering a system of exercise that helped alleviate his pain, but that couldn't be supported by his injured shoulder. "So I would do the exercise," he said, and feel better, but then the shoulder would give out and I would have to rest for a week. Then I would do it again and it would help, and the same thing would happen. So with the needed rest, my shoulder muscles would get weaker and I would have to start over again. It's either one or the other, and there's a very fine razor's edge between the two. And it requires very close attention not to slip and get cut on that edge. For the normal person, that level of attention isn't necessary, but for me, if I slip and don't get to that level of attention, the consequence is very impactful. It can be disastrous. People don't get that you have to be so careful.

So in this upsidedown world, you must stop exercising *before* you get tired, and instead of making yourself clean your house, you must be disciplined in walking past the messes. You must close your eyes to the disorder around you—knowing that if you give in to the intense temptation to work, to clean, to organize, you will pay dearly in long-term pain or fatigue.

The same is true for a fun night out (or in) with friends or other social events. The soul and heart are nurtured but the payment is often dear and sometimes even in the midst of festivities, though you may be enjoying yourself on one level, your body is hurting so much you may ask yourself, "Is this really worth it?" The people around you don't have a clue about the hoops you have jumped through to get there, nor about your plummeting energy level, nor the fear you carry that whatever small well of energy you do have left will dry up before you realize what is happening, leaving you with no way to gracefully extricate yourself from the social web in which you are suddenly caught. This has happened to me so many times that I feel shame in even acknowledging it.

And what do you say when people ask you how you are? The polite thing, of course, is to say, "Fine, and how are you?" But normal people, who are feeling the way you feel, are usually allowed to say, "I feel bad," or at least to acknowledge that they are not feeling well. But if you say how you're really feeling, people will be distressed, or if it's a day when you're feeling not terrible, but just bad, it begins to sound like whining because that's how you always feel. And anyway, you get tired of it. So you either lie and say you're fine, or crank out some banal euphemism. My friend, who deals with chronic pain, and I compared notes one day on some of the answers we have used: "Fair,"

"I can't complain (no one will listen anyway)," "Do you want the long story or the short story?" "I'm good, but my body feels like shit."

Putting Your Life on Hold

You may see that your life is not working and that you need to cut down on your activities. So you begin to cut out all unnecessary things, but then you realize that almost *nothing* is necessary. This can lead to putting your life on hold.

If you are ill, you stay in bed. If you are dealing with a short-term crisis or long-term commitment (such as law school or nursing a loved one), you take care of things and then collapse in a heap at night exhausted. You don't do anything extra. The fun things—just hanging out, calling a friend to chat, the impromptu picnic, almost everything social—are the first to go, and the last to be reinstated. Then there's the next tier of postponing—bills that don't need to be paid right away, food you like to eat but can do without, calling your mom who you realize is not getting any younger, or a friend you haven't talked to in a while, etc.

With a chronic illness, if you did the thing that any sensible "normal" person would do when they were feeling like you are feeling, the life that goes on hold could stay there, on ice, indefinitely. In the meantime, the clock is ticking. The sand is passing through the hourglass. The years are passing, and your life is passing with them. I saw this happening to me. As the months turned into years and I went from doctor to doctor, from treatment to treatment, searching for a cure, searching for that magic bullet that was going to give me my life back, I saw the life I had slipping through my fingers. I wasn't willing to continue to let that happen. So after a while I began to do things that sane, sensible, "normal" people would not do.

I went to parties when I was dead on my feet. I played with my kids even though I was hurting badly. I looked for ways to add joy to my life, even if it meant I was going to be doing an activity that almost any person in a condition like mine would never think of attempting. I found myself faced with choices that no one "should" have to make: get myself clean or go out to some fun event; take care of important business or make myself supper; stop at the store to get some much needed supplies or change into something cooler when it's 85 degrees and I am wearing long underwear, a turtleneck, and wool sweater; abandon a project that is three-fourths done and into which I have put considerable work and time (in which case it will be as if I hadn't done it at all) or risk having a relapse. I do not regret my choices.

Hitting the Wall

Once, I was in the middle of freezing corn, when I hit my wall. "Hitting my wall" for me means STOP in neon letters. The corn was half cobbed, many ears still full of corn but scalded and ready for the cobber. The rest was cobbed in a huge bread bowl ready to be simply put in freezer bags and into the freezer for a cold winter night when freezer corn—the way we do it, from garden to freezer within an hour or so—tastes like summer: sweet, tender, and warm.

Granted, the choice I made to go ahead with the freezing project was speculative to begin with, but it was not *stupid*. In strict terms of "should" and "shouldn't" from the viewpoint of my health, I "shouldn't" have done it. However, the stark truth that some ridiculously easy task, like putting corn into freezer bags, was just too hard for me was, at that point, simply unacceptable to me. It seemed so absurd, so unreasonable that I struggled against it with all the strength of my being.

Changing from a Goal-Oriented to a Feeling-Oriented Life

These are hard lessons and bring one face-to-face with deep existential questions. What does it mean to be human? What is the importance of doing? Is it in the doing—or is it in the result? If I am forced to throw my milk away, have I wasted my time? These absurd situations are like zen koans, putting me in the squeeze, hitting me on the head. They make no sense in the normal way of sense-making. The only way to make sense of them is to embody the moment—to do things simply for the sake of doing them. This forces us to look again at our attachment to results. It forces us to turn from a life focused on getting something accomplished to a life focused on being; from a goal-oriented life to a feeling-oriented life. And on an even deeper level, it brings us face-to-face with all of our beliefs about what our life was supposed to look like and to essentially give them up, because obviously, life doesn't look anything like these pictures. It forces us to enter the world of not knowing, a world where we have no idea of what will or can happen.

A woman I'll call Natalie, from my Attitudinal Healing Center wellness group, was dealing with a relatively new chronic illness, which had turned her life upside-down. She was perhaps five months into it. The doctors were confused about what she had, but were beginning to settle on a rheumatoid arthritis-type illness from which she suffered considerable pain.

She had had some respite as a result of chemotherapy, which caused her pain to go away for a time. She thought it was going away for good. She thought she had her life back. She made plans. She made commitments. She began to live her life again as if she were a well person. But the pain came back, and her world came crashing down around her. She had to break her commitments, cancel her plans, renege on the lease she had signed for an office for her new life. The agonizing truth was dawning that perhaps this pain was permanent. Perhaps she had a chronic condition. Perhaps she would have to live with this pain for the rest of her life. "I have been in denial," she said, "but now I'm beginning to see the truth. I'd rather stay in denial than to have this brutal honesty. I don't want it. I don't like it. But this is what I have."

There was something so touching, so real, about this woman who sat there acknowledging the truth that was descending upon her like an unwanted guest. Her authenticity, as she sat with this raw truth, was poignant and open. The immediacy was palpable—a place that was somehow holy. And it seemed an open door through which all of us, to some extent, could enter with her into that holy state. In spite of herself, someone in her was accepting this honesty. Someone was opening to this truth in spite of her protestations that she would rather have denial. Though she didn't like it, she saw that there was something there for her in that realness, in that truth.

This, I think, was the beginning of a turning for her—a turning that is forced upon many of us with chronic illness and other kinds of loss. It is a difficult—actually an excruciating turning—but an essential one, a turning we must have if we want to live a more open and authentic life. It is the turning away from life as we think it "should" be to life as it is, from the life that seems to always need to go somewhere to the life that is right here now—the place that knows itself from inside out. The place is here. This is the new order. The Kingdom of Heaven is at hand, not some place that we have to get to.

Yearning for a "Normal Life"

When I have been at my worst, in bed, unable to do anything except think and meditate, or sometimes, not even that, the feeling of isolation is often extreme. I yearn for contact with another person. "If only my thoughts could go directly into the brain of the person with whom I want to communicate," I've thought. I've imagined a world in which that would be possible—some future world in which electrodes could be attached to your brain and thoughts could be sent out for people like me who couldn't talk. But I don't live in that future world—I live in this one, a world in which to communicate with someone you have to actually say the words. And I don't always have the energy for that. A well person cannot possibly imagine what a gift it is to simply be able to talk when one wants to.

Through the ups and downs of chronic illness, I have wanted desperately to have some kind of normal life—to do something creative or useful, or to have some kind of social activity in my life, so I push myself to my limits to try to do that. But then I often find myself gritting my teeth to make myself "enjoy" those experiences I have worked so hard to have. This can be humiliating. I say to myself, "You're supposed to be having fun, but if people really knew the extent to which you are stretching yourself just to be here—at a party or a restaurant—just to have a conversation that is meant to be relaxing and entertaining, they would wonder if you were crazy." They would say, "For Pete's sake, go lie down."

On one level I would have to agree—having fun "should not" be so hard. One "shouldn't" have to make oneself miserable to have a good time. But the drive to live is a strong one and people will go to extreme lengths to "have a life," which may mean different things to different people.

Once I was hurting so badly and was so exhausted I could barely walk. Yet I had been looking forward to a certain poetry event for weeks. I said to my friend as I drove away, "I asked myself, 'If I knew I was going to die tomorrow, would I go?' and the answer was 'Yes!'" He replied with a laugh, "Yes, even though going might make that event more likely."

The Paradox of Illness:
Nourishment of the Soul vs. Taking Care of the Body

And laughter? Yes, it's good medicine and very important for healing and well-being, but it uses incredible amounts of energy. I have had to stop myself from laughing many times because laughing can use up to a whole day's worth of energy in five minutes. Sometimes, however, I do it anyway—damn the consequences. Sometimes the nourishment of the spirit has to take precedence.

With all these new rules under which chronic illness forces us to live, we constantly find ourselves in paradoxes. We want to be who we were. We think we still want all those things we wanted when we were well. We plan and scheme and manipulate our lives so that somehow we can have them, but then find we can't enjoy them. We want to be with people yet find that it is just too much—it moves too fast, we can't keep up. We become exhausted and need to be alone, yet we do not want to be alone.

This is the dilemma, this cacophony of mixed messages can be very confusing both to you and to the person or persons with whom you are in relationship. There may be a person in you saying "Yes, yes, I want to be here, I want to talk with you, to discuss all the important issues of life with you, and explore the deep work of the soul. I want to make stupid jokes with you, laugh with you, make small talk, and do all the silly and unimportant things that humans do together."

But at the same time your body may be screaming, "I can't do this. I don't want to do this. I am just too tired, too sick and I hurt too much. I just want to lie down, to be alone, to have peace and quiet, to rest." And the "I" who makes the decisions about what the body does may be saying, "If I make myself do this to satisfy my emotional needs, the payment in bodily pain and suffering or disability will just be too much for too long, but if I don't do this, I will be so sad or depressed or so incredibly bored that I may feel that my life is not worth living." Stephen Levine in his book, *Healing into Life and Death* (p. 52), said, "Perhaps it is the conflict between these qualities of eagerness and despair that such deep fatigue arises to limit our healing."

Once, my friend called me the day before a planned party with our support group. It was to be an excursion to our former facilitator's house about 1¼ hours away. She was in tears and wracked with conflict about whether to risk the trip. She had been in bed for five days with severe pain from a setback in her RSD.

Her body was so on edge that the noise of the pages turning in the book her partner was reading nearly sent her up the wall. The vibrations and jostling from the trip and sitting up in the car, along with the stress of the gathering and social interactions, would put her in danger of a further setback. "I'm scared," she confided.

> I was suicidal for three days and I just don't want to go back there. I could use the endorphins and the support of the group, I love going to Kathy's, but my body says no—I need to stay in bed. When I was well, my spirit and my body wanted the same things, but now my body doesn't usually want what my spirit wants.

All of this may seem a little grim and it can be, but the absurdity of this upside down world can also lead to a lightening up, to a point where everything becomes so absurd you just have to laugh. And it can take you to a place where you are finally willing to try something new, or perhaps simply to surrender to what is.

Driving my car, I often experience a wild series of emotions. In one instant I am feeling sorry for myself and thinking how pathetic and sad it is that I am so desperate for energy, that I am driving down the road sweating but too exhausted to take off my sweatshirt or even roll down the car window.

Then I am laughing at myself because I realize that, of course, I am in this position because I insist on doing things I "shouldn't" be doing. If I were "sensible," I would be at home doing nothing—resting. The next instant I weep with grief for my lost life. And just one more layer down is the wise observer who encompasses all these feelings with a deep compassion for this soul who loves life and just keeps on trying to live it against all odds.

I begin to sing from my gut with an oldie on the radio and within one minute my throat muscles hurt so badly I am forced to stop. Again a kaleidoscope of feelings cascade over me. Sadness, grief, and loss over yet one more thing I love that I must give up, and finally another opening into a kind of open-hearted joy and thankfulness for the deep connection and love of life, the goodness of life, to which these feelings of loss and grief point. So I see that even in this confusion—in the heart of this deep conflict—lie the seeds of opening to a deeper truth, a deeper kind of happiness.

Everyone at some point must give things up in life, but hasn't it been a blast? One minute of life, of true opening and joy, seems to make it all worthwhile. Jung called the heart "the place of the coincidence of opposites," and Joseph Chilton Pearce claimed that, if we go deeply enough into the heart, the personal drops away and we find ourselves in the Big Heart, the collective heart of the universe, the place where there are no boundaries and no separation. So perhaps all these confusing and seemingly conflicting feelings are helping us to drop into that deep heart place out of which we emerge into the universal soul.

Inventing Your Life

It seems that my most intense, most real, most "successful" moments of practice (which incidentally are also usually my most joyful moments) come during times of crisis, when my physical, mental, emotional or environmental conditions are at their worst. When I am at the end of my rope and nothing seems to work, when all my ideas or preconceived notions of practice or even of life are for naught, I must invent my practice, my life, myself, *moment by moment*. So here I can finally enter beginner's mind—the mind Shunryu Suzuki tells us we must have—limitless mind, the mind of possibility. There can be real opening! In the midst of chemotherapy for my breast cancer, I wrote in my journal one day:

> I'm spinning down, down into the center of myself—this cancer, this chemotherapy, this sickness is stripping me of everything, stripping all away until I am empty. I'm sick to death of spirituality and high thoughts. I want nothing to do with meditation or talking about spiritual things, and when others bring them up, I feel disdain. All I want is aliveness, vitality, love, play. I wonder why I should feel so, when the whole thrust of my life over the past thirty years has been the spiritual life—the inner path.

That "aliveness, vitality, love [and] play" I crave at those times of extremity *are* the true spirituality I seek. Meditation is often simply an attempt to get to that place but is actually one more step removed from it than the state I am in when I feel that emptiness. And "talking about spiritual things" is ... well, *talking about* them—not *experiencing* them.

When I separate out spirituality from life, I have created an artifice—a false God like the golden calf of the ancient Egyptians. We're all just spinning in this crystal sphere we call life and every particle of it is spiritual and every particle of it is not spiritual. It is essence—it is being—it is God. It is simply "what is." Teilhard de Chardin, the Christian mystic, said, " Nothing here below is profane for those who know how to see. On the contrary, everything is sacred."

When Jim Dreaver had his third stroke he said,

> I could perceive everything coming in, but when I searched for words, it was difficult. In my mind, [I] had to learn to rethink, in some ways, [to] rethink myself.
>
> A stroke is a strange disease, because it really cripples the brain function temporarily. At my worst, I couldn't think, I just survived inch by inch through the day ... learning to do everything again. The teaching is that we're not our story, we're not this person we take ourselves to be. And what is interesting is that I had the stroke and none of my deepest inner experience changed. Nothing touches that, the stroke, or rheumatoid arthritis or whatever. My fundamental well-being doesn't depend on circumstances.

Tectonic Plates Are Moving

Sometimes, when we have a big upheaval in our life, it can create an opening for change. And we make changes that have nothing to do with those required by the upheaval. There are no formulas for this because the nature of this opportunity is that you have the chance to experience reality, and reality is always inventing itself from moment to moment.

A friend of mine recently separated from his wife of twenty-five years. It was very traumatic for him. One would think that was enough to deal with, but he suddenly found himself questioning his relationship to his work. He saw that he had fallen into a "let's just make it through" attitude toward his work, trying to just tough it out until retirement, even though he was not happy in his job. He saw that he had compromised his values because it just seemed overwhelming to try to make a change. But now that he was in such pain from the loss of his marriage, this other area of his life that was out of alignment could suddenly no longer be ignored.

In the physical/geological world, there are huge tectonic plates under the surface of the earth that float on molten lava. Sometimes there is tension because they are pushing in different directions and they hold each other back. Sometimes the tension gets to be too much and suddenly there is movement—an earthquake or volcanic eruption. Things come back into balance.

I think we are like that. Under the surface if there are tensions, eventually something has to give, and when it does, all hell breaks loose. It affects everything, and suddenly all the other aspects of our lives that were out of alignment are shifting too. When we get a chronic illness or life-threatening disease or have some huge loss that shakes our world, everything else in our life that was held together by a stitch and a song comes tumbling out of our virtual closets and lands at our feet.

"Good things come in bunches" as do bad. So when things begin to go wrong, it seems the entire universe conspires against us and all our old ghosts come back to haunt us. There are a few logical reasons which could be offered to explain this, I suppose. When we're weak, we are less able to handle inner and outer stresses. Things that we would normally slough off are blown out of proportion and become problems. Add to that the fact that when we're more sick, we can do less: thus we have more time to think, and what was the side show often becomes the main attraction.

More importantly, we have time and space to *feel*. There is nothing to cover over raw feelings: the helplessness of a life out of control; the sorrow of a life that will never meet our expectations; or perhaps finally having to face the real truth of the situation we are in—that our marriage has been in deep trouble for years or that we truly cannot bear to stay working at our present job for another minute. And even deeper are the forces, huge and elemental, that are beyond our human understanding—the tectonic plates and their slow inexorable movement.

The statistical odds for parents of a profoundly handicapped child staying together drop by 50% after the child is born. Another fact is that 75% of marriages in which one partner has a chronic medical condition will end in divorce (Pitzele, 1986, 64). That figure jumps to 80% when it comes to parents of murdered children (Press Democrat, USA Weekend, June 6-8, 1997, p. 8). I don't know what the statistics are for chronically ill or disabled single people getting married, but my guess is that it would be pretty low. My friend John, after describing that the pain in his joints, which went on for years and years, felt like hot glass had been poured into them, said:

> I didn't have very much social life. The little I had was just barely tolerable. It's really hard to be present, really hard to be there, engaging, taking on the lessons of relationship. I mean I've got this big lesson pounding me on my back all day long. I don't need another intense lesson. I can just barely handle this one.

He added simply, "I've been single a lot."

The statistics may seem disheartening, yet I think there is more here than meets the eye. For singles, yes, it is much harder to find a partner, but on the other hand, it forces us to look deeper—to look beyond the more superficial attractions that often bring people together. And as for the high divorce rate among couples besieged by illness or tragedy, it may appear that the illness or loss has "caused" the break-ups. While this may be partly true due to the incredible stresses placed on a marriage under these conditions, the harder and deeper truth may be that many of these marriages were already in trouble and these stresses simply made it impossible to cover over the rifts with niceties or distractions.

The stress of illness can cause problems or shine a light on problems that are already there in other kinds of relationships as well, as when my friend Jane had to go back and live with her mom again as a young adult. Being homebound caused her friendships to dry up and she became completely dependent on her mom for all her emotional and social needs.

> Because I was so dependent on her and we were living together again, issues from childhood that had never gotten worked out were triggered, one of them being that ever since I was young she would always have drinks at night. I always had this really strong sense that she was betraying me when she would have any alcohol—that she's supposed to be there a hundred percent all the time and, if she's not, then I'm somehow endangered, and I'm resentful of that.
>
> There we were living together and I was as dependent or more than I was as a kid. I didn't have any friends—I didn't have any—there were so few people to talk to. My mom had always been my buddy too, so I'd look forward to her coming home ... just to talk. But a few hours into being home, there were a few drinks and I wouldn't be not interested in talking to her any more. I didn't even want to be around her.
>
> I would go to bed early and just cry and cry that "I want my mom, I want my friend, and she betrayed me." That was something that came up in therapy quite a bit.
>
> [And my mom] had tons of guilt ... she would always go to the first session with me. And one of the first things she would talk about was guilt at why she didn't see this coming, that all the signs [were there] if you looked back through my life, and she could have done something to prevent this from getting so bad.

Life has a tendency to get really basic and, as has been noted previously, brutally honest when illness or loss strikes. This is not necessarily a bad thing. In my own case, I saw how chronic illness brought to the forefront everything that was wrong in my marriage. What could formerly hide in the camouflage of a busy life became a glaring neon sign amid the simple realities of life with chronic illness. For both my husband and myself, our most painful difficulties with each other presented themselves, saying, "Deal with me NOW." This was very hard. I used to ask God, the universe, my husband, whoever I could think of to ask, "Could there be a worse time to bring this up?"

It seemed almost as if all of these beings and forces were colluding and saving up these painful topics and experiences to present to me in my most vulnerable moments. When I took a closer look, I saw that I too was part of that collusion. It is a common story—a strange one, but the condition, it seems, of being human—that the times when we are most in need of love and understanding and mercy are the very times our judgment of ourselves is the harshest. And yes, we can learn to offer ourselves loving kindness—we must do this—but we cannot, nor would it even be desirable even if we could, keep ourselves from experiencing the pain that is being uncovered.

In hindsight, of course, I see that everything in my marriage happened in the only way that it could have. I remembered the lessons I had learned working with experiencing—how my low energy level actually allowed for less suppression, and this was a *good* thing, even though it felt bad. I also understood that these incredible stresses were pushing on my husband, my children, and all the people closest to me in my life as much as they were pushing on me. The lava had to flow out—there was nowhere else for it to go. I also believe that these underground forces were bigger than any of us, and the end result after the painful sliding and grinding has been a deeper harmony, a deeper understanding, and an opening to a level of peace that was not possible before.

Finding New Resources

We hold so tightly to our view of reality, to our beliefs of what we think life is about, of what we believe we need to be happy. We have been on the same program all our lives and we are sure it is the only one because it is the only one we know. But this view of reality is so narrow, so small. There is a huge world of experience both within and outside of ourselves that is waiting to be discovered. It is like owning a computer with thousands of programs, but we only use one because we don't know how to use the others—we don't even know how to get into them. Illness or other seemingly adverse life experiences can help us to access these undiscovered territories. If the program we have been using suddenly stops working, we are forced to look for new ways of doing, of seeing, of being.

If we could just relax into our experience—stop our frantic thrashing for one moment—and look around at where we are, we may discover that it is not so bad after all, that in fact this new world is rich and deep, flush with adventure, intensity, joy, and experiences of a completely new kind. If we open to it, we realize that this has always been here but we have never seen it. It's like discovering a tropical island in your back yard. At the very least, we will discover resources that we never knew we had and ways of seeing and being that are different.

John, in desperation over the pain in his back, went to a ten-day meditation retreat to try to get some perspective. A fine-tuned concentration practice beginning with acute and continuous awareness of a spot on his upper lip and expanding to various parts of the body finally led to the exact point of pain in his back.

He shared part of his experience with me:

> It was eleven hours of meditation every day for ten days. You can sit any way you want. I sat in a chair. So you sit with your eyes closed for ten days. You're totally confronted. What happened was, my awareness was pulled along what I believe to be the meridian that that pain spot was on, and I had a journey inside my body from one end of that meridian to the other and back, to the point where it was so mind-blowing, that it left me in a state of wonder for hours. It was a shift. This was a direct experience of inner energy in the body that could have been there all along, that I had no awareness of previously.
>
> I don't have much awareness of it now, either. It takes a lot of work to get to that point. But what it did was help me to get out of feeling completely powerless, or completely at the affect of what was going on. It gave me insight. It gave me a kind of spiritual dimension of the experience of pain. And then it became more and more apparent, as it had already been somewhat apparent, that this experience was my teacher. I had a hard time embracing that, but it became a little easier to embrace it and not be so angry and frustrated about it. I became more able to be a witness of it than a victim.

It seems we've got everything backwards. We think we can use spiritual practice to make our lives better. But really the whole purpose of our lives is to use them to wake up to the perfection of life as it is. We think we need love, but the only real need we have is to love because love is what we are.

The Smile

Slowly over the years of a relentless "in-your-face" kind of suffering, I saw that I was changing. The situation that had taken away so many of the things that had brought me joy in life was bringing me, it seemed, to a place of much deeper joy: the kind of joy I never thought possible, the kind of joy that is not dependent on things or conditions. With these realizations came the dawning of a new thought—a breathless thought—an unthinkable thought—that hovered at first for a moment at a time in the corner of my mind just out of reach. It was an awareness, a feeling—almost a hope at first—that perhaps there is nothing to fear after all, that life is really benevolent.

If this "bad" thing, my illness, could turn out to be "good," perhaps *all* things could have unseen benefits. *All* things, in their essence, are good. Anything that happens is *really* okay. I don't have to be afraid. The universe is not out to get me, but to heal me. I am safe. Life will bring me what I need and I don't need to fret and choose.

This, to the conditioned mind, body and heart, is revolutionary. It turns all existing ideas and feelings on their heads. It is like a breath of pure air in a smoggy land—one that I was, at first, afraid to take in. The idea that I no longer needed to brace my body and my very being against a hostile world was so foreign, so far out, that I struggled against the sheer absurdity of the idea.

But as the truth dawned and I began, bit by bit, to relax into it, a smile began to spread like a light across my face and shone into my very heart. This was not a thought, but an experience. This was not something I could or needed to talk myself into. It came only after much suffering and struggling through the muck, trying, trying to make things different, to make things better. The change was slow, like dense fog soaking in year after year until I was wet through. Finally I settled into the mud and allowed myself to feel its warm therapeutic qualities. The new order, it turns out, is not some future world with electrodes in my brain to allow me to fulfill some desire, but simply a new way of seeing and being in this very life I have, a willingness to be here, now, in the miracle of life as it is. And when someone asks me how I am, I can say "good," without the slightest hesitation or twinge of regret.

CHAPTER 20

Moving On

Impermanence

BEING ILL OR FACING DEATH, however useful on our path, does not guarantee that we will open spiritually. A sick person can be just as miserable as a busy well person, in fact even more so. When we are well, our busyness keeps us from our true heart; when we are sick, buying into our wretchedness can keep us from experiencing the simple joy of being. We add layers of suffering onto the simple aches and pains that exist in our bodies in just this moment: fear, embarrassment, wanting, despair, worry.

Three major things seem to get in the way of peace and to cause suffering:
1. Resisting what is.
2. Attaching meaning to experience.
3. Living in the past or the future instead of staying with now.

If I stay simply with the body, with the sensations of just this much, just this moment, my experience is never really all that bad. What makes it bad is the looking back—when I say to myself, "See how long you've been sick? How long you've been struggling?" It is remembering the thrill of using the body and the simple joy of doing, and longing for that again. It is the looking into the future, to what lies ahead—suffering and death, because surely yes, we will all die.

So I suffer when I go to some imagined future and make up a story about what will happen, instead of staying with the truth of this moment, which may be that I'm too tired to go to an event. And I suffer more when I believe the thoughts that go along with that story: "I'll *never* be able to do the things that normal people do—I'll *never* have a relationship. I can't have fun in my life. I can't go to parties. I can't go for walks. I can't even talk."

These words come from the fear place. It is the fear that life is over now—that there will be no more moments of doing those things that have seemed to bring joy in the past. I add the embarrassment of facing others and not being able to say, "I'm doing better. I feel good." It is the fear that I will be a downer to others, that I am spiritually inept because I haven't been able to heal myself, that there is something I am supposed to be doing and I am not doing it—something that could heal me. So again, there is shame and the sense of responsibility but with no clue as to what step to take. I keep doing all these things and none of them seem to be working. I keep coming up against a brick wall—thus I feel like a failure, like my friends are all rooting for me and I am letting them down.

There is the fear that eventually they will all give up on me, go back to their lives of living, and I will be left alone in this no man's land between life and death. I compare myself to others, adding more suffering. They hike, dance, talk, party, work, sing—I can't. These are all stories I have told myself from time to time, instead of simply lying on the grass experiencing the wind blowing through the trees and my hair. What a waste of time—precious time.

Even when we are able to open to our pain and the messenger of death, to the little bird that sits on our shoulders reminding us that life is fleeting, and even when we are able to listen to what they have to teach us about living and loving fully and joyously now, we can manage to turn that very opening into one more obligation, one more prison. I saw this happen in the midst of my struggle with breast cancer. I wrote in my journal one day:

> This pain in my legs and chest is scary. (My oncologist wants me to have a chest x-ray and a bone scan). But it's also my path and I definitely know that—though sometimes I forget. I've been seeing recently how I've gotten off track. No matter how hard I try to guard against it, it seems that the ego takes every good thing and turns it for its own uses.
>
> So while the cancer has turned me, opened me to the possibility that exists of living more deeply in the moment, of living my life more fully, more joyously, of doing things that I really want to do and not delaying them, not putting them off until I have things "more together" and of

finally opening to my power, I see the subtle turning of these wonderful things into a race against death.

So instead of living joyously and freely in the moment, taking time to do the things that I love, as this little messenger on my shoulder has taught me to do, I sometimes find myself in a race—doing the things I love, but in such a way—squeezing them in before I die, and squeezing out the joy along with it.

Many who have had a brush with death, or whose lives have been changed dramatically and apparently irrevocably by chronic illness, have experienced great openings in their lives. When our hearts crack open to that place of love and peace, it may seem that we are changed forever. But the Buddha taught that nothing is forever—the only thing that is permanent is impermanence. This is the condition of life.

Jane experienced anxiety when she began to wonder if the lessons and gifts that had come to her as a result of her illness would disappear once she "got things together" and became more enmeshed in the world of doing and accomplishment.

> When I started going back to college, more things had become easier. I had a boyfriend. My life was gaining the semblance of something normal. I remember going through a phase of being terrified of realizing that [my illness] was an opportunity because my life had become so small and so simplified that I could really have these perspectives and these insights that weren't par for the course. At my everyday writing sessions, I [had] really [been feeling] like I was getting a very large perspective.
>
> But as my life became more involved in the world [again], not only did I not have the motivation [anymore], because I didn't have the need to keep reasserting the purpose of my existence, but I also didn't have the constant questioning of existence that had somehow helped me to stay connected to my spirituality.
>
> I got really scared that somehow I was losing a piece of myself or something that was a really special gift.

A woman in my meditation group shared how her life had changed dramatically when she experienced cancer many years ago. As a teacher she had suddenly found herself speaking from a place of deep authenticity and love, unconcerned about what people would think of her. Her students noticed the difference and were excited and enlivened in her classes. Slowly, over the years, she lost some of that aliveness, that sense of living on the edge. For her there is a sense of longing for the vitality, the aliveness, that arose out of the realization of impending death.

An even more poignant example of that kind of longing was the story of a woman I'll call Marty who was part of my chronic illness support group. During the course of our time together, several of us developed cancer. Marty was diagnosed with ovarian cancer. They gave her a fifty-fifty chance to live. Marty is a no-nonsense kind of women with a very energetic and strong inner self, who knows how to go after what she wants. When she learned she had cancer, she went through chemotherapy, always claiming she was fine with a smile on her face, saying she felt good—even through the chemo and the loss of all her hair.

And when she came out the other side, a number of months after she had been declared cancer free, she came to group one day in tears and begged us not to hate her for what she was going to say. "I want the cancer to come back," she exclaimed through her tears.

> When I had cancer, life was so simple: there was no worrying about making myself look good for a possible lover; no urgency to look for a new house and struggle with mortgage brokers; no worry about having enough money to pay the mortgage or losing my job; no dealing with problems at work or with acquaintances. There was only doing what I had to do to survive one minute at a time, drinking in the love being showered on me by my dear family and friends, and appreciating each precious moment of life.

When she finished talking, my heart went out to her and I knew exactly what she was talking about. I remembered the bittersweet taste of that edge upon which I had walked during my brush with breast cancer—the intense aliveness of it—the dancing trees and the exquisite clarity of birdsong—the dropping away of all superfluous worries, and I too longed for that place.

So we see that, though life-threatening or chronic illnesses are very valuable in helping us to wake up to the joy and the preciousness of this life, we cannot hold on to these realizations or experiences any more than we can hold on to life itself. Even our epiphanies can lead to a new clinging and a new way to avoid opening to each moment as it presents itself, and can get in the way of and actually block a new and deeper understanding from entering. The moment a great truth is realized, the mind begins to harden around it—to make it into some "Eternal Truth." The ego tricks us and takes over our understanding to use for its own aggrandizement. The freedom we momentarily experience is turned into another device to keep us in chains. Earl Balfour wrote:

> Our highest truths are but half truths;
> Think not to settle down forever in any truth.
> Make use of it as a tent in which
> to pass the summer night,
> But build no house of it or it will be your tomb.

The Usefulness of a New Identity (and Giving It Up)

When we have done our work with forgiveness, "experiencing" and opening to grief etc., and have allowed our illness or loss to soften and open us, we may notice that we have acquired a new identity. At some point, especially if we have spent a bit of time in a quality support group that focuses on feelings, the above-mentioned practices and accepting ourselves as we are, the identity of being a sick, disabled or depressed person may not look so bad.

Our false friends have dropped away, the quality of our new friends has increased in the sense of being authentic, real, compassionate, and true, and we ourselves have been moved along in the same direction. Our spiritual journey has most likely been greatly enhanced—jolted into tenth gear—if we had one, or initiated if we didn't. Though we can't do many of the things we used to be able to do and have lost many of our old identities, we have gained other qualities and identities, some of which may have more value and be of more use to us in the long run than some of the ones we lost.

Jane, who had pretty much been in the basement self-esteem-wise, was greatly helped by her new identity of "agoraphobic," when she was able to accept herself as she was:

> I really loved the doctor that led [our] group and he, more than anyone else I'd ever heard, spoke these names; he called you an agora-

phobic and spoke in terms of "us agoraphobics." He was really pushing this identity. It was interesting. He had adjectives for phobics—they are highly creative, sensitive, passionate—like it's this group of people that have these specific qualities and that they are somehow set apart from the rest of the human population. It's like we're a different breed. And I really dug that. It helped me a lot. And it helped explain things; it helped to justify certain things and [say,] "All right, this is what I am, and I'm somebody."

In illness, many of the identities we had as a well person are stripped away. We are left empty and lost, wondering who we are. As the teachings begin to ripen, a certain pride may begin to develop and illness itself can become a badge of courage we wear in the world. Illness can become the identity to which we cling. This is not a bad thing. It may be an important, though hopefully temporary, step to help support us as we leave our old life of materialism and perhaps a "poor me" mentality behind.

The world reinforces these attachments. People often tell me how courageous I am. Sometimes I buy into the story and begin to think of myself as "special" because I deal with such hard things. But most of the time these days I have the presence of mind to know that I am no more courageous than anyone dealing with the hardballs life sometimes sends. Anyone who is thrown into the ocean naturally swims for his life.

We may also be tantalized by the feeling of specialness because of what we have learned from our hardships—how "light" we have become, how "empty," how free of attachments. There's the trickster again showing us how stuck we still are in attachments—attachments to our non-attachment! On the other side of the spectrum, if we have not learned to open to the teachings illness and loss can bring, we may take on the identity of the poor victim. On the spiritual path, these identities and attachments, as with all others, must eventually be relinquished.

Letting Go of the Messenger

There is much to learn from illness and loss. Both have been my teacher, an awesome one, for twenty-four years. In my apprenticeship,

I have learned incredible lessons and have journeyed with others who have also shared the myriad and priceless lessons they have received, many of them chronicled in this book. At some point, however, it became clear that it was time to move on.

The Buddhist Ox Herding Pictures begin with an old man alone in a field and mountains in the distance. It moves on to a picture that looks similar to the first. In between we see the old man seemingly stalking, then catching, then taming and riding a giant white bull. I feel that my own spiritual path, and probably that of many others, especially in relation to illness and loss, has followed a parallel design. One major difference, of course, is that in our case, the bull (our spiritual lessons in the guise of our pain and loss) was stalking *us*. In any case, whether it be bull, spiritual teacher, illness or loss as teacher, LSD, or teachings of any kind that we cling to, we must give them up if we want to be free. Then we are back to a very simple life: ourselves, mountains, sky, and trees, that looks very different, and yet the same, as when we started out.

So we see that in the journey with illness and loss, some may become too attached as they begin to realize the power in this teaching. Illness as teacher, as hard-driving taskmaster, as kind and loving mentor, even as temporary identity, serves us well in terms of the positive qualities and spiritual movement it has engendered in us, but there's a danger of becoming too dependent on our teacher. It can become a crutch.

Jane released her identity of "agoraphobic" slowly, almost without realizing it, but some of her friends didn't. This created difficulties in their relationships.

> I'd been leading up to what felt like a normal life. Though I had limits within the life I had constructed for myself, I started feeling less agoraphobic, but I also had a little bit of guilt because [of a friend I had made during that time]. Although her life had also expanded incredibly, she was still really, really, attached to being agoraphobic.
>
> Even though she wouldn't use it as an excuse, it was still really important to her. Every time she did something that she used to not be able to do, even though she'd done it fifty times, [she'd] articulate: "Wow, I'm an agoraphobic and I can do this now." That was important for me for a long time too, and then at some point it just wasn't any more. I don't know why. But it just wasn't and it didn't give me anything.

And so I remember there being tension between us. I think there was this stance [for her] of: "How can you not fear something? That's who you are! How can you not see yourself that way?" But I didn't.

Moving on can create its own difficulties. We recognize again (of course) that we are never "home free," and adjusting to life as simply "a person" is another stage that must be approached with consciousness and humility. Jane continued:

After I got to New Jersey, I was really depressed and having a hard time. I didn't have anxiety, which was amazing, and I noted that. But I was just lonely and depressed and my life felt weird and meaningless and confused.

So I found a therapist through the psychology department at school and I told him one day, "You know, I'm wishing that I had anxiety because then I could go to an agoraphobia work group." And I realized right then that I didn't really know how else to get support. That had been so useful for me [when] I did have that sense of support, that sense of pride, and I needed that. I needed something. I needed community. And I was alone.

As soon as I heard myself say that, something caught and it was like, "Whoa! That is really interesting. I'm almost wishing to be sick." And so then I went through this period of realizing it was a conscious decision at that point. "I really know that I am not agoraphobic. That's not my experience of myself anymore."

This is how we grow. When something has outlived its usefulness, it's time to let it go. Sometimes it will fall away on its own if we let it. Sometimes we need to make a conscious decision to let it go. This is the natural way of things. When we continue to hold onto something or someone after it has done its job, or say, in the case of children or others dependent on us, after they've grown enough and learned enough to be independent, we're starting down a dangerous path. We're choosing consciously to limit or stunt our own or their future growth.

Any teacher or any tool we use to achieve a goal or to learn something must, at some point, be given up. We must stand on our own feet. We must trust our own inner wisdom and take one step further into the unknown. There is a Buddhist saying, "If you meet the Buddha in the road, kill him." I think this means that we must be willing to give up our dear teacher and friend to *become* the teaching. Kwong Roshi once said, "There are ten thousand openings." We begin to see that illness is just one of them. We must finally move from an illness-based teaching to a life-based teaching.

For me, the deep healing process became, at a certain point, more important than whatever state of health my body happened to be in. I simply began noticing that I was no longer focused on bodily health or illness, even as teaching, but more on "What is true for me now? What direction do I need to go?" The process seems to have moved on without much fanfare. Though illness still teaches me continuously, it is within the larger context of life.

And should we be through with our grief as well? Should we release it and move on? Sometimes we think we should and believe that we can. Sometimes when we have worked really hard and have reached states of great openness, love and clarity, we think we have moved on from grief for good.

We have done good work. We have surrendered to our grief and moved through it. We have seen fantastic things, experienced amazing grace, and pure joy, seen through the delusions of attachment, the beguiling sirens of comfort and desire, known the truth of who we are (which is Love). We have reaped the rewards of practice—our willingness to learn from our discomfort, pain, fatigue, and despair—our willingness to be with our illness and our life in whatever form it takes. We have taken the plate that was offered us and eaten heartily and we think that meal is done—that we have left grief behind. Well, "Big Surprise," as Stephen Levine would say.

There's a famous painting of heaven and hell in which those near the top of the ladder, who are just on the verge of being welcomed into the heavenly realms, fall off into the fire of hell. This is an all too graphic reminder of what can happen to a person who becomes complacent or arrogant, who begins to feel that he/she has done the work and should therefore be able to relax and reap the rewards of that work.

I have gone deep into my grief and learned amazing lessons. I have thought, "This time when I get better, I'm going to remember my lesson. I'm going to attend to my inner voice." But as much as I feel I've learned my lessons, as deep as I know I have gone, as sure as I am that I will never forget, that I will always see and appreciate life in this way—I have learned over the years that this is sadly not true.

I have found that when I begin to get a little better, when I begin to be able to accomplish things again, to take care of the things that "need" to be taken care of, when I begin to have more energy to live my life, the paradox is that I often "live" my life less. I find myself caught up in doing, in accomplishing. I begin to miss the essential and wonderful moments of my life. It is not that I haven't been changed. I have and I will never be quite the same. But real aliveness and truth are an edge we walk moment by moment.

There have been times when I have experienced states of such deep peace that I thought it could never be shaken again. But then grief steals back to my house like a thief in the night. We may think we are finished, but some new, perhaps seemingly benign event can throw us back or provide us that opportunity to finally open to the pocket of grief that has stayed hidden—until now, and without which we cannot be whole.

One evening I was enjoying the scene in the movie *The Horse Whisperer*, when Robert Redford and Kristin Scott Thomas are galloping across an open expanse of beautiful countryside. The grief that welled up inside me was sudden and fierce—it hit me like a Mack truck. Tears flowed like gushing springs. Sobs wracked my body.

I hadn't been able to ride a horse in nearly twenty years, but my body remembered. I could feel the wind whipping my face, the strong supple body of my horse beneath me, the power of moving through and being part of a magnificent world. I knew with near certainty that never again would I know the pure joy of that experience in this body. There I was sitting in a movie theater, watching two people enjoy each other and the beautiful countryside, and I was sobbing uncontrollably. I tried to get a grip. I didn't want to ruin the movie for others, but it was very hard.

Yet I also knew that having the grief was not a bad thing and that it was my work in that moment. And that, I think, is the crucial difference in me after having done my work with grief and loss. By simply opening to and allowing the feeling of grief and loss to just be in my body, and by bringing some loving kindness to myself around the poignancy of the feeling, it could move through me like a great storm and pass on, leaving fertile ground for new growth. We must continually be open to experiencing the healing power of grief. And of course, we need to continue to examine the stories we still harbor about who we think we should be and how our lives should be. In this case, I needed to see the vestiges of mind that still believed I need to have certain experiences to be happy.

So if we think we will learn our lesson, and then be a changed person forever more, we're probably mistaken. If we feel that tragedy, sickness or hardship are somehow mistakes or aberrations that were never meant to happen, this also, I believe, is misguided. Life knows just what to do at any one moment. The erroneous assumption is that being sick is bad. Slowly the realization has dawned on me: illness has value in and of itself.

Life as Teacher

If illness is so wonderful, why don't we choose it? Why don't we do things intentionally to be ill? Sometimes I think we do, perhaps because we unconsciously know that we need the teachings that illness will bring. But in the big picture, illness is no better than health, and health is no better than illness. It may seem at times that illness, hardship, austere Lenten practices, or sitting in long meditation retreats are more perfect or "pure" than "ordinary" life. But is a tree greater than the seed? The father than the child? Perfection is inherent in each moment.

The teaching is that each state of existence is wonderful unto itself, and serves the needs of the moment as well as some larger design beyond our comprehension. When I am well and in life, certain kinds of experiences are available to me. When I am ill or in pain, other experiences are available to me. One is not better than the other. They are both good. With that realization I can just flow with it. I can rest in that truth. I don't have to worry and think, "Oh, I need to do this or that, because if I don't, I'm going to get sick."

Barbara Rhodes, JDPSN, a guiding dharma teacher of the Kwan Um School of Zen, wrote,

> Whether we perceive our experiences as joyful or painful doesn't matter. The more we awaken, the less we make distinctions. We gradu-

ally stop thinking in terms of opposites (good and bad, health and illness) and simply are with each moment in a clear and open relationship. Our healing, our growth, come from being open and awake. Our discomfort, our suffering, come from defending and protecting our delusional separate selves.

This is the healing process—awakening to the original wholeness of life. Open and present in this moment, the thought of healing disappears; healing is a human idea. There is only being in an intimate relationship with the conditions and situations in our lives (1991, 10).

So our ceaseless choosing is unnecessary, futile, and causes needless suffering. What we *can* do is learn to tune in on a more and more subtle level to the wisdom of the body, to the wisdom of the inner voice or divine child—to listen when our body or innate wisdom tells us that it needs something or needs to be away from something. Slowly, we learn to distinguish the demands and alarmist fear-based warnings of the false ego from the signals of our deep basic knowing.

Modern peoples tend to separate the spiritual, psychological, and material worlds. Lionel Corbett, a Jungian psychotherapist and author of *The Religious Functions of the Psyche*, says that we're immersed in a field of consciousness and that the psyche and the material world are continuous, not separate. Jung himself claimed that whatever we do not make conscious will manifest in the material world. We project onto others that which we need to see or manifest in ourselves—that is the shadow, the unclaimed part of ourselves.

Whatever door we enter—as we go deeper and deeper into it—we see that all these things we think of as separate, eventually meet. Scientists have discovered that, as they go deeper and deeper into matter, there is nothing there—only energy—so again we come round to Suzuki's assertion: there is no other way but this way. Eventually all ways meet.

And our personal stories, whether heroic, tragic or pathetic, in the end, are still just stories—fairy tales, like Rumplestiltskin's heroine spinning her straw into gold, like the stories we have told ourselves all of our lives about who we are and what we can and can't do, what we should and shouldn't do. There's no real substance to any of these stories. They're all spun out of the infinite flow of creation issuing from the mouth of the uncreated—the dance of Leela. Gold out of straw? What a story! We are already gold.

Appendix

A Simple Loving Kindness Meditation
(to be read slowly to a friend or to oneself)

SIT OR LIE IN A COMFORTABLE POSITION. Take a few deep breaths and drop into your body. Experience the gravity of your body; feel it sinking into whatever surface you are sitting or lying on. Read the meditation slowly to yourself, have someone read to you, or record it to play back for yourself.

Sitting comfortably, allow the attention to come gradually to the breath.
The breath, coming and going all by itself, deep within the body.
Take a few moments to allow the attention to gather within.
Experience the rhythm of the breath.

Turning gently within, begin to direct toward yourself feelings of loving kindness, relating to yourself as though you were your only child. Silently in the heart say, "May I dwell in the heart. May I be free from suffering. May I be healed. May I be at peace."

Just feel the breath breathing into the heart space as we relate to ourselves with mercy and loving kindness.
Allow the heart silently to whisper the words of mercy that heal, that open. "May I dwell in the heart. May I be free from suffering. May I be healed. May I be at peace."
Allow a willingness to be healed to converge in your heart. Whispering to yourself, send feelings of well-being to you.

"May my heart flower. May I know the joy of my own true nature. May I be healed into this moment. May I be at peace."

Repeating gently with each in-breath into the heart, "May I dwell in the heart." With each out-breath, "May I be free from suffering."

With the next in-breath, "May I be healed."

With the following out-breath, "May I be at peace."

Repeating these words slowly and gently with each in-breath, with each out-breath, not as a prayer but as an extending of a loving well-being to yourself.

Noticing whatever limits this love touching yourself, this mercy, this willingness to be whole, to be healed.

"May I dwell in the heart. May I be free from suffering. May I be healed. May I be at peace."

Continue with the rhythm of this breath, this deepening of merciful joy and loving kindness drawn in with each breath, expanding with each exhalation.

"May my heart flower. May I be free from suffering. May I be whole. May I be at peace."

Let the breath continue naturally as mercy for yourself, for this being within, deepening as it expresses itself.

Though at first these may only feel like words echoing from the mind, gently continuing, a feeling of warmth is drawn in with each breath, a sense of patience developing with each exhalation.

Drawing in warmth, expanding patience.

Room to live, room to heal.

"May I dwell in the heart. May I be at peace."

Each breath deepening the nurturing warmth of relating to oneself with loving kindness and compassion. Each exhalation deepening in peace, expanding into the spaciousness of being, developing the deep patience that does not wait for things to be otherwise, but relates with loving kindness to things as they are.

"May my heart flower. May I be free from suffering. May I be healed. May I be at peace."

Allowing the healing in with each breath. Allowing yourself to heal into your true spacious nature.

Continuing for a few breaths more, this drawing in, this opening to loving kindness. Relating to yourself with great tenderness, sending well-being into your mind and body, embracing yourself in these gentle words of healing.

Now gently bring to mind someone for whom you have a feeling of warmth and kindness.

Picturing this loved one in your heart, with each in-breath whisper to them, "May you dwell in your heart. May you be free from suffering. May you be healed. May you be at peace."

With each breath drawing them into your heart, "May you dwell in your heart, may your heart flower."

With each out-breath filling them with your loving kindness, "May you be free from suffering."

With the next inhalation drawing their heart closer to yours, "May you be healed."

With the following out-breath extending to them a wish for their well-being, "May you be at peace."

Continuing to breathe them into your heart, whispering silently to yourself, to them, "May your heart be ever open. May you be free from suffering. May you be healed into this moment. May you be at peace."

Continue the gentle breath of connection, the gentle whisper of your wish for their happiness and wholeness.

Let the breath be breathed naturally, softly, lovingly into the heart, coordinated with your words, with your concentrated feelings of loving kindness and care.

"May you dwell in your heart. May you be freed of any suffering. May you be healed wherever healing is called for. May you know the deepest levels of peace."

Send them your love, your compassion, your care.

Breathing them in and through your heart.

"May you dwell in the open heart. May you be free from suffering. May you be healed. May you know your deepest joy, your greatest peace."

And as you sense them in your heart, sense this whole world that wishes so to be healed, to know its true nature, to be at peace.

And in your heart with each in-breath, with each out-breath, whisper, "May all beings be free of suffering. May all beings be at peace."

Let your loving kindness reach out to all beings as it did to your loved one, sensing all beings in need of healing, in need of the peace of their true nature.

"May all beings be at peace. May all beings be healed of their suffering."

"May all sentient beings, to the most recently born, be free of fear, free of pain. May all beings heal into their true nature. May all beings know the absolute joy of absolute being."

"May all beings everywhere be healed and whole. May all beings be free of suffering."

The whole world, like a bubble floating in your heart, embraced by your loving kindness.

Each breath drawing in the love that heals the world, that deepens the peace we all seek.

Each breath feeding the world with the mercy and compassion, the warmth and patience, that quiets the mind and opens the heart.

"May all beings dwell in their heart. May all beings be free from suffering. May all beings be healed. May all beings be at peace."

Let the breath come softly. Let the breath go gently. Wishes of well-being and mercy, of care and loving kindness, extended to this world we all share.

"May all beings be free of suffering. May all beings dwell in the heart of healing. May all beings be at peace."

The Forgiveness Meditation
(to be read slowly to a friend or to oneself)

Begin to reflect for a moment on what the word "forgiveness" might mean. What is forgiveness? What might it be to bring forgiveness into one's life, into one's mind?

Begin by slowly bringing into your mind, into your heart, the image of one person at a time for whom you have some resentment. Gently allow a picture, a feeling, a sense of this person to gather there. Gently invite him/her into your heart just for this moment.

Notice whatever fear or anger may arise to limit or deny his/her entrance and soften gently all around it. No force. Just an experiment in truth which invites this person in.

And silently in your heart say to this person, "I forgive you." Open to a sense of his/her presence and say, "I forgive you for whatever pain you may have caused me in the past, intentionally or unintentionally, through your words, your thoughts, your actions. However you may have caused me pain in the past, I forgive you."

Feel for even a moment the spaciousness relating to that person with the possibility of forgiveness.

Let go of those walls, those curtains of resentment, so that your heart may be free, so that your life may be lighter.

"I forgive you for whatever you may have done that caused me pain, intentionally or unintentionally, through your actions, through your words, even through your thoughts, through whatever you did—through whatever you didn't do. However the pain came to me through you, I forgive you. I forgive you."

It is so painful to put someone out of your heart. Let go of that pain. Let him/her be touched for this moment at least with the warmth of your forgiveness.

"I forgive you. I forgive you."

Allow that person to just be there in the stillness, in the warmth and patience of the heart. Let him/her be forgiven. Let the distance between you dissolve in mercy and compassion.

Let it be so.

Now, having finished so much business, dissolved in forgiveness, allow that being to go on his/her way. Not pushing or pulling from the heart, but simply letting this person be on his/her own way, touched by a blessing and the possibility of your forgiveness.

And now gently, giving yourself whatever time is necessary, allow the other person to dissolve as you invite another in.

Now gently bring into your mind, into your heart, the image, the sense, of someone who has resentment for you. Someone whose heart is closed to you.

Notice whatever limits him/her entrance and soften all about that hardness. Let it float.

Mercifully invite him/her into your heart and say to him/her, "I ask your forgiveness."

"I ask your forgiveness."

"I ask to be let back into your heart. That you forgive me for whatever I may have done in the past that caused you pain, intentionally or unintentionally, through my words, my actions, even through my thoughts."

"However I may have hurt or injured you, whatever confusion, whatever fear of mind caused you pain, I ask your forgiveness."

And allow yourself to be touched by his/her forgiveness. Allow yourself to be forgiven. Allow yourself back into his/her heart.

Have mercy on you. Have mercy on him/her. Allow him/her to forgive you.

Feel his/her forgiveness touch you. Receive it. Draw it into your heart.

"I ask your forgiveness for however I may have caused you pain in the past. Through my anger, through my lust, through my fear, my ignorance, my blindness, my doubt, my confusion. However I may have caused you pain, I ask that you let me back into your heart. I ask your forgiveness." Let it be. Allow yourself to be forgiven.

If the mind attempts to block forgiveness with merciless indictments, recriminations, judgments, just see the nature of the unkind mind. See how merciless we are with ourselves. And let this unkind mind be touched by the warmth and patience of forgiveness.

Let your heart touch this other heart so that it may receive forgiveness, so that it may feel whole again.

Let it be so.

Feel forgiveness now as it touches you.

If the mind pulls back, thinks it deserves to suffer, see this merciless mind. Let it sink into the heart. Allow yourself to be touched by the possibility of forgiveness.

Receive the forgiveness.

Let it be so.

And now gently bid that person adieu and with a blessing let him/her be on his/her way, having even for a millisecond shared the one heart beyond the confusion of seemingly separate minds.

And now gently turn to yourself in your own heart and say, "I forgive you," to yourself.

It is so painful to put ourselves out of our hearts.

Say, "I forgive you" to yourself.

Calling out to yourself in your heart, using your own first name, say, "I forgive you" to you.

If the mind interposes with hard thoughts, such as that it is self-indulgent to forgive oneself, if it judges, if it touches you with anger and unkindness, just feel that hardness and let it soften at the edge. Let it be touched by forgiveness.

Allow yourself back into your heart. Allow yourself to be forgiven by you.

Let the world back into your heart. Allow yourself to be forgiven.

Let forgiveness fill your whole body.

Feel the warmth and care that wishes for your own well-being. Seeing yourself as if you were your only child, let yourself be bathed by this mercy and kindness. Let yourself be loved. See your forgiveness forever awaiting your return to your heart.

How unkind we are to ourselves. How little mercy. Let it go. Allow yourself to embrace yourself with forgiveness. Know that in this moment you are wholly and completely forgiven. Now it is up to you just to allow it in. See yourself in the infinitely compassionate eyes of the Buddha, in the sacred heart of Jesus, in the warm embrace of the Goddess.

Let yourself be loved. Let yourself be love.

And now begin to share this miracle of forgiveness, of mercy and awareness. Let it extend out to all people around you.

Let all be touched by the power of forgiveness. All those beings who have also known such pain. Who have so often put themselves and others out of their hearts. Who have so often felt so isolated, so lost.

Touch them with your forgiveness, with your mercy and loving kindness, that they too may be healed, just as you wish to be healed.

Feel the heart we all share filled with forgiveness so that we all might be whole.

Let the mercy keep radiating outward until it encompasses the whole planet—the whole planet floating in your heart, in mercy, in loving kindness, in care.

"May all sentient beings be freed of suffering, of their anger, of their confusion, of their fear from suffering."

Whole world floating in the heart. All beings freed of their suffering. All beings at every level of reality, on every plane of existence, may they all be freed of their suffering. May they all be at peace.

May we heal the world, touching it again and again with forgiveness. May we heal our hearts and the hearts of those we love by merging in forgiveness, by merging in peace.

Stephen Levine

Notes

1. The way we use situations, and experiences in our lives to wake up to a new way of being as well as disciplines such as meditation or chanting that we use to increase our awareness are referred to in this book as "practices" or simply "practice." "The work" or "work on myself" may be used in the same way.
2. Responsive Sympathetic Dystrophy—an illness causing severe pain in the sympathetic nervous system.
3. The Bohemian, 04,26,06, Patricia Henely.
4. Meditation practice that does not focus on anything specific, but is very wide and inclusive of everything.
5. See appendix.
7. Sisyphus: In Greek mythology, Sisyphus was an evil king of Corinth. After he died, he was condemned in the underworld to roll a huge stone uphill, which always fell back before he could reach the top, at which time he would have to start all over. From *Probert Encyclopaedia*.
8. Ibid.
9. Chakra—Originating from within the ancient yoga systems of India, chakras refer to spinning vortices of energy created within us by the interpenetration of consciousness and the physical body. Through this combination, chakras become *centers of activity for the reception, assimilation and transmission of life energies*. Technically, the word is from the Sanskrit language and translates as *wheel* or *disk*. We can think of them as spheres of energy radiating from the central nerve ganglia of the spinal column. There are seven major chakras within each of us, arranged vertically from the base of the spine to the top of the head, centered more or less, through the middle of our body. (from the *Sevenfold Journey*, Anodea Judith and Selene Vega; pp. 6-7).

Bibliography

Albom, Mitch. *Tuesdays with Morrie*. New York, London, Toronto, Sydney, Auckland: Doubleday, 1997.

Anthony (Metropolitan) and LeFebvre, Georges. *Courage to Pray*. London and New York Darton, Longman and Todd, 1973 or St Vladimir's Seminary Press, 1984.

Barks, Coleman. *Feeling the Shoulder of the Lion*. Boston & London: Shambhala Publications, Inc., 1991, 2000.

Barrows, Anita and Macy, Joanna. *Rilke's Book of Hours*. Translation. New York: Riverhead Books, 1996.

Bauby, Jean-Dominique. *The Driving Bell and the Butterfly: A Memoir of Life and Death*. New York: Vintage Books, 1997.

Beck, Charlotte Joko. *Nothing Special*. San Francisco: Harper, 1993.

Benoit, Herbert. *The Supreme Doctrine*. Brighton, UK: Sussex Academic Press, 1995.

Bly, Robert. *Versions. The Kabir Book: Forty-Four of the Ecstatic Poems of Kabir*. Toronto: The Seventies Press. 1977.

Bonheim, Jalaja. *Aphrodite's Daughters*. New York: Fireside, 1997.

Cameron, Julia with Bryan, Mark. *The Artist's Way*. New York: G. P. Putnam's Sons, 1992.

Casey, Caroline W. *Making the Gods Work for You*. New York: Three Rivers Press, 1998.

Chopich, Erica and Paul, Margaret. *Healing Your Aloneness*. San Francisco: Harper & Row, 1990.

Coleman, Barks and Mayne, John. Trans. *The Essential Rumi*. Translation. New York: HarperCollins Publishers, 1995.

Goldberg, Natalie. *Writing Down the Bones*. Boston and London: Shambhala Publications, 1986.

Healey, Terry, *At Face Value: My Triumph Over a Disfiguring Cancer*. Caveat Press, 2006.

Hendricks, Harville, *Getting the Love You Want: A Guide for Couples*. New York: Henry Holt, 2007

Judith, Anodea, and Vega, Selene. *The Sevenfold Journey.* The Crossing Press, 1993.

Jung, C. G. *Letters Vol. 1: 1906 –1950.* Edited by Gerhard Adler and Aniela Jaffe, translated by R.F.C. Hull, Bollingen Series XCV, Princeton University Press.

Kapleau, Philip, ed. *The Three Pillars of Zen: Teaching, Practice, Enlightenment.* Boston: Beacon, 1967.

Klaus, Marshall H. M.D., and Klaus, Phyllis H. C.S.W. *Your Amazing Newborn.* Persens Books. Reading, MA, 1998.

Ladinsky, Daniel. *The Subject of Love: 60 Wild and Sweet Poems of Hafiz.* Pumpkin House Press, SC, 1996.

Levine, Stephen. *Healing into Life and Death.* New York, London, Toronto, Sydney, Auckland: Doubleday, 1987.

Ouspensky, P. D. *In Search of the Miraculous.* New York. Harcourt, Brace and Company, Inc., 1949.

Pearce, Joseph Chilton. *Magical Child.* New York. E.P. Dutton, 1977.

Pema Chödrön. *The Places That Scare You.* Boston & London: Shambhala Publications, Inc., 2001.

Pema Chödrön. *The Wisdom of No Escape.* Boston & London: Shambhala Publications, Inc., 1991.

Pema Chödrön. *Start Where You Are.* Boston & London: Shambhala Publications, Inc., 1994.

Pema Chödrön. *When Things Fall Apart.* Boston & London: Shambhala Publications, Inc., 1997.

Pitzele, Sefra Kobrin. *We Are Not Alone: Learning to Live with Chronic Illness.* New York: Workman Publishing, 1986.

Rhodes, Barbara. *A Thousand Eyes, A Thousand Hands: Primary Point, an International Journal of Buddhism*, Vol.8, #2, Summer 1991.

Ruskin, John. *Emotional Clearing.* New York: R. Wyler & Company, 1993.

Sharp, Joseph. *Living Our Dying.* New York: Hyperion, 1996.

Suzuki, Shunryu. *Zen Mind, Beginner's Mind: Informal Talks on Zen Meditation and Practice.* New York & Tokyo: John Weatherhill, Inc., 1983.

About the Author

DIANE LARAE BODACH began her spiritual practice in 1969, first in a Gurdjieff community, then as a student of Zen. Her path deepened after becoming chronically ill in 1980, and transformed even further when she was diagnosed with breast cancer in 1999. Diane died of cancer in her home in Santa Rosa, California on September 18, 2007, having been a spiritual practitioner for almost forty years. She was also a talented poet, artist and musician, mother of two daughters, and beloved friend to many.

CPSIA information can be obtained at www.ICGtesting.com
Printed in the USA
LVOW090318270612

287837LV00001B/64/P